Readings in Global Health

Readings in Global Health

ESSENTIAL REVIEWS FROM THE

NEW ENGLAND JOURNAL OF MEDICINE

Edited by David J. Hunter and Harvey V. Fineberg

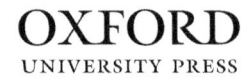

OXFORD

UNIVERSITY PRESS

OXFORD
UNIVERSITY PRESS

Oxford University Press is a department of the University of
Oxford. It furthers the University's objective of excellence in research,
scholarship, and education by publishing worldwide.

Oxford   New York
Auckland   Cape Town   Dar es Salaam   Hong Kong   Karachi
Kuala Lumpur   Madrid   Melbourne   Mexico City   Nairobi
New Delhi   Shanghai   Taipei   Toronto

With offices in
Argentina   Austria   Brazil   Chile   Czech Republic   France   Greece
Guatemala   Hungary   Italy   Japan   Poland   Portugal   Singapore
South Korea   Switzerland   Thailand   Turkey   Ukraine   Vietnam

Oxford is a registered trademark of Oxford University Press
in the UK and certain other countries.

Published in the United States of America by
Oxford University Press
198 Madison Avenue, New York, NY 10016

Library of Congress Cataloging-in-Publication Data
Readings in global health : essential reviews from the New England journal
of medicine / edited by David J. Hunter and Harvey V. Fineberg.
p. ; cm.
Includes bibliographical references and index.
ISBN 978-0-19-027122-0 (alk. paper)
I. Hunter, David J., editor.   II. Fineberg, Harvey V., editor.   III. Massachusetts
Medical Society.   IV. New England journal of medicine.
[DNLM: 1. Global Health—Collected Works.   2. Public Health—Collected
Works. WA 530.1]
RA441
362.1—dc23
2015027837

1 3 5 7 9 8 6 4 2
Printed in the United States of America
on acid-free paper

To Leona and Mary

We also dedicate this book to the late Tony McMichael, a pioneer
in environmental and occupational epidemiology, and the health
effects of climate change.

{ CONTENTS }

PART III **Noncommunicable Diseases: Introduction**

PART IV **Health System Responses: Introduction**

PART V **Global Institutional Responses: Introduction**

EPILOGUE

{ CONTRIBUTORS }

Lindsey R Baden, M.D.
Division of Infectious Diseases
Brigham and Women's Hospital
Harvard Medical School
Boston, Massachusetts

Anne E. Becker, M.D., Ph.D.
Department of Global Health and
    Social Medicine
Harvard Medical School
Department of Psychiatry
Massachusetts General Hospital
Boston, Massachusetts

Zulfiqar A. Bhutta, M.B., B.S., Ph.D.
Centre for Global Child Health
Hospital for Sick Children (SickKids)
Toronto, Canada
Center of Excellence in Women
    and Child Health
Aga Khan University
Karachi, Pakistan

Robert E. Black, M.D.
Institute for International Programs
Bloomberg School of Public Health
Johns Hopkins University
Baltimore, Maryland

Lincoln Chen, M.D.
China Medical Board
Cambridge, Massachusetts

Nigel Crisp, M.A.
House of Lords
London, United Kingdom

Majid Ezzati, Ph.D.
School of Public Health
Imperial College London
London, United Kingdom

Anthony S. Fauci, M.D.
National Institute of Allergy and
    Infectious Diseases
National Institutes of Health
Bethesda, Maryland

Harvey V. Fineberg, M.D., Ph.D.
Gordon and Betty Moore Foundation
Palo Alto, California

Julio Frenk, M.D., M.P.H., Ph.D.
Office of the President
University of Miami
Miami, Florida

Lawrence O. Gostin, J.D.
O'Neill Institute for National and
    Global Health Law
Georgetown University Law Center
WHO Collaborating Center on Public
    Health Law and Human Rights
Washington, District of Columbia

Debarati Guha-Sapir, Ph.D.
WHO Collaborating Center for
    Research on the Epidemiology of
    Disasters
Institute of Health and Society
University of Louvain
Brussels, Belgium

Donald R. Hopkins, M.D., M.P.H.
Carter Center
Atlanta, Georgia

David J. Hunter, MBBS, MPH, ScD
Office of the Dean
Harvard T.H. Chan School of Public
    Health
Boston, Massachusetts

Prabhat Jha, M.D., D.Phil.
Center for Global Health Research
St. Michael's Hospital and Dalla Lana
    School of Public Health
University of Toronto
Toronto, Canada

**Rupa Kanapathipillai, MBBS, FRACP,
MPH, DTM&H**
Infectious Diseases Physician
Editorial Fellow New England
    Journal of Medicine
Boston, Massachusetts

Arthur Kleinman, M.D.
Department of Global Health and
    Social Medicine
Harvard Medical School
Boston, Massachusetts
Department of Anthropology
Harvard University
Cambridge, Massachusetts

**Olive Kobusingye, M.Med.
(Surg), M.P.H.**
Makerere University College of
    Health Sciences
Kampala, Uganda
Institute for Social and Health
    Sciences
University of South Africa
Johannesburg, South Africa

Jennifer Leaning, M.D.
Francois-Xavier Bagnoud Center for
    Health and Human Rights
Harvard T.H. Chan School of
    Public Health
Boston, Massachusetts

Alan D. Lopez, Ph.D.
University of Melbourne
School of Population and
    Global Health
Carlton, Victoria, Australia

**Anthony J. McMichael, M.B., B.S.,
Ph.D. (dec.)**
National Centre for Epidemiology and
    Population Health
Australian National University
Canberra, Australia

Anne Mills, D.H.S.A., Ph.D.
London School of Hygiene and
    Tropical Medicine
London, United Kingdom

Suerie Moon, M.P.A., Ph.D.
Forum on Global Governance
    for Health
Harvard Global Health Institute
John F. Kennedy School of
    Government
Cambridge, Massachusetts

David M. Morens, M.D.
National Institute of Allergy and
    Infectious Diseases
National Institutes of Health
Bethesda, Maryland

**Christopher J.L. Murray,
M.D., D.Phil.**
Institute for Health Metrics and
    Evaluation
University of Washington
Seattle, Washington

Gary J. Nabel, M.D., Ph.D.
Sanofi
Cambridge, Massachusetts

Robyn Norton, Ph.D., M.P.H.
George Institute for Global Health
University of Oxford
Oxford, United Kingdom
University of Sydney
Sydney, Australia

Richard Peto, F.R.S.
Clinical Trial Service Unit and
    Epidemiological Studies Unit
Nuffield Department of
    Population Health
University of Oxford
Oxford, United Kingdom

Peter Piot, M.D., Ph.D.
London School of Hygiene and
    Tropical Medicine
London, United Kingdom

Thomas C. Quinn, M.D.
National Institute of Allergy and
    Infectious Diseases
National Institutes of Health
Bethesda, Maryland

K. Srinath Reddy, M.D., D.M.
Public Health Foundation of India
New Delhi, India
World Heart Foundation
Geneva, Switzerland

Elio Riboli, M.D.
School of Public Health
Imperial College London
London, United Kingdom

Armand G Sprecher MD MPH
Public Health Specialist
Médecins Sans Frontière
Operational Center of Brussels

Devi Sridhar, Ph.D.
WHO Collaborating Centre for
    Population Health Research
    and Training
University of Edinburgh
Edinburgh, United Kingdom
Blavatnik School of Government
University of Oxford
Oxford, United Kingdom

{ INTRODUCTION }

"Global Health" is a relatively recent construct, largely replacing and extending concepts embedded in prior terms such as "Tropical Medicine" and
"International Health." We have adopted a working definition of Global Health
as "Public Health for the world". In this view, everyone in the world is the relevant
population, and Global Health seeks to prevent and treat the diseases that compromise good health anywhere in the world. A brief review of the origin and evolution of the concept of Global Health may cast light on some of the institutions
and impulses still intrinsic to the study of Public Health for the world.

A number of leading academic institutions in global health, such as the London
School of Hygiene and Tropical Medicine and the Institute of Tropical Medicine in
Antwerp, bear names that indicate their origins in the colonial era. Not only did the
colonial powers have an interest, variously interpreted, in the health of the populations they ruled, they also encountered a wide range of diseases that were not present, or rarely encountered, in their home countries. The study of these diseases, the
development of treatments, the medical care of the colonizers, and in some countries the medical care of the colonized, became known as Tropical Medicine. The
Figure I.1 shows the Google Ngram usage of this term in books since 1850, showing
use of the term starting in the 19th century and increasing in the first half of the
20th century, with a gradual decline since then. The colonizers also brought novel
diseases to the colonies, diseases such as measles and tuberculosis that could have a
devastating effect on non-immune populations. For instance, in what we might now
consider the international transfer of risks, diseases such as smallpox were exported
to the Americas, while tobacco was imported to Europe. Colonial medical services
varied widely in quality and orientation – from an exclusive focus on the health
needs of colonizers before and after their tours of duty, to those that tried to improve
sanitation and health conditions among the colonized. Missionary medical systems
existed in parallel to these systems, and were often the major means of projecting
contemporary medical and surgical practice into the colonies.

With the wave of decolonization after the Second World War, new international institutions concerned with health came into being. Foremost among these
was the World Health Organization, founded in 1948, building on predecessor
organizations such as the International Sanitary Bureau that became the Pan
American Health Organization, and the Health Organization of the League
of Nations. Around this time use of the term "international health" increased
sharply, peaking in the 1950's, but still being the predominant term at the end of
the 20th century. "International Health" is often considered as having some of
the connotations of "international aid", with the suggestion it is the study of how
"developed" countries could help improve health conditions in what were called

"less developed" countries, now characterized as "developing" countries. Under the rubric of international health vigorous debates took place on how to best achieve gains in health in developing countries, with large philosophical differences that continue in policy debates today.

In 1978, at the Alma Ata conference, delegates convened by the WHO endorsed the concept of "Health for All" by 2000, with the main vehicle for achieving this goal to be the extension of universal access to primary health care. This "horizontal" approach was soon challenged by the notion of "selective primary health care", the concept of a more limited "package" of "cost-effective" interventions that focused on more "vertical" programs that were said to offer better value for money spent than the more comprehensive approach to primary health care. This more focused approach appealed to donors looking for the low hanging fruit in terms of improving child health, one expression of which was the GOBI package promoted by UNICEF, comprising growth monitoring, oral rehydration therapy, breast-feeding and immunizations.

Another international institution, the World Bank, emerged as a major force in discussions about health, notably with the publication of the World Development Report in 1993[1]. Previously the World Bank had been involved more indirectly, as it pressured countries that needed loans in the economic downturn of the 1980's to undertake "structural adjustment" policies that cut public spending, often resulting in restriction of funds to health systems that relied mainly on government funding. One strategy, promoted by the World Bank and others, was the "user fee" movement, based on the idea that by charging patients "small" fees to access health services, local revenue would be generated to maintain these services. Over time, evidence showed that even very small user fees deterred the poor from accessing health services, and modified policies were put in place exempting some services such as childhood immunizations and treatment for sexually transmitted diseases.

Such approaches as charging patients for services in order to pay for health care and limiting services to those that are most cost-effective, have been challenged by a variety of activists and researchers who have documented unintended and negative effects of these policies. The proponents of more comprehensive approaches argue that health care is a human right and that governments are responsible for ensuring the provision of at least basic health services, at least for the poorest of the poor. What constitutes the services that are "basic" and to which every individual has a right, and how these are financed, is subject to much debate. Some critics of more timid approaches to health and health care argue that a prior assumption that resources are fixed constrains our ability to imagine new methods of financing and care delivery that bring expanded resources to specific problems[2].

What has been termed the "golden age" of global health dawned at the end of the 20th century and the beginning of the 21st, with influential reports such as the Commission on Macroeconomics and Health[3] making the case that broad spending in setting the conditions for better health and the treatment of disease could be seen as an investment that would pay off by increasing rates of economic growth. This coincided with the rapid rise of the term "global health" which became the predominant term in the early 2000's (Figure I.1). The discovery in the mid-1990's

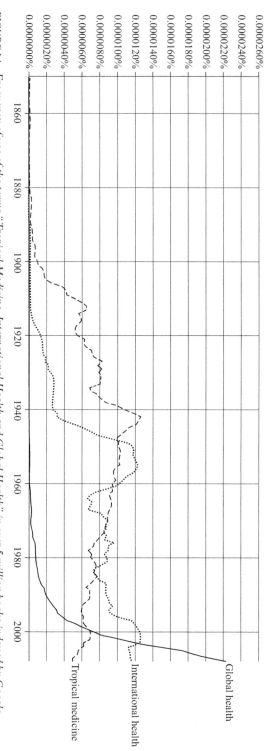

FIGURE I.1: *Frequency of use of the terms "Tropical Medicine, International Health and Global Health" in over 5 million books indexed by Google*

that HIV could be effectively managed with combinations of antiretroviral drugs, initially only available at great expense in developed countries, led to the institution of the US PEPFAR program and the Global Fund on HIV, Tuberculosis and Malaria, and dramatically increased funding to treat these diseases in developing countries, and the creation of a two-tier (in reality multiple tiers) system for funding antiretroviral drugs. The emergence of the Bill and Melinda Gates Foundation, with an annual budget for global health in 2010 almost 75% as large as the WHO budget, has brought new resources and influence to the field. The Millenium Development Goals, established by the United Nations in 2000, committed the world to attempt to reach several health-related morbidity and mortality reduction targets by 2015. Between 1990 and 2013, development assistance for health increased about 5.5-fold to about $31 billion[4], although a stagnation in the rate of increase began in 2010 after the global financial crisis.

If this truly represents a "golden age" for global health, the world nevertheless faces daunting health challenges. Even for AIDS, the disease with most focus, funding and demonstrable achievements, UNAIDS estimated that in 2012 almost two-thirds of people eligible for treatment worldwide were not receiving it[5]. In 2011 in about 46 million of the 135 million live births, women were not attended by a skilled birth attendant[6]. Very large disparities in access to health care exist across the globe, and in many countries that have made progress in providing health care to urban dwellers, little progress has been made in rural areas. New global threats to health have emerged, notably the impacts of Climate Change, and the threat of emerging and re-emerging infections is ever-present. The global movement towards Universal Health Coverage[7] invites many questions about quality and depth of coverage, the place of cost-effectiveness analyses, the limits of health care, and how health systems are to be administered and paid for.

This very brief and selective history illustrates the emergence of Global Health as a field. In the chapters that follow, leaders in the field summarize areas of progress and changing needs. We hope these reviews are informative and inspiring to those with an interest in global health and that they convey a sense of opportunity and challenge for future leaders in the field.

References

1. WDR 1993: Investing in Health. The World Bank and Oxford University Press. 1993.
2. Reimagining Global Health. Paul Farmer (Editor), Arthur Kleinman (Editor), Jim Kim (Editor), Matthew Basilico (Editor). California Series in Public Anthropology
3. World Health Organization. Macroeconomics and health: Investing in health for economic development. Report of the Commission on Macroeconomics and Health. Geneva, World Health Organization, 2001. Available from: http://whqlibdoc.who.int/publications/2001/924154550x.pdf
4. Dieleman JL, Graves CM, Templin T, et al. Global health development assistance steady in 2013 but did not align with recipients' disease burden. Health Aff (Millwood). 2014 May;33(5):878–86.
5. UNAIDS. 2013 Global Fact Sheet. Available from: http://www.unaids.org/en/media/unaids/contentassets/documents/epidemiology/2013/gr2013/20130923_FactSheet_Global_en.pdf
6. United Nations. Millennium Development Goals and Beyond. Available from: http://www.un.org/millenniumgoals/
7. World Health Organization. Universal health Coverage. Available from: http://www.who.int/universal_health_coverage/en/

A Global View of Health

AN UNFOLDING SERIES

Harvey V. Fineberg
and David J. Hunter

This book is a series based on review articles on global health originally published in the *New England Journal of Medicine*.[1] This series demonstrates that local health and local health care are linked to sources of ill health elsewhere in the world. Today, not only health problems are global but so are lessons, insights, and fresh solutions regarding such problems, which flow in all directions. The series is built around articles that explain the need for global health, the challenges to achieving it, and the solutions to problems related to it.

The meaning of the term *global health* has evolved over time.[2,3] In developing this series, we adopted the concept of global health as "public health for the world." Public health focuses on the health of populations, as distinct from medicine's focus on the health of individuals. In addition to the population-level determinants that are central to public health, the health of populations owes much to the effective delivery of clinical care; it also depends on how medical activities affect it. Notably, according to our definition of global health, the distinction between domestic health and foreign health is dissolved. The notion of public health for the world condenses the definition offered by the Institute of Medicine's Expert Committee on the US Commitment to Global Health in 2008:[4]

> Global health is the goal of improving health for all people in all nations by promoting wellness and eliminating avoidable diseases, disabilities, and deaths. It can be attained by combining clinical care at the level of the individual person with population-based measures to promote health and prevent disease. This ambitious endeavor calls for an understanding of

health determinants, practices, and solutions, as well as basic and applied research concerning risk factors, disease, and disability.

The changing definitions of global health, as well as the transition from previously used terms—such as *tropical medicine, international health*, and *geographic medicine*—reflect new demographic, economic, and political realities.[5,6] Older divisions of the world into developed and developing countries, or into north and south, are less salient in the interconnected, globalized world of 2015. During the past 50 years, infant mortality has fallen by more than 60%, total fertility rates have halved, the growth rate of the world population has diminished by half since a peak in the late 1960s, and the average life expectancy worldwide has increased by almost 20 years.[7] The result of these changes will be an aging world population, which will herald age-related changes in the burdens of disease. Economic power, including the capacity of countries to fund health systems and disease-prevention activities, is increasing most rapidly in formerly poor countries in East Asia, South Asia, and Latin America. In sub-Saharan Africa, many of the demographic changes are emerging more gradually, but rates of economic growth in this region are among the fastest in the world. Challenges to global health are huge, and the disparities between and within countries are vast; however, the connectivity of global trade, travel, and skilled labor and our collective exposure to transnational threats, such as climate change and pandemics, have necessitated a more global approach to improving the health of populations. Diseases of global importance—such as injuries, noncommunicable diseases, and mental health—can be partitioned according to their differential geographic and temporal effects. Assessing these effects requires metrics to measure the global burden of disease. Pandemic diseases, such as HIV/AIDS and influenza, are quintessentially global in character, whereas some problems are best understood in terms of the population at risk, as in the area of maternal and child health. Global forces such as globalization and climate change, as well as personal behavior involving risk factors such as tobacco use, excessive alcohol consumption, and poor diet, affect health in all countries.

Solutions to global health problems depend on new technologies, such as safer, more effective, and more practical vaccines, and on improved capacities and resources, such as workforce and training; they will also depend on better-designed health care systems, systems to promote population health, and improved global governance. Coordinated action across countries will often be needed in response to disasters and violence. For some infectious and parasitic diseases, the ultimate global solution could be disease eradication.

Although the series does not attempt to cover every topic in global health comprehensively, we invited the authors to summarize key examples of problems and their potential solutions and to present major themes and current priorities in this field. We hope the series will be of keen interest to health professionals at all levels who seek a deeper appreciation of global health as well as to experienced practitioners of modern public health for the world.

References

1. Hopkins DR. Disease eradication. *N Engl J Med* 2013;368:54–63.
2. Olds GR. Geographic medicine: a new movement within international health. *Acad Med* 1989;64:190–192.
3. Brown TM, Cueto M, Fee E. The World Health Organization and the transition from "international" to "global" public health. *Am J Public Health* 2006;96:62–72.
4. Institute of Medicine, Committee on the U.S. Commitment to Global Health. *The U.S. Commitment to Global Health: Recommendations for the Public and Private Sectors*. Washington, DC: National Academies Press, May 2009.
5. Bryant JH, Harrison PF. *Global health in Transition: A Synthesis: Perspectives from International Organizations*. Washington, DC: National Academy Press, 1996.
6. International health. *Br Med J* 1925;2:578–579.
7. Department of Economic and Social Affairs. *Population Division. World Population Prospects: The 2010 Revision*. New York, NY: United Nations, 2011.

PART I

Global Disease Patterns and Predictions

INTRODUCTION

One of the earliest examples of the use of data to predict disease patterns was the analysis of death records in London by John Graunt, published in *Natural and Political Observations Made upon the Bills of Mortality* in 1662. Graunt was motivated in part by the desire to create a system to predict outbreaks of the bubonic plague. He is credited with developing the first life tables, subsequently improved upon by others, including the astronomer Edmund Halley. In this case the linkage of the heavens with disease risk was personified in the scientist, a step ahead of astrologers scanning the skies for omens and portents of disease.

Most developed countries established methods to monitor the vital statistics of their populations in order to anticipate the need for public services. The registration of causes of death is a critical source of information on the patterns of disease between and within populations over time. Despite being subject to changes in the practice of physicians in certifying causes of death and the changes over time in disease taxonomies, death records are the best single source for the systematic enumeration of disease patterns. It is estimated that in 2005 about 18.8 million deaths (about 36%) of an estimated 51.7 million deaths worldwide were captured by registration systems that included certification of the medical cause of death.[1] The other 64% would have had to be reconstructed from a wide variety of records, relying on substantial assumptions.

Although specific countries have kept detailed records showing major national trends, such as the greater than 50% reduction in age-adjusted rates of death from cardiovascular disease in the United States since 1950, statistics for the entire world were limited and disjointed prior to the publication of the *Global Burden of Disease* study in 1990.[2] This study provided global estimates of deaths due to more than 120 diseases or injuries.[2] Years

of life lost from various causes were also calculated, a metric that gives more weight to death earlier in life, along with disability-adjusted life years, a measure of the morbidity associated with diseases and injuries. The review by Murray and Lopez describes the 2010 update on the global burden of disease, which includes data on 261 diseases and injuries. Region- and country-specific data now allow comparisons between countries that can inform policies, and trends over time within countries permit the assessment of the impact of policy changes. Just below the surface of these predictions are a range of value judgments such as how to weight the relative disabilities caused by different diseases and injuries and whether a death at an older age should be discounted relative to a death at a younger age. Some diseases are major causes of morbidity but much lesser causes of mortality, and disease-specific advocates can cherry-pick the data for the elements that rank "their" disease more highly. Although it may appear that the collection and interpretation of statistics on human health is a dry and dispassionate actuarial exercise, choices made by the statisticians can have a large impact on the interpretation and policy implications of the results.

Projections of future disease burdens can be made by combining demographic predictions with information about the prevalence of risk factors. These predictors may be confounded by large-scale shocks such as pandemics, economic crises, and wars. An increasingly likely influence on health is that posed by climate change, addressed in the article by the late Tony McMichael in this volume. As the UN Intergovernmental Panel on Climate Change[2] has moved from discussing the mitigation of climate change to the question of how to adapt to its effects, the manifold unpredictable consequences for human health must be part of planning for the future. Populations in low-lying areas on coasts are an immediate concern. As ecologies change, the range of disease vectors will change as well. Access to water may become more difficult in some areas and less difficult in others. Long-standing patterns of agriculture will change. Given the inevitability of at least some of these consequences, climate change will be an important component of future planning for health. The prospects of social disruption, costs to human health, and environmental degradation warrant more concerted attention and action to moderate the sources of climate change and to prepare for its consequences.

References

1. Lozano R, Naghavi M, Foreman K, et al. (2012). Global and regional mortality from 235 causes of death for 20 age groups in 1990 and 2010: a systematic analysis for the Global Burden of Disease Study 2010. *Lancet* 380(9859):2095–2128.
2. United Nations Intergovernmental Panel on Climate Change (2014). Climate change 2014: mitigation of climate change. Available at: http://mitigation2014.org/

Measuring the Global Burden of Disease

Christopher J.L. Murray
and Alan D. Lopez

It is difficult to deliver effective and high-quality care to patients without know-ing their diagnoses; likewise, for health systems to be effective, it is necessary to understand the key challenges in efforts to improve population health and how these challenges are changing. Before the early 1990s, there was no com-prehensive and internally consistent source of information on the global bur-den of diseases, injuries, and risk factors. To close this gap, the World Bank and the World Health Organization launched the Global Burden of Disease (GBD) Study in 1991.[1] Although assessments of selected diseases, injuries, and risk fac-tors in selected populations are published each year (e.g., the annual assessments of the human immunodeficiency virus [HIV] epidemic[2]), the only comprehensive assessments of the state of health in the world have been the various revisions of the GBD Study for 1990, 1999–2002, and 2004.[1,3–10] The advantage of the GBD approach is that consistent methods are applied to critically appraise available information on each condition, make this information comparable and system-atic, estimate results from countries with incomplete data, and report on the bur-den of disease with the use of standardized metrics.

The most recent assessment of the global burden of disease is the 2010 study (GBD 2010), which provides results for 1990, 2005, and 2010. Several hundred investigators collaborated to report summary results for the world and 21 epi-demiologic regions in December 2012.[11–18] Regions based on levels of adult mortality, child mortality, and geographic contiguity were defined. GBD 2010 addressed a number of major limitations of previous analyses, including the need to strengthen the statistical methods used for estimation.[11] The list of causes of the disease burden was broadened to cover 291 diseases and injuries. Data on 1160 sequelae of these causes (e.g., diabetic retinopathy, diabetic neuropathy, amputations due to diabetes, and chronic kidney disease due to diabetes) have been evaluated separately. The mortality and burden attributable to 67 risk fac-tors or clusters of risk factors were also assessed.

GBD 2010, which provides critical information for guiding prevention efforts, was based on data from 187 countries for the period from 1990 through 2010. It includes a complete reassessment of the burden of disease for 1990 as well as an estimation for 2005 and 2010 based on the same definitions and methods; this facilitated meaningful comparisons of trends. The prevalence of coexisting conditions was also estimated according to the year, age, sex, and country. Detailed results from global and regional data have been published previously.[11–18]

The internal validity of the results is an important aspect of the GBD approach. For example, demographic data on all-cause mortality according to the year, country, age, and sex were combined with data on cause-specific mortality to ensure that the sum of the number of deaths due to each disease and injury equaled the number of deaths from all causes. Similar internal-validity checks were used for cause-specific estimates related to impairments such as hearing loss and vision loss, anemia, heart failure, intellectual disability, infertility, and epilepsy when there were substantial data on the overall levels of the impairment.

Although GBD 2010 provides the most comprehensive and consistent assessment of global data on descriptive epidemiology, there remain many limitations. There were insufficient data on many diseases, injuries, and risk factors from many countries. Estimates depended on sophisticated statistical modeling to address sparse and often inconsistent data.[13,16,19,20] All outcomes were measured with 95% uncertainty intervals, which captured uncertainty from sampling, non-sampling error from the study designs or diagnostic methods, model parameter uncertainty, and uncertainty regarding model specification. This combined assessment of uncertainty was meant to communicate the strength of the evidence available for a particular condition in a particular place.

To compare the burden of one disease with that of another, it is necessary to consider the age at death and life expectancy of persons affected by each disease and to take account of the degree of disability (e.g., discomfort, pain, or functional limitations) imposed by each condition on those who live with the disease. In GBD 2010, years of life lost due to premature death were computed by multiplying the numbers of deaths by the life expectancy at the time of death in a reference population; this reference population was chosen as a population with a life expectancy at birth of 86.0 years, according to the lowest observed mortality in age groups for each sex.[11] A death at 1 year of age represents 85.2 years of life lost, and a death at 25 years of age represents 61.4 years of life lost. The same reference life expectancy at birth is used for males and females.[11] Because of a huge variation in severity, it is not very meaningful to compare the number of persons in the world with disorders as different as eczema, dental caries, scabies, major depression, multiple sclerosis, and tuberculosis. In GBD 2010, various sequelae were compared with the use of disability weights that were derived from surveys of the general population in five countries and an open Internet survey.[14] These surveys used pairwise comparisons and questions on population health equivalence, which ask respondents to assess improvements in health produced by various interventions that change disability or prevent premature death, to generate disability weights on a scale from 0.0 to 1.0, with 0.0 indicating ideal health and 1.0

indicating a state of health equivalent to death.[14] Years lived with disability were computed as the prevalence of a sequela multiplied by the disability weight for that sequela. Because years of life lost and years lived with disability were measured in units of healthy life lost, they were reported with the use of a comprehensive summary metric—disability-adjusted life-years (DALYs). In the lexicon of GBD 2010, disability is synonymous with any short-term or long-term health loss. In response to the recommendations of a panel of philosophers and ethicists, DALYs in GBD 2010 were not discounted or weighted according to age.[11]

Different metrics highlight different aspects of the health status of a population. Table 2.1 shows metrics for the United States, including the set of specific conditions that account for the 10 leading causes of death, years of life lost, years lived with disability, and DALYs. The numerical value for each metric and the rank for that cause across all causes listed in GBD 2010 are shown. These data provide various perspectives on the leading health problems in the United States. Large numbers of DALYs due to low back pain, other musculoskeletal disorders, neck pain, and osteoarthritis, along with DALYs due to vision loss, hearing loss, and anemias, highlight how metrics that capture all short-term or long-term decreases in health functioning yield a distinctive perspective. In the United States, the top 10 causes of the burden of disease as assessed with the use of DALYs include cardiovascular diseases (ischemic heart disease and stroke), chronic obstructive pulmonary disease (COPD), one type of cancer (of the trachea, bronchus, or lung), three musculoskeletal disorders (low back pain, other musculoskeletal disorders, and neck pain), major depressive disorder, diabetes, and road-traffic injury.

Some Key Findings from GBD 2010

Many findings in this study of 291 types of diseases and injuries and 67 risk factors in 187 countries over time have policy implications. In 1990, there were 2497 million global DALYs; this number decreased slightly, to 2482 million DALYs, in 2010. The steady volume of DALYs masks major changes in the distribution of the burden according to age, sex, country, and cause. On the basis of population growth alone, we would have expected the number of DALYs to increase by 37.9%; the small overall decrease of 0.6% was largely due to progress in reducing DALY rates according to age and sex.

Table 2.2 shows the 25 leading causes of DALYs in the world in 2010 in order, as well as the rank and number of DALYs in 1990. The leading causes included communicable diseases, noncommunicable diseases, and some injuries. The major causes of death in children in low-income countries in 1990, including lower respiratory tract infections, diarrhea, malaria, complications of preterm birth, and neonatal encephalopathy, were among the top 15 DALYs in 2010. In addition, HIV infection and the acquired immune deficiency syndrome (HIV–AIDS) and tuberculosis remained in the top 15 causes of DALYs. Noncommunicable diseases such as ischemic heart disease, stroke, COPD, and diabetes—which

TABLE 2.1 Top 10 Causes of Death, Years of Life Lost from Premature Death, Years Lived with Disability, and Disability-Adjusted Life-Years (DALYs) in the United States, 2010

Cause of Death	Deaths (N = 2664)		Years of Life Lost (N = 45,145)		Years Lived with Disability (N = 36,689)		DALYs (N = 81,835)	
	Rank	No. (%) in thousands	Rank	No. (%) in thousands	Rank	No. (%) in thousands	Rank	No. (%) in thousands
Ischemic heart disease	1	563 (21.1)	1	7165 (15.9)	16	685 (1.9)	1	7850 (9.6)
Chronic obstructive pulmonary disease	5	154 (5.8)	4	1913 (4.2)	6	1745 (4.8)	2	3659 (4.5)
Low back pain	—	—	—	—	1	3181 (8.7)	3	3181 (3.9)
Cancer of the trachea, bronchus, or lung	3	163 (6.1)	2	2988 (6.6)	73	45 (0.1)	4	3033 (3.7)
Major depressive disorder	—	—	—	—	2	3049 (8.3)	5	3049 (3.7)
Other musculoskeletal disorders	36	14 (0.5)	37	254 (0.6)	3	2603 (7.1)	6	2857 (3.5)
Stroke	2	172 (6.5)	3	1945 (4.3)	17	629 (1.7)	7	2574 (3.1)
Diabetes mellitus	6	86 (3.2)	7	1392 (3.1)	8	1165 (3.2)	8	2557 (3.1)
Road-traffic injury	12	44 (1.7)	5	1873 (4.1)	26	373 (1.0)	9	2246 (2.7)
Drug-use disorders	27	19 (0.7)	15	841 (1.9)	7	1295 (3.5)	10	2136 (2.6)
Neck pain	—	—	—	—	4	2134 (5.8)	11	2134 (2.6)
Alzheimer's disease and other dementias	4	158 (5.9)	9	1192 (2.6)	12	830 (2.3)	12	2022 (2.5)
Anxiety disorders	—	—	—	—	5	1866 (5.1)	13	1866 (2.3)
Self-harm	16	37 (1.4)	6	1457 (3.2)	121	6 (<0.05)	14	1463 (1.8)
Cirrhosis of the liver	11	50 (1.9)	8	1233 (2.7)	98	16 (<0.05)	15	1249 (1.5)
Chronic kidney disease	9	60 (2.3)	16	780 (1.7)	22	410 (1.1)	17	1191 (1.5)
Colorectal cancers	8	64 (2.4)	10	1074 (2.4)	56	73 (0.2)	18	1147 (1.4)
Lower respiratory tract infections	7	85 (3.2)	11	1032 (2.3)	62	61 (0.2)	20	1093 (1.3)
Asthma	61	4 (0.2)	57	100 (0.2)	10	932 (2.5)	24	1032 (1.3)
Osteoarthritis	—	—	—	—	9	994 (2.7)	25	994 (1.2)
Other cardiovascular and circulatory diseases	10	57 (2.1)	17	765 (1.7)	34	213 (0.6)	26	979 (1.2)

TABLE 2.2 Global DALYs Caused by the 25 Leading Diseases and Injuries in 1990 and 2010

Cause	2010		1990	
	Rank	DALYs (95% UI) in thousands	Rank	DALYs (95% UI) in thousands
Ischemic heart disease	1	129,795 (119,218–137,398)	4	100,455 (96,669–108,702)
Lower respiratory tract infections	2	115,227 (102,255–126,972)	1	206,461 (183,354–222,979)
Stroke	3	102,239 (90,472–108,003)	5	86,012 (81,033–94,802)
Diarrhea	4	89,524 (77,595–99,193)	2	183,543 (168,791–197,655)
HIV–AIDS	5	81,549 (74,698–88,371)	33	18,118 (14,996–22,269)
Malaria	6	82,689 (63,465–109,846)	7	69,141 (54,547–85,589)
Low back pain	7	80,667 (56,066–108,723)	12	56,384 (38,773–76,233)
Preterm birth complications	8	76,980 (66,210–88,132)	3	105,965 (88,144–120,894)
Chronic obstructive pulmonary disease	9	76,779 (66,000–89,147)	6	78,298 (70,407–86,849)
Road-traffic injury	10	75,487 (61,555–94,777)	11	56,651 (49,633–68,046)
Major depressive disorder	11	63,239 (47,894–80,784)	15	46,177 (34,524–58,436)
Neonatal encephalopathy*	12	50,163 (40,351–59,810)	10	60,604 (50,209–74,826)
Tuberculosis	13	49,399 (40,027–56,009)	8	61,256 (55,465–71,083)
Diabetes mellitus	14	46,857 (40,212–55,252)	21	27,719 (23,668–32,925)
Iron-deficiency anemia	15	45,350 (31,046–64,616)	14	46,803 (32,604–66,097)
Sepsis and other infectious disorders in newborns	16	44,236 (27,349–72,418)	17	46,029 (25,147–70,357)
Congenital anomalies	17	38,890 (31,891–45,739)	13	54,245 (45,491–69,057)
Self-harm	18	36,655 (26,894–44,652)	19	29,605 (23,039–37,333)
Falls	19	35,406 (28,583–44,052)	22	25,900 (21,252–31,656)
Protein-energy malnutrition	20	34,874 (27,957–41,662)	9	60,542 (50,378–71,639)
Neck pain	21	32,651 (22,783–44,857)	25	23,107 (16,031–31,890)
Cancer of the trachea, bronchus, or lung	22	32,405 (24,401–38,327)	24	23,850 (18,839–29,837)
Other musculoskeletal disorders	23	30,877 (25,858–34,650)	29	20,596 (17,025–23,262)
Cirrhosis of the liver	24	31,026 (25,951–34,629)	23	24,325 (20,653–27,184)
Meningitis	25	29,407 (25,578–33,442)	18	37,822 (33,817–44,962)

*The category of neonatal encephalopathy includes birth asphyxia and birth trauma.

primarily cause premature death—were among the top 15 causes of DALYs; disabling conditions such as low back pain and major depressive disorder were also leading causes. Low back pain, for example, affects 10% of the world population and ranges from mild to quite severe. Three types of injuries were among the top 25 causes of DALYs; road-traffic injuries, which caused the most DALYs, increased by 33% between 1990 and 2010. A comparison of data from 1990 with data from 2010 shows some profound shifts. In general, communicable, maternal, neonatal, and nutritional conditions decreased in absolute terms (both in numbers of DALYs and rates) and relative to noncommunicable diseases; the notable exceptions were malaria and HIV–AIDS. The burden of noncommunicable diseases, both from the causes of years of life lost and the causes of years lived with disability, has been increasing in terms of the absolute number of years of life lost and years lived with disability and in terms of the share of the total burden over the two decades, with the largest increases associated with diabetes.

The burden of disease attributable to risk factors is shown in Table 2.3. The leading risk factors changed substantially, and there were major shifts in the burden of disease between 1990 and 2010. In 1990, the leading risk factor was childhood underweight, which was ranked 8th among the risk factors evaluated in 2010, representing an absolute decrease in DALYs of 61%. Other major decreases were observed in the burden attributable to household air pollution (from 2nd to 3rd rank), suboptimal breast-feeding (defined as nonexclusive breast-feeding for up to 6 months of life and discontinued breast-feeding between 6 and 23 months of life) (5th to 14th rank), unimproved sanitation (15th to 26th rank), vitamin A deficiency (17th to 29th rank), zinc deficiency (19th to 31st rank), and unimproved water sources (22nd to 34th rank). Conversely, increases in attributable DALYs of more than 30% occurred for the following risk factors: obesity (high body-mass index), a high fasting plasma glucose level, a high-sodium diet, a diet low in whole grains, drug-use disorders, and lead exposure. The list of leading risk factors includes multiple components of diet, each of which were evaluated in isolation; taken together, all components of diet and physical inactivity accounted for 10.2% of global DALYs in 2010. The burden attributable to tobacco smoking (including exposure to secondhand smoke) remained roughly constant (6.3% of DALYs in 2010) from 1990 to 2010 because of decreased smoking in high-income countries and increased smoking in developing regions, most notably in East Asia.

THREE GLOBAL DRIVERS OF RAPID TRANSITIONS IN GLOBAL HEALTH

Three broad transitions explain much of the changing pattern in global health: demographic changes, changes in causes of death, and changes in causes of disability. Demographic effects on the burden of disease include both the increase in the numbers of people and the effect of an increasing average age of the population. As part of GBD 2010, investigators measured the change from 1990 to 2010 in the burden of disease expected on the basis of increases in population size and

TABLE 2.3 Global DALYs Attributable to the 25 Leading Risk Factors in 1990 and 2010

Risk Factor	2010		1990	
	Rank	DALYs (95% UI) in thousands	Rank	DALYs (95% UI) in thousands
High blood pressure	1	173,556 (155,939–189,025)	4	137,017 (124,360–149,366)
Tobacco smoking, including exposure to secondhand smoke	2	156,838 (136,543–173,057)	3	151,766 (136,367–169,522)
Household air pollution from solid fuels	3	108,084 (84,891–132,983)	2	170,693 (139,087–199,504)
Diet low in fruit	4	104,095 (81,833–124,169)	7	80,453 (63,298–95,763)
Alcohol use	5	97,237 (87,087–107,658)	8	73,715 (66,090–82,089)
High body-mass index	6	93,609 (77,107–110,600)	10	51,565 (40,786–62,557)
High fasting plasma glucose level	7	89,012 (77,743–101,390)	9	56,358 (48,720–65,030)
Childhood underweight	8	77,316 (64,497–91,943)	1	197,741 (169,224–238,276)
Exposure to ambient particulate-matter pollution	9	76,163 (68,086–85,171)	6	81,699 (71,012–92,859)
Physical inactivity or low level of activity	10	69,318 (58,646–80,182)	—	—
Diet high in sodium	11	61,231 (40,124–80,342)	12	46,183 (30,363–60,604)
Diet low in nuts and seeds	12	51,289 (33,482–65,959)	13	40,525 (26,308–51,741)
Iron deficiency	13	48,225 (33,769–67,592)	11	51,841 (37,477–71,202)
Suboptimal breast-feeding	14	47,537 (29,868–67,518)	5	110,261 (69,615–153,539)
High total cholesterol level	15	40,900 (31,662–50,484)	14	39,526 (32,704–47,202)
Diet low in whole grains	16	40,762 (32,112–48,486)	18	29,404 (23,097–35,134)
Diet low in vegetables	17	38,559 (26,006–51,658)	16	31,558 (21,349–41,921)
Diet low in seafood n–3 fatty acids	18	28,199 (20,624–35,974)	20	21,740 (15,869–27,537)
Drug use	19	23,810 (18,780–29,246)	25	15,171 (11,714–19,369)
Occupational risk factors for injuries	20	23,444 (17,736–30,904)	21	21,265 (16,644–26,702)
Occupation-related low back pain	21	21,750 (14,492–30,533)	23	17,841 (11,846–24,945)
Diet high in processed meat	22	20,939 (6982–33,468)	24	17,359 (5137–27,949)
Intimate-partner violence	23	16,794 (11,373–23,087)	—	—
Diet low in fiber	24	16,452 (7401–25,783)	26	13,347 (5970–20,751)
Lead exposure	25	13,936 (11,750–16,327)	31	5,365 (4534–6279)

the aging of the world population. The effects of population growth alone would increase the number of DALYs from all causes, but because population growth was largest in sub-Saharan Africa, it would differentially increase DALYs caused by communicable, maternal, neonatal, and nutritional diseases by 47.6%, those caused by noncommunicable diseases by 27.8%, and those caused by injuries by 32.6%. The increasing mean age of the population, however, decreased the number of DALYs from communicable, maternal, neonatal, and nutritional diseases by 22.2% but increased DALYs associated with noncommunicable diseases by 19.1%. Demographic change (population growth and aging) is the key driver of increases in the burden of noncommunicable diseases; at the global level, age-specific rates of nearly all conditions are actually decreasing.

The second major transition is the change in age-specific and sex-specific rates of death associated with diseases and injuries. From 1990 to 2010, in the aggregate category of communicable, maternal, neonatal, and nutritional diseases, DALYs decreased by 52.1% because of decreases in age-specific and sex-specific rates of death—notably, this overall decrease occurred despite the increases in DALYs due to HIV–AIDS and smaller increases in DALYs due to malaria over this period. This decrease may be related to a combination of increasing levels of maternal education, improved delivery of preventive and medical care with key forms of technology, increasing income per capita, and increasing health expenditures, including development assistance for public health and medical care.[21–24] Decreases in global DALYs due to noncommunicable diseases were more modest, at 22.4%, because of lower age-specific and sex-specific rates of noncommunicable diseases and were even more modest for injuries (20.2%). At a slightly more detailed level, changes in age-specific and sex-specific rates of DALYs led to a 33.6% decrease in global DALYs due to cardiovascular causes and a 24.0% decrease in age-specific and sex-specific global cancer rates. These decreases in the face of the increasing prevalence of some risk factors such as obesity and tobacco use suggest the important role of other factors, including better prenatal care and early-childhood interventions, prevention and treatment provided by health systems, and improvements in socioeconomic status. Although the decreases in rates of noncommunicable diseases and injuries are small, the decreases indicate that the relative importance of noncommunicable diseases and injuries as a share of causes of death will increase. Progress in reducing global age-specific and sex-specific rates of death associated with all three major groups of causes (communicable diseases, noncommunicable diseases, and injuries) is reflected in the increase from 1990 to 2010 in the global life expectancy at birth from 62.8 years to 67.5 years for men and from 68.1 years to 73.3 years for women. Both demographic change and change in age-specific and sex-specific mortality drive the shift toward a larger fraction of the burden due to noncommunicable diseases. Figure 2.1A shows the fraction of the total burden from noncommunicable diseases according to country in 2010. In most of Latin America, North Africa, the Middle East, Southeast Asia, and East Asia, the substantial majority of the

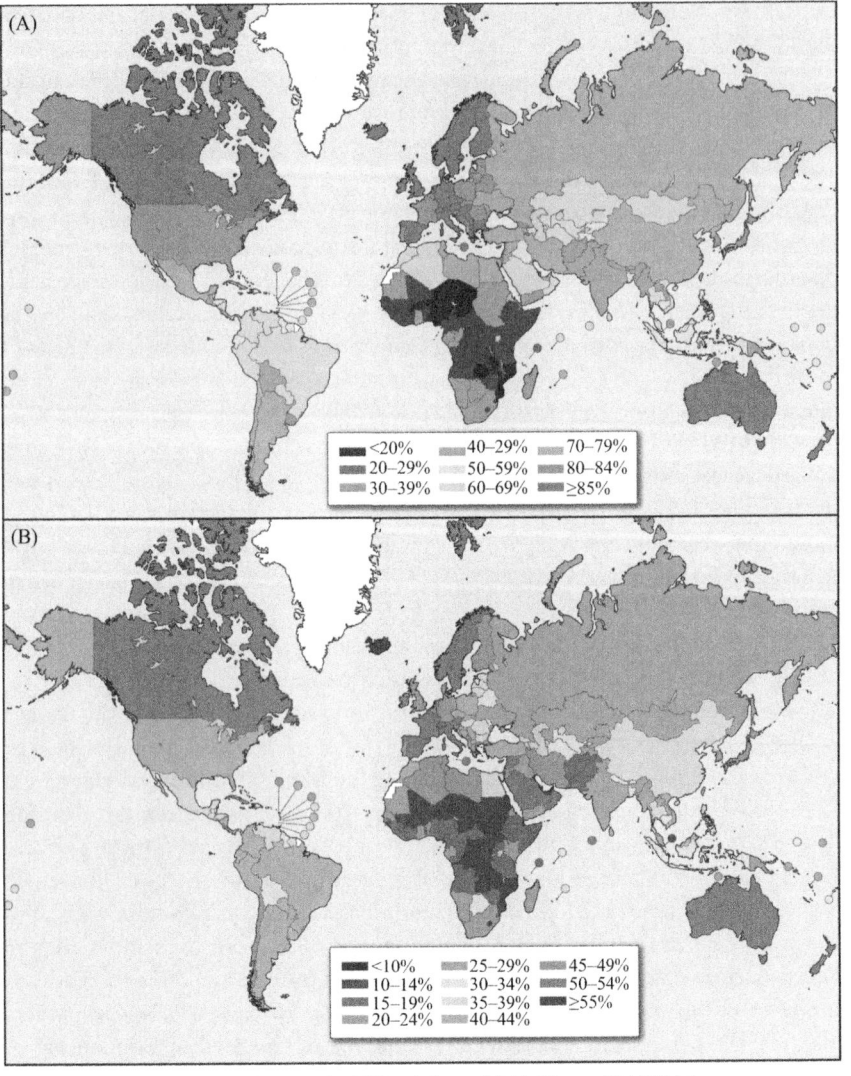

FIGURE 2.1 **Percentage of Total Disability-Adjusted Life-Years (DALYs) in
2010 According to Country** *Panel A shows the percentage of total DALYs due to
noncommunicable diseases in each country. Noncommunicable diseases are defined in the
hierarchical list of causes[11] in the Global Burden of Disease 2010 study and include the
following major cause groups: cancers; cardiovascular and circulatory diseases; chronic
respiratory diseases; cirrhosis; digestive diseases; neurologic conditions; mental and
behavioral disorders; diabetes; urogenital, blood, and endocrine diseases; musculoskeletal
diseases; and other noncommunicable diseases such as congenital anomalies and skin
diseases. Panel B shows the percentage of total DALYs due to years lived with disability
per country.*

burden was from noncommunicable diseases. Even in South Asia, the fraction due to noncommunicable diseases was more than 40%.

The third transition is a profound shift toward a greater fraction of the burden of disease from disability than from premature death. Of the top 25 causes of years lived with disability, only COPD, diabetes, road-traffic injury, ischemic heart disease, tuberculosis, and diarrhea are also among the top 25 causes of years of life lost. Simply put, what ails most persons is not necessarily what kills them. Major groups of disorders that cause disability include musculoskeletal disorders, mental disorders and substance abuse, neurologic conditions, anemias, vision loss, hearing loss, diabetes, and skin diseases. Age-specific and sex-specific prevalence rates of nearly all these conditions are stable or decreasing only slightly, and the rates of some conditions, such as diabetes, are increasing. Stable or increasing rates combined with population growth and aging lead to substantial increases in the number of years lived with these disabling conditions. Overall, there is a progressive shift toward a larger share of the burden of disease from disability. Figure 2.1B shows the fraction of the burden attributable to disability in 2010 according to country; more than 40% of the disease burden in many developed countries, much of Latin America, North Africa, the Middle East, and parts of Southeast Asia was from disability. The fraction of the burden from years lived with disability increased from 1990 to 2010 in nearly all countries. Disabling conditions cause a substantial loss of healthy life and are costly for health systems to manage.[25,26]

The three major transitions account at a broad level for much of the change in global health, but they do not explain the entire story. There are marked regional and national divergences from this general pattern. The development of large HIV epidemics in eastern sub-Saharan Africa and southern sub-Saharan Africa has had an enormous effect on the burden of disease in those regions. Interpersonal violence is among the top 5 causes of the disease burden in Guatemala, Honduras, El Salvador, Colombia, Venezuela, Ecuador, Bahamas, Mexico, Jamaica, and Brazil. It is also among the top 5 causes of the burden in South Africa, Lesotho, Namibia, Botswana, and Swaziland. Malaria is a leading cause of the disease burden in areas from West Africa to Madagascar where malaria is hyperendemic (defined as parasitemia in >50% of the population) or mesoendemic (defined as parasitemia in 10 to 50% of the population). There is a particularly large burden of diabetes in Central America, the Caribbean, North Africa, the Middle East, and Oceania. The demographic changes, changes in mortality associated with disease and injuries, and changes in causes of disability, combined with local variations in the disease burden, have led to important differences among countries. Thirteen different causes (HIV–AIDS, diarrhea, lower respiratory tract infections, malaria, preterm birth conditions, ischemic heart disease, stroke, major depressive disorder, diabetes, low back pain, road-traffic injury, violence, and natural disasters) account for the leading causes of disease and injury burden in at least 1 country. A similar assessment of the leading risk factor according to country shows that eight different risk factors account for the leading cause of attributable DALYs across countries. These risk factors are alcohol use (in 22 countries), high body-mass index (in

32 countries), suboptimal breast-feeding (in 2 countries), a high fasting plasma glucose level (in 3 countries), household air pollution (in 14 countries), high systolic blood pressure (in 59 countries), smoking (in 24 countries), and childhood underweight (in 31 countries).

GBD 2010 RESULTS FOR BENCHMARKING

An important dimension of GBD 2010 is the capacity to use consistent data and metrics to compare the health outcomes of one nation with those of other countries. Comparisons over time and across nations help to place local performance in health improvement in context; this analysis has already been published in the United Kingdom.[27] For example, the age-standardized mortality or DALY rates in each country can be computed and then ranked across the 187 countries. These rankings provide information on how a country is doing relative to other countries. Changes in these ranks provide insights into relative performance. Figure 2.2 shows the leading causes of death in the United States and the associated rank of the age-standardized mortality in 1990 and 2010, with 95% uncertainty intervals. Ranks are a relative measure; a higher (worse) rank may be due to increasing age-standardized rates or to decreases that are smaller than those in other nations. This figure shows that for the leading causes of death, the United States has the best global performance with respect to stroke and the worst relative performance with respect to lung cancer and Alzheimer's disease. Significant

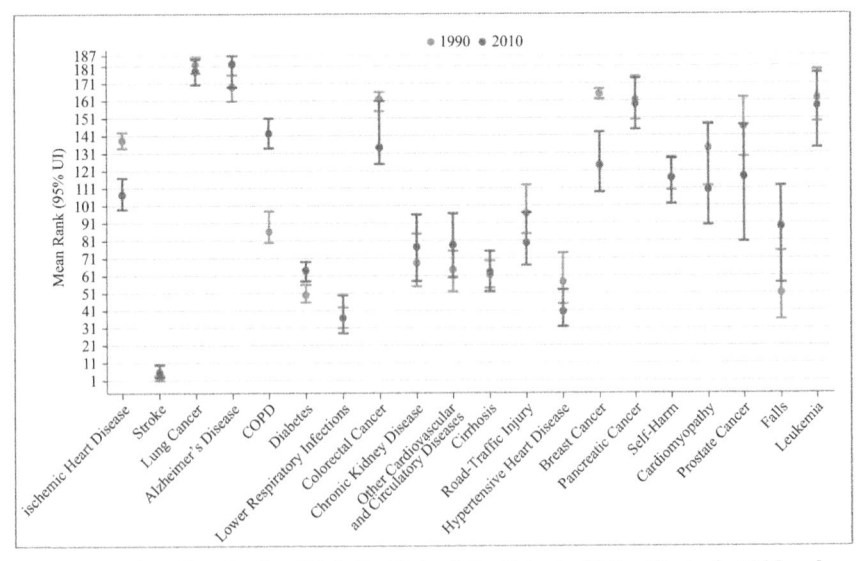

FIGURE 2.2 **Age-Standardized Relative Rate of Death in the United States in 1990 and 2010, as Ranked among 187 Other Countries** *Ranks for the 20 leading causes of death in the United States are shown. Rank 1 is the lowest age-standardized mortality across the 187 countries, and rank 187 is the highest. I bars indicate 95% uncertainty intervals (UIs). COPD denotes chronic obstructive pulmonary disease.*

improvements in relative rank are shown for ischemic heart disease and breast cancer. Significant decreases in relative performance are shown for COPD and diabetes. Data and analyses are lacking to elucidate the drivers of these changes in relative performance, such as the contributions of medical care, public health, or trends in risk factors. Such benchmarking, however, provides a high-level synopsis of diseases for which the United States is achieving good outcomes and those for which it is not. Similar comparative assessments could be conducted within a country across units such as states or counties[28-34] to shed light on disparities.

Future Development

Quantifying the burden of disease provides useful input into health policy dialogues and identifies conditions and risk factors that may be relatively neglected and others for which progress is not what was expected. Nevertheless, estimates of disease burden can only improve as further data are collected and methods are refined. Going forward, we plan to release regular GBD study updates annually as new data or major new studies are released. With each revision, the entire time series from 1990 forward will be reassessed so that meaningful comparisons over time will be possible. Everyone—consumers, health professionals, researchers, and decision makers—will have access to assessments based on the latest available evidence. Continuous revisions will also facilitate the incorporation of scientific feedback on how to improve the estimation for any particular disease, injury, or risk factor in countries. With time, we hope that the definitions, methods, and estimation techniques from the GBD study effort will also be widely used to understand patterns of health within countries that are differentiated according to geographic region, social class, or race or ethnic group.

References

1. World Bank. World Development Report 1993—investing in health: world development indicators. Oxford, United Kingdom: Oxford University Press, 1993.
2. Global report: UNAIDS report on the global aids epidemic. Joint United Nations Programme on HIV/AIDS (UNAIDS), 2010 (http://www.unaids.org/globalreport/documents/20101123_GlobalReport_full_en.pdf).
3. Murray CJ, Lopez AD. Mortality by cause for eight regions of the world: Global Burden of Disease Study. Lancet 1997;349:1269-76.
4. Idem. Regional patterns of disability-free life expectancy and disability-adjusted life expectancy: Global Burden of Disease Study. Lancet 1997;349:1347-52.
5. Idem. Global mortality, disability, and the contribution of risk factors: Global Burden of Disease Study. Lancet 1997;349:1436-42.
6. Idem. Alternative projections of mortality and disability by cause 1990-2020: Global Burden of Disease Study. Lancet 1997;349:1498-504.

7. Murray CJL, Ferguson BD, Lopez AD, Guillot M, Salomon JA, Ahmad O. Modified logit life table system: principles, empirical validation, and application. Popul Stud 2003;57:165–82.
8. Salomon JA, Murray CJL. The epidemiologic transition revisited: compositional models for causes of death by age and sex. Popul Dev Rev 2002;28:205–28.
9. Salomon JA, Tandon A, Murray CJL. Comparability of self rated health: cross sectional multi-country survey using anchoring vignettes. BMJ 2004;328:258.
10. The World Health Report 2000—health systems: improving performance. Geneva: World Health Organization, 2000.
11. Murray CJL, Ezzati M, Flaxman AD, et al. GBD 2010: design, definitions, and metrics. Lancet 2012;380:2063–66.
12. Wang H, Dwyer-Lindgren L, Lofgren KT, et al. Age-specific and sex-specific mortality in 187 countries, 1970–2010: a systematic analysis for the Global Burden of Disease Study 2010. Lancet 2012;380:2071–94.
13. Lozano R, Naghavi M, Foreman K, et al. Global and regional mortality from 235 causes of death for 20 age groups in 1990 and 2010: a systematic analysis for the Global Burden of Disease Study 2010. Lancet 2012;380:2095–128.
14. Salomon JA, Vos T, Hogan DR, et al. Common values in assessing health outcomes from disease and injury: disability weights measurement study for the Global Burden of Disease Study 2010. Lancet 2012;380:2129–43.
15. Salomon JA, Wang H, Freeman MK, et al. Healthy life expectancy for 187 countries, 1990–2010: a systematic analysis for the Global Burden of Disease Study 2010. Lancet 2012;380:2144–62. [Erratum, Lancet 2013;381:628.]
16. Vos T, Flaxman AD, Naghavi M, et al. Years lived with disability (YLDs) for 1160 sequelae of 289 diseases and injuries 1990–2010: a systematic analysis for the Global Burden of Disease Study 2010. Lancet 2012;380:2163–96.
17. Murray CJL, Vos T, Lozano R, et al. Disability-adjusted life years (DALYs) for 291 diseases and injuries in 21 regions, 1990–2010: a systematic analysis for the Global Burden of Disease Study 2010. Lancet 2012;380:2197–223.
18. Lim SS, Vos T, Flaxman AD, et al. A comparative risk assessment of burden of disease and injury attributable to 67 risk factors and risk factor clusters in 21 regions, 1990–2010: a systematic analysis for the Global Burden of Disease Study 2010. Lancet 2012;380:2224–60.
19. Foreman KJ, Lozano R, Lopez AD, Murray CJ. Modeling causes of death: an integrated approach using CODEm. Popul Health Metr 2012;10:1.
20. Naghavi M, Makela S, Foreman K, O'Brien J, Pourmalek F, Lozano R. Algorithms for enhancing public health utility of national causes-of-death data. Popul Health Metr 2010;8:9.
21. Gakidou E, Cowling K, Lozano R, Murray CJL. Increased educational attainment and its effect on child mortality in 175 countries between 1970 and 2009: a systematic analysis. Lancet 2010;376:959–74.
22. Preston SH. The changing relation between mortality and level of economic development. Int J Epidemiol 2007;36:484–90.
23. Building a future for women and children: the 2012 report. Washington, DC: World Health Organization and UNICEF, 2012.

24. Financing global health 2012: the end of the Golden Age? Seattle: Institute for Health Metrics and Evaluation, 2012.

25. Yelin E, Callahan LF. The economic cost and social and psychological impact of musculoskeletal conditions. Arthritis Rheum 1995;38:1351–62.

26. Coyte PC, Asche CV, Croxford R, Chan B. The economic cost of musculoskeletal disorders in Canada. Arthritis Care Res 1998;11:315–25.

27. Murray CJL, Richards MAR, Newton JN, et al. UK health performance: findings of the Global Burden of Disease Study 2010. Lancet 2013;381:997–1020.

28. Schopper D, Pereira J, Torres A, et al. Estimating the burden of disease in one Swiss canton: what do disability adjusted life years (DALY) tell us? Int J Epidemiol 2000;29:871–77.

29. Kominski GF, Simon PA, Ho A, Luck J, Lim Y-W, Fielding JE. Assessing the burden of disease and injury in Los Angeles County using disability-adjusted life years. Public Health Rep 2002;117:185–91.

30. Zhou S-C, Cai L, Wan C-H, Lv Y-L, Fang P-Q. Assessing the disease burden of Yi people by years of life lost in Shilin county of Yunnan province, China. BMC Public Health 2009;9:188.

31. Friedman C, McKenna MT, Ahmed F, et al. Assessing the burden of disease among an employed population: implications for employer-sponsored prevention programs. J Occup Environ Med 2004;46:3–9.

32. Hsairi M, Fekih H, Fakhfakh R, Kassis M, Achour N, Dammak J. Années de vie perdues et transition épidémiologique dans le gouvernorat de Sfax (Tunisie). Sante Publique 2003;15:25–37.

33. Dodhia H, Phillips K. Measuring burden of disease in two inner London boroughs using Disability Adjusted Life Years. J Public Health (Oxf) 2008;30:313–21.

34. Kulkarni SC, Levin-Rector A, Ezzati M, Murray CJL. Falling behind: life expectancy in US counties from 2000 to 2007 in an international context. Popul Health Metr 2011;9:16.

Globalization, Climate Change, and Human Health

Anthony J. McMichael

The global scale, interconnectedness, and economic intensity of contemporary human activity are historically unprecedented,[1] as are many of the consequent environmental and social changes. These global changes fundamentally influence patterns of human health, international health care, and public health activities.[2] They constitute a syndrome, not a set of separate changes, that reflects the inter-related pressures, stresses, and tensions arising from an overly large world population, the pervasive and increasingly systemic environmental impact of many economic activities, urbanization, the spread of consumerism, and the widening gap between rich and poor both within and between countries.

In recent decades, international connectivity has increased on many fronts, including the flow of information, movements of people, trading patterns, the flow of capital, regulatory systems, and cultural diffusion. These exponential increases in demographic, economic, commercial, and environmental indexes have been labeled the Great Acceleration.[3] Remarkably, the resultant environmental effects are now altering major components of the Earth system.[4,5] The current geologic epoch is being called the Anthropocene (successor to the Holocene epoch)[5,6] in recognition of the global force that *Homo sapiens* has become, pushing or distorting Earth's great natural global systems beyond boundaries considered to be safe for continued human social and biologic well-being.[4,7] The loss of biodiversity, the greatly amplified global circulation of bioactive nitrogen compounds, and human-induced climate change have already reached levels that are apparently unsafe.[4]

These changes pose fundamental threats to human well-being and health.[4,7] For example, a positive relationship has been observed between regional trends in climate (rising temperatures and declining rainfall) and childhood stunting in Kenya since 1975, indicating that as projected warming and drying continue to occur along with population growth, food yields and nutritional health will be impaired.[8] These human-induced climatic changes often act in concert with

environmental, demographic, and social stressors that variously influence regional food yields, nutrition, and health. Furthermore, at the current level of global connectedness and interdependence, the environmental impact of human activity has a wider geographic range, although its influence may be offset somewhat by more effective global alerts and more rapid distribution of food aid. The extreme heat and wildfires in western Russia in the summer of 2010 destroyed one third of that country's wheat yield, and the subsequent ban on exported grain contributed to a rise in the price of wheat worldwide, exacerbating hunger in Russia (where flour prices increased by 20%) and in low-income urban populations in countries such as Pakistan and Egypt.[9,10] On the economic front, the recent global financial crisis has underscored the domino-like interdependence of national economies.

Effects of Globalization on Population Health

Global influences on population health such as those described above transcend the more specific, focused frame within which international health issues are addressed.[2] The processes of global change are more systemic, involving disruption or depletion (not merely local pollution). Remediating or adapting to these changes requires an understanding of dynamic systems, their complexity and associated uncertainties, and coordinated policy responses across relevant sectors. The relationships between these pervasive processes of change and human health are shown in Figure 3.1.

DEMOGRAPHIC CHANGES

Population growth is often overlooked in the discourse on global change, including its relation to the mitigation (abatement) of climate change, to which the contribution of global emissions is obvious.[11] The projections by the United Nations that today's population of 7 billion will increase to 9.3 billion by 2050[12] should reactivate the debate about whether we can succeed in pursuing realistic objectives for a healthy climate without curtailing the actual number of humans pressing on the environment. Furthermore, the negative-feedback loop of excessive population pressure on regional environments (involving soil exhaustion, water depletion, and the loss of various wild animal and plant food species) not only exacerbates various ongoing worldwide environmental and ecologic changes but also entrenches conditions of poverty and disadvantage. In these latter circumstances, fertility rates tend to remain high.

Some additional increase in the world population is inevitable in countries with high fertility rates, given the demographic flywheel momentum of populations weighted toward the young. Meanwhile, moderate gains have been made in facilitating education for girls, although progress in this, as well as in the provision of adequate education about reproduction and reproductive choice, remains slow in many low-income countries.[13] Where unplanned pregnancy rates remain high (e.g., Timor-Leste and Nigeria), so do risks to maternal and child health.

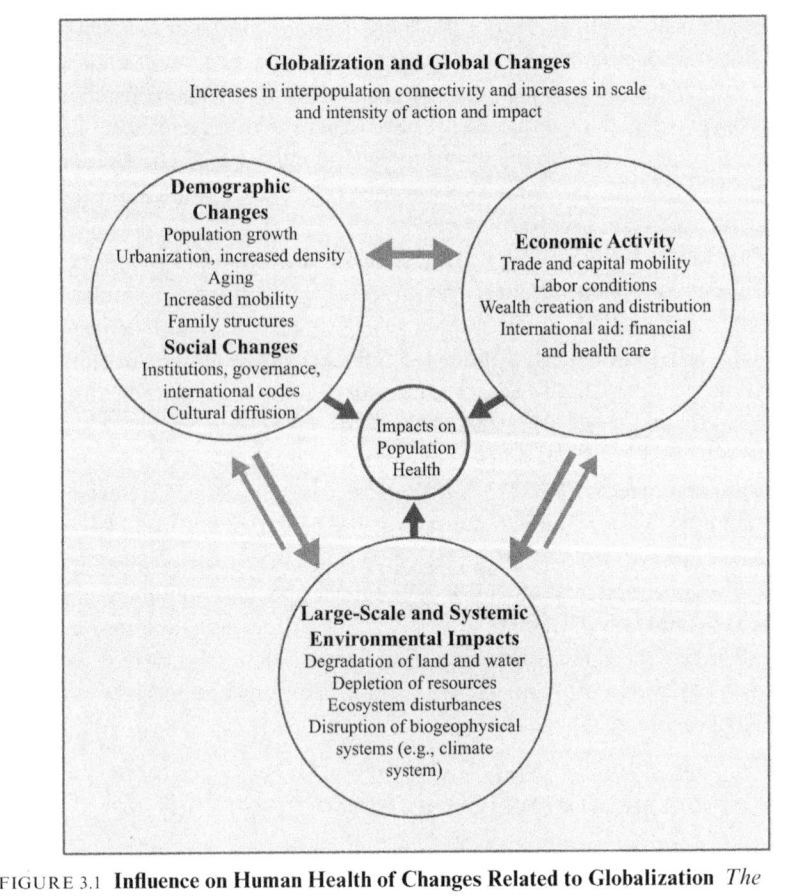

FIGURE 3.1 **Influence on Human Health of Changes Related to Globalization** *The figure is a schematic representation of the three major domains—social, economic, and environmental—within which globalizing processes and changes are occurring. Shown are their main components, the two-way interactions between them, and the central fact that all three domains influence the conditions for and levels of population health. In particular, changes in population size, distribution, mobility, levels and types of economic activity, and global flows of capital and labor all have consequences for the environment, including the recent rapid increase in greenhouse-gas emissions as the primary cause of current climate change. Those great contemporary environmental changes have diverse and far-reaching consequences for human health.*

SOCIAL CHANGES AND ECONOMIC ACTIVITY

Many other aspects of globalization influence population health,[2] including the accelerated emergence of new infectious diseases,[14,15] the near-ubiquitous rise in the rates of obesity and associated noncommunicable diseases as daily bodily energy budgets (food energy input vs. physical energy output) shift into surplus,[16] the spread of cigarette marketing, the effects of climate change,[17,18] increases in resistance to antimicrobial agents, and health risks in the workplace due to the

deregulation of international labor markets.[2] Looming large in the background as additional determinants of health are the persistent, even increasing, disparities in wealth, education, autonomy, and social inclusion.[19] There are, of course, certain aspects of globalization that are beneficial to health, such as the enhanced flow of information, improvements in internationally coordinated vaccination programs and systems to respond to infectious diseases, and a greater capacity for long-distance responses to disasters.

Adverse global influences on health, such as rising food prices and extended ranges of some infectious diseases, have also impeded attainment of the United Nations Millennium Development Goals.[20] Future global health goals must be better integrated with the fundamental influences of poverty, inequity, illiteracy, climate change, land-use patterns, and food insecurity on health. After the Rio+20 Conference (2012), the Millennium Development Goals are to be replaced by Sustainable Development Goals in 2016, reflecting the principle set forth at the original Rio Declaration on Environment and Development (1992) that concern for humans must be at the center of sustainable development. Nevertheless, concern for human health is not yet near that center. This reflects the continuing misperception of what health means and the dominance of a narrow, clinically based view that seemingly does not take into account the fundamental need, in improving population health, to address the poor fit between environmental and sociocultural conditions and basic human biologic and psychological needs.

ENVIRONMENTAL AND ECOLOGIC CHANGES

The deep-seated, essentially ecologic risks to population health cannot be countered effectively at the local level alone. Climate change induced by human activities, for example, is due to the globally aggregated excess of greenhouse emissions. Primary prevention of health problems arising from such global environmental and sociodemographic changes therefore requires coordinated international policy, supplemented by more local policy-making and action. For example, the World Trade Organization should give greater priority to averting the adverse health and environmental effects of international free trade.[21] There is also a need for instruments similar to the WHO Framework Convention on Tobacco Control[1,22] and the WHO Global Outbreak Alert and Response Network, in relation to the emergence of infectious diseases,[23] as well as the United Nations Environmental Programme Montreal Protocol to protect the ozone layer.[24]

The following four examples describe other environmental and ecologic changes on a global scale that will increasingly influence the world's health. First, the probability that new strains of influenza virus will emerge is increasing, particularly in the rural villages of Southeast Asia and East Asia.[14,25] The risk increases with population growth; the juxtaposition of traditional backyard pig, chicken, and duck farming with intensified commercial poultry production; and environmental changes that affect the flight paths of migrating wild birds.

Second, the decline in available seafood protein (which is important for many low-income coastal populations) is a threat to health and reflects the unprecedented combination of ocean warming, acidification (due to increased uptake of carbon dioxide), deoxygenation,[26] destruction of coastal fish nurseries, and overfishing.[27]

Third, diverse health risks are posed by the deprivation, displacement, and conflict that result from shortages of fresh water.[8,28] Many populations, such as those in Bangladesh, Vietnam, Egypt, and Iraq, live downstream on great rivers that traverse several countries. In many cases, river flows are threatened by the loss of glacier mass and snowpack due to global warming and by the increased diversion of flow by neighbors upstream.

Finally, the need to maintain food supplies and adequate nutrition for the increasing world population presents a major challenge.[29] Global food production also faces pressures as a result of reduced yield due to land degradation, water shortages, and climate change and the rising demand for animal foods among middle-income populations. Furthermore, agriculture (especially livestock production) accounts for around one fourth of global greenhouse-gas emissions.[30] Thus, there are growing pressures to transform food production (e.g., more mixed cropping and inclusion of acceptable genetically modified crops), distribution, and consumption. Since the environmental, particularly climatic, effects of producing red meat from methane-producing ruminants (e.g., cattle, sheep, and goats) are so great, thought needs to be given to the question of whether production of this protein source will need to be curtailed—while allowing a sufficient increase to ensure safe childhood nutrition in the many poorer populations, which currently consume levels of red meat that are lower than those in the overconsuming rich populations by a factor of 10.[30] The global food security issue is further complicated by the ongoing land grab in eastern Africa and elsewhere by richer countries seeking investment opportunities and self-insurance against future land, food, and biofuel shortages (e.g., Middle Eastern oil-producing states, China, and South Korea).[31]

These four examples also confirm that, in a world of global and systemic changes, these individual changes for the most part do not impinge on population health in isolation; instead, they typically act jointly and often interact. Specific examples are discussed in the next section, which reviews the health risks posed by climate change.

Global Climate Change

Global climate change is part of the larger Anthropocene syndrome of human-induced global environmental changes. These include land degradation, ocean acidification, and disruptions and depletions of the stratospheric ozone concentration, soil fertility, fresh-water resources, biodiversity stocks and ecosystem functioning, and global nitrogen and phosphorus cycles.[4] Greenhouse emissions from fossil fuel–based power generation and transport and from the

agriculture and mining sectors increase the heat-retaining capacity of the lower atmosphere, resulting in global warming (see the interactive graphic available at NEJM.org). In addition, deforestation and ocean saturation have added to greenhouse warming by reducing the capacity of terrestrial and marine environments to absorb extra carbon dioxide (the main greenhouse gas) from the atmosphere. Also contributing to such warming are any ongoing natural variations in climate caused by cosmologic and geologic influences.[32]

Most of the global warming since 1950 (an increase of 0.7°C) has been the result of human activity.[32] Annual global emissions of carbon dioxide have increased over the past decade, as have the rates of sea-level rise, the loss of Arctic sea ice, and the number of extreme weather events.[33] Without substantial and prompt international action to abate these emissions, average global temperatures (relative to the year 2000) are likely to rise by 1 to 2°C by 2050 and by 3 to 4°C by 2100, including increases of up to 6 to 7°C at high northern latitudes.[33,34] Additional warming of another 0.7°C is locked in from the extra radiative energy already absorbed by the lower atmosphere and, in turn, by the oceans, though not yet manifested as surface warming. An average rise of 4°C would return Earth's temperature to a level not experienced for 10 million to 20 million years.[35]

Rainfall patterns will also change, with rainfall increasing in some regions and seasons and decreasing in others. Modeling consistently projects an increase in regional aridity, and in the geographic range and severity of droughts, during this century.[36] The frequency, and perhaps intensity, of extreme weather events is also expected to increase in most regions—and may well have already begun to do so.[37]

Effects of Climate Change on Human Health

The complex nature of climate change and its environmental and social manifestations results in diverse risks to human health.[17,18,38] A three-way classification of these risks and causal pathways is shown in Table 3.1.[39]

TABLE 3.1 Categories of Climate-Change Risks to Health, According
to Causal Pathway

Risk Category	Causal Pathway
Primary	Direct biologic consequences of heat waves, extreme weather events, and temperature-enhanced levels of urban air pollutants
Secondary	Risks mediated by changes in biophysically and ecologically based processes and systems, particularly food yields, water flows, infectious-disease vectors, and (for zoonotic diseases) intermediate-host ecology
Tertiary	More diffuse effects (e.g., mental health problems in failing farm communities, displaced groups, disadvantaged indigenous and minority ethnic groups) Consequences of tension and conflict owing to climate change–related declines in basic resources (water, food, timber, living space)

Our current, rather skewed knowledge of climate–health relationships has come from epidemiologic studies of health risks in relation to differences and extremes in temperature and from quasicyclical climatic events such as the El Niño–Southern Oscillation phenomenon. However, most of the health risks will arise from climatic influences on environmental systems and social conditions that affect food yields, water supplies, the stability of infectious disease patterns, and the integrity of natural and human-built protection against natural disasters (including forest cover, windbreaks, mangroves, vulnerable constructed seawalls, and urban water-drainage systems) and from the adverse health consequences of social disruption, displacement of communities, and conflict situations.[18,38]

Key examples of these types of causal paths are shown in Figure 3.2. Many of the indirect effects of climate change will be simultaneously influenced by other global changes and socio-demographic pressures that act in conjunction with climate change. Food yields and, hence, nutritional status reflect changes not only in climate[40] but also in water supplies, soil fertility, nitrogen levels, biodiversity (e.g., pollinators and pest predators), and the health and vitality of farm workers.

It is not surprising that the health effects of climate change will be predominantly adverse.[38] After all, human biology, domesticated food sources, and culture in general have evolved over many millennia within the usual prevailing climate. Furthermore, populations everywhere will be vulnerable to increasingly severe extreme weather events.

Some beneficial health effects are expected to occur, at least in the earlier stages of climate change.[38] In some temperate zones, milder winters may lead to fewer wintertime deaths from myocardial infarction and stroke, and in some low-latitude regions, hotter and drier conditions may reduce mosquito survival and, hence, mosquito-borne infection.

Populations living in diverse social, economic, and physical conditions will be affected differently by climate changes.[18,38] Low-income and remote populations are more vulnerable to physical hazards, undernutrition, diarrheal and other infectious diseases, and the health consequences of displacement. Populations on low-lying islands and in coastal areas, such as Bangladesh, are vulnerable to increased storm surges and flooding as the sea level rises. In Arctic circumpolar regions, communities may undergo enforced changes in diet as land and marine animal populations migrate or decline and as access to traditional food sources becomes physically more difficult.[41]

The likely future effects of climate change on various health outcomes have been modeled with the use of plausible scenarios of future climate change that have been agreed on internationally. For example, in temperate countries, as summers become hotter and heat waves more severe, modeling indicates that, from around mid-century, additional heat-related deaths will progressively overwhelm the number of deaths averted as a result of milder winters.[42,43] Such estimates of the extreme effects of weather will improve as the modeling of changes in climatic variability under climate-change conditions improves and as researchers take better

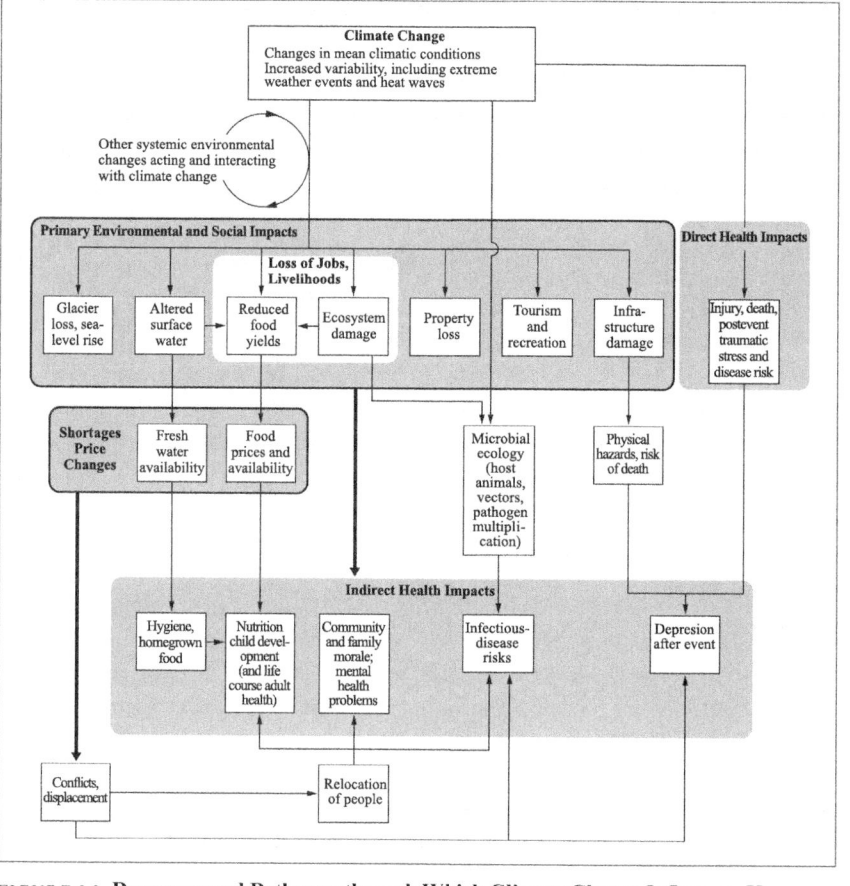

FIGURE 3.2 **Processes and Pathways through Which Climate Change Influences Human Health** *The direct health impacts of climate change are shown in the upper right part of the figure, most of them due to amplified extreme weather events. All the other, less direct health impacts, shown in the lower part of the figure, are mediated by the primary environmental and social impacts of climate change. These include the five categories of indirect health impacts and the tertiary effects on health and survival that arise from more diffuse disruptions, dislocations, and conflicts, which are likely to increase in future decades and are indicated by upward-pointing arrows.*

account of physiological, behavioral, and technological adaptation by populations over time.

In China, the modeling of medium-scenario warming indicates that the transmission zone of freshwater snail–mediated schistosomiasis will extend northward, putting another 20 million people at risk by 2050.[44] Such model-based estimation of the direction and approximate extent of likely change in health risks is an important resource for decision-making about both climate-change abatement and localized adaptation.

Meanwhile, an important research task is to identify ongoing changes in health risks and outcomes that can be reasonably attributed to recent climate change. Given the multivariate causation of most human health outcomes, attribution is rarely simple.[45] Nevertheless, over the past decade, observed changes in some health outcomes, viewed collectively, suggest a climate signal (Box 3.1).[18,38,46]

Health Risks and Benefits of Climate-Change Mitigation and Adaptation

The mitigation of climate change is a crucial first-order task for the world. However, while governments continue to wrestle with this unprecedented, complex political and ethical task, the more immediate challenge for the health sector is to identify the main regional health threats posed by climate change and ensure the development of risk-lessening adaptations.

ADAPTATION STRATEGIES

Adaptation capacities and strategies will differ greatly among populations. They will be particularly important where the rates of preexisting disease (e.g., childhood diarrhea and malnutrition) are already high and therefore, in absolute terms, would become considerably higher because of the multiplier effects of climate change. Effective adaptive strategies will mostly require collaboration among diverse government sectors, research disciplines, and communities.

During heat waves, deaths and hospitalizations predominate among the elderly, patients with chronic cardiorespiratory disease, and persons living in low-grade housing. Early heat wave–warning systems, community caregiver schemes for vulnerable persons, well-insulated housing, and educational advice

---

BOX 3.1 Indicators of Early Health Effects of Climate Change

Increases in annual numbers of deaths and hospitalizations due to extreme heat, observed in a range of high-income and low-income countries

Increases in rates of injuries and deaths due to the rising frequency of weather disasters in many regions

Extensions in the geographic range of several vector-borne infectious diseases or their vectors, including tickborne encephalitis in Sweden, the tick vector of Lyme disease in eastern Canada, and malaria in the western Kenyan highlands

Although less certain, increases in the tempo of coastal outbreaks of cholera relative to the warming of coastal waters and El Niño events

Increases in the price of some staple foods, especially in vulnerable, food-insecure regions, leading to nutritional deprivation in low-income households

---

from primary health care providers would lower this risk. Meanwhile, longer-term planning is needed to climate-proof urban residential areas.[47]

HEALTH BENEFITS OF CLIMATE-CHANGE MITIGATION

One favorable aspect of efforts to mitigate climate change is that local health gains will quickly accrue to populations that undertake such efforts.[48] Awareness of this potential health dividend—in addition to the longer-term global health benefits—should strengthen support for such actions.

Health benefits will result from mitigating actions that address modes of transport, housing-design standards, energy generation, and agricultural systems (including livestock production). In many poor populations, improvements in environment-related technologies will help to replace indoor-polluting cooking fuels with low-carbon fuels, and improvements in reproductive literacy will lead to fewer, better-spaced pregnancies; both types of improvement reduce pressures on the climate system.[11] All these actions will directly reduce well-known risk factors for disease and premature death (e.g., air pollution, sedentary living, and dietary excesses).[48] Innovative urban design can have wide-ranging positive effects with regard to energy use, greenhouse-gas emissions, the effects of urban heat islands, patterns of physical activity, social relations, and community cohesion.

Challenges for the Health Sector

The health sector has important roles to play in relation to climate-change abatement and adaptation strategies for lessening unavoidable risks to health (Table 3.2).[49,50] Such strategies would include the "greening" of health care institutions and participation in national health impact assessments and in intersectoral planning of sustainable energy systems, transportation, and urban design. National delegations to international policymaking meetings that address global trends and threats (e.g., the annual conferences convened under the United Nations Framework Convention on Climate Change) should include representatives from, or at least substantive briefing by, the formal health sector.

Conclusions

Rapid globalization has brought new, large-scale influences to bear on patterns of human health. Various global-scale changes—economic, social, demographic, and environmental (particularly climatic)—are linked, for example, to the increased prevalence of obesity, changes in regional food yields, the emergence of infectious diseases, the spread of cigarette smoking, and the persistence of health disparities.

TABLE 3.2 Role of the Health Sector in Climate-Change Mitigation (Primary
Prevention) and Adaptation (Preparedness, or Secondary Prevention)*

Goal and Generic Action	Suggested Strategies
Mitigation of climate change	
Carry out health impact assessment of mitigation strategies	Conduct epidemiologic research to estimate and document changes in health outcomes that result directly from mitigation actions
Limit the carbon (and other environmental) footprint related to the health care system	Design buildings, transport services, and facilities to achieve energy efficiency, in terms of energy sources and use, and to minimize waste
Enlist health professional organizations and government health departments	Educate the public about risks to health from climate change and explain that mitigating actions can confer additional, local health benefits
Include physicians and other health care workers as citizens	Participate in wider public discussion and moderate personal behaviors
Adaptation to lessen health risks	
Provide adequate health care facilities and services	Improve facilities for handling increased patient volume resulting from extreme weather events and ensure adequate stocks of vaccine
Anticipate necessary surge capacity (e.g., for major heat waves, fires, epidemics)	Coordinate with emergency-services agencies and ambulance facilities and consider morgue capacity
Reinforce and extend public health programs to provide a foundation for dealing with most types of climate-related health effects	Develop early-warning systems (e.g., for heat waves, floods, and possible epidemics); programs for infectious-disease surveillance and analysis, vaccination, and vector control (e.g., mosquitoes, ticks); support for vulnerable communities; and mental health services (e.g., for postevent trauma and depression)
Educate and train the health workforce	Develop programs that prepare health care workers to contribute to public education and to be on the alert for unexpected diagnoses
Engage in broader collaboration with other sectors	Institute policies for creating green spaces in cities (to promote physical and mental health); develop housing design and insulation to optimize health protection; consider livestock and wild animals as possible risks for infection

*The listed adaptation activities are intended to reduce health risks on the local and regional levels.

Undertaking primary prevention at the source to reduce health risks resulting from these global influences is a formidable challenge. It requires conceptual insights beyond the conventional understanding of causation and prevention, as well as political will, trust, and resources. The complexities of policies to mitigate human-induced climate change are clear. Meanwhile, additional resources and strategies will be needed to reduce the health risks related to global change that have already arisen or are now unavoidable. For populations to live sustainably and with good long-term health, the health sector must work with other sectors in reshaping how human societies plan, build, move, produce, consume, share, and generate energy.

References

1. Lee K, Yach D, Kamradt-Scott A. Globalization and health. In: Merson MH, Black RE, Mills AJ, eds. Global health diseases, programs, systems and policies. Burlington, MA: Jones and Bartlett Learning, 2012:885–913.

2. Labonté R, Mohindra K, Schrecker T. The growing impact of globalization on health and public health practice. Annu Rev Public Health 2011;32:263–83.

3. Hibbard KA, Crutzen P, Lambin EF, et al. The great acceleration. In: Costanza R, Graumlich LJ, Steffen W, eds. Sustainability or collapse? An integrated history and future of people on earth: Dahlem Workshop Report 96. Cambridge, MA: MIT Press, 2007:417–46.

4. Rockström J, Steffen W, Noone K, et al. A safe operating space for humanity. Nature 2009;461:472–75.

5. Barnosky AD, Hadly EA, Bascompte J, et al. Approaching a state shift in Earth's biosphere. Nature 2012;486:52–58.

6. Crutzen PJ. Geology of mankind: the Anthropocene. Nature 2002;415:23.

7. McMichael AJ, Butler CD. Promoting global population health while constraining the environmental footprint. Annu Rev Public Health 2011;32:179–97.

8. Grace K, Davenport F, Funk C, Lerner AM. Child malnutrition and climate in Sub-Saharan Africa: an analysis of recent trends in Kenya. Appl Geogr 2012;35:405–413.

9. Hernandez MA, Robles M, Torero M. Fires in Russia, wheat production, and volatile markets: reasons to panic? Washington, DC: International Food Policy Research Institute, 2010 (http://www.ifpri.org/sites/default/files/wheat.pdf).

10. Welton G. Oxfam research report: the impact of Russia's 2010 wheat export ban. June 2011 (https://www.oxfam.org/sites/www.oxfam.org/files/rr-impact-russias-grain-export-ban-280611-en.pdf).

11. Smith KR, Balakrishnan K. Mitigating climate, meeting MDGs, and moderating chronic disease: the health co-benefits landscape. Health Ministers Update 2009:59–65(http://www.thecommonwealth.org/files/190381/FileName/4-KirkSmith_2009.pdf).

12. World population prospects, the 2010 revision. New York: United Nations Department of Economic and Social Affairs, May 2011 (http://esa.un.org/unpd/wpp/index.htm).

13. Butler CD, McMichael AJ. Population health: where demography, environment and equity converge. J Public Health (Oxf) 2010;32:157–58.

14. Weiss R, McMichael A. Social and environmental risk factors in the emergence of infectious diseases. Nat Med 2004;10:Suppl:S70–76.

15. Jones KE, Patel NJ, Leyy MA, et al. Global trends in emerging infectious diseases. Nature 2008;451:990–93.

16. Beaglehole R, Bonita R, Horton R, et al. Priority actions for the non-communicable disease crisis. Lancet 2011;377:1438–47.

17. Epstein PR. Climate change and human health. N Engl J Med 2005;353:1433–36.

18. McMichael AJ, Lindgren E. Climate change: present and future risks to health, and necessary responses. J Intern Med 2011;270:401–413.

19. Marmot M, Friel S, Bell R, Houweling TAJ, Taylor S. Closing the gap in a generation: health equity through action on the social determinants of health. Lancet 2008;372:1661–69.

20. Haines A, Cassels A. Can the millennium development goals be attained? BMJ 2004;329:394–97.
21. Drager N, Fidler DP. Foreign policy, trade and health: at the cutting edge of global health diplomacy. Bull World Health Organ 2007;85:162.
22. Shibuya K, Ciecierski C, Guindon E, Murray C. WHO Framework Convention on Tobacco Control: development of an evidence based global public health treaty. BMJ 2003;327:154–57.
23. Global Outbreak Alert and Response Network (GOARN). Geneva: World Health Organization (http://www.who.int/csr/outbreaknetwork/en).
24. Tripp JTB. UNEP Montreal Protocol: industrialized and developing countries sharing the responsibility for protecting the stratospheric ozone layer. N Y Univ J Int Law Polit 1987-1988;20:733–52.
25. Perdue ML, Swayne DE. Public health risk from avian influenza viruses. Avian Dis 2005;49:317–27.
26. Keeling RE, Körtzinger A, Gruber N. Ocean deoxygenation in a warming world. Ann Rev Mar Sci 2010;2:199–229.
27. Pauly D, Watson R, Alder J. Global trends in world fisheries: impacts on marine ecosystems and food security. Phil Trans R Soc Lond B Biol Sci 2005;360:5–12.
28. Moore S. Climate change, water and China's national interest. China Security 2009;5:25–39.
29. Beddington JR, Asaduzzaman M, Clark ME, et al. What next for agriculture after Durban? Science 2012;335:289–90.
30. McMichael AJ, Powles J, Butler CD, Uauy R. Food, livestock production, energy, climate change and health. Lancet 2007;370:1253–63.
31. Scheidel AH, Sorman A. Energy transitions and the global land rush: ultimate drivers and persistent consequences. Glob Environ Change 2012;22:588–95.
32. Climate change 2007: the physical science basis: contribution of Working Group I to the Fourth Assessment Report of the Intergovernmental Panel on Climate Change. Cambridge, United Kingdom: Cambridge University Press, 2007.
33. National Oceanic and Aeronautical Agency. State of the Climate in 2011. Asheville, NC: NOAA, 2012 (http://www.ncdc.noaa.gov/bams-state-of-the-climate/2011.php).
34. Meinshausen M, Meinshausen N, Hare W, et al. Greenhouse-gas emission targets for limiting global warming to 2 degrees C. Nature 2009;458:1158–62.
35. Hansen JE, Sato M. Paleoclimate implications for human-made climate change. New York: NASA Goddard Institute for Space Studies and Columbia University Earth Institute, 2008 (http://arxiv.org/abs/1105.0968).
36. Dai A. Drought under global warming: a review. New York: John Wiley, 2010.
37. Coumou D, Rahmstorf S. A decade of weather extremes. Nat Climate Change 2012;2:491–96.
38. Confalonieri U, Menne B, Akhtar R, et al. Human health. In: Parry ML, Canziani OF, Palutikof JP, van der Linden PJ, Hanson C, eds. Climate change 2007: impacts, adaptation and vulnerability: contribution of Working Group II to the Fourth Assessment Report of the Intergovernmental Panel on Climate Change. Cambridge, United Kingdom: Cambridge University Press, 2007:391–431.
39. Butler CD, Harley D. Primary, secondary and tertiary effects of eco-climatic change: the medical response. Postgrad Med J 2010;86:230–34.
40. Lobell DB, Field CB. Global scale climate—crop yield relationships and the impacts of recent warming. Environ Res Lett 2007;2:014002.

41. Evengård B, McMichael AJ. Vulnerable populations in the Arctic. Glob Health Action 2011;4:3–5.

42. Knowlton K, Lynn B, Goldberg RA, et al. Projecting heat-related mortality impacts under a changing climate in the New York City region. Am J Public Health 2007;97:2028–34.

43. Bambrick H, Dear K, Woodruff R, Hanigan I, McMichael AJ. The impacts of climate change on three health outcomes: temperature-related mortality and hospitalisations, salmonellosis and other bacterial gastroenteritis, and population at risk from dengue. Garnaut Climate Change Review, 2008; 1–47. (http://garnautreview.org.au/CA25734E0016A131/WebObj/03-AThreehealthoutcomes/$File/03-A%20Three%20health%20outcomes.pdf).

44. Zhou X-N, Yang G-J, Yang K, et al. Potential impact of climate change on Schistosomiasis transmission in China. Am J Trop Med Hyg 2008;78:188–94.

45. Rosenzweig C, Karoly D, Vicarelli M, et al. Attributing physical and biological impacts to anthropogenic climate change. Nature 2008;453:353–57.

46. McMichael AJ, Bertollini R. Risks to human health, present and future. In: Richardson K, Steffen W, Liverman, D, eds. Climate change: global risks, challenges and decisions. Cambridge, United Kingdom: Cambridge University Press, 2011:114–16.

47. Hunt A, Watkiss P. Climate change impacts and adaptation in cities: a review of the literature. Clim Change 2011;104:13–49.

48. Haines A, McMichael AJ, Smith KR, et al. Public health benefits of strategies to reduce greenhouse gas emissions: overview and implications for policymakers. Lancet 2009;374:2104–114.

49. Costello A, Abbas M, Allen A, et al. Managing the health effects of climate change. Lancet 2009;373:1693–733.

50. Pencheon D. Health services and climate change: what can be done? J Health Serv Res Policy 2009;14:2–4.

PART II

Infectious Diseases

INTRODUCTION

Historically, few global phenomena have posed an existential threat to humanity as severe as the possibility of a highly lethal infectious disease pandemic. Since ancient times, plagues have been a powerful deterrent of human progress and well-being, and pandemic influenza remains a constant menace. Although direct experience of the great 1918 "Spanish flu" epidemic is limited to an ever-decreasing number of nonagenarians and centenarians, the ongoing risk is highlighted by the appearance from time to time of highly lethal flu variants as well as other dangerous, emerging infections. The scientific reality is periodically hyped in the popular mind by apocalyptic science fiction films in which wide swaths of humanity are wiped out by an ever-expanding fatal infection.

The early roots of the public health movement are grounded in the mitigation of infectious diseases via environmental changes (e.g., draining the marshes to eliminate malaria in Boston), quarantine, pest control (e.g., control of rats in cities), the provision of clean water (e.g., the classic studies of John Snow on cholera in London), sanitation (e.g., departments of sanitary engineering in the first schools of public health), and better housing and nutrition. Substantial declines in many infectious diseases were seen prior to specific medical interventions; for instance, mortality from tuberculosis in the United Kingdom dropped in a steady and almost linear fashion for a full century prior to the introduction the bacille Calmette-Guérin (BCG) vaccine and streptomycin.[1] Much of the continued existence of some infectious and parasitic diseases in developing countries is due to the failure or inability to implement these century-old interventions in impoverished, underserved, far-flung rural areas and in rapidly growing urban slums.

Medical historians point to a period after the Second World War when the introduction of antibiotics and the widespread availability of vaccines led to a growing belief that infectious diseases were, if not actually

conquered, well on their way to being conquered. The famous declaration that "It is time to close the book on infectious diseases, and declare the war against pestilence won" now turns out to have been misattributed. It was long credited to US Surgeon-General William Stewart, who actually said (in the speech often referenced as the source of the quote) that "Warning flags are still flying in the communicable disease field."[2] Although it is possible to find strong statements in the literature about the relative *decline* in the importance of infectious diseases as major sources of mortality in developed countries, these are often linked to reminders of the continued vigilance needed to prevent a recrudescence of these diseases and the fact they were eliminated only in some regions and not eradicated globally. Nonetheless, there were voices who felt that too many infectious disease specialists were being trained in the United States, and trainees who were worried that they were about to enter a "disappearing" field.[3] Subsequent events, notably the emergence of HIV/AIDS, put infectious diseases back on center stage. Indeed, the global response to AIDS, notably the emergence of large-scale programs to provide hitherto unavailable drugs to people and countries that could not afford them at developed-country prices, has been credited with the invention of the "global health movement as we know it today."[4]

Of course even the triumphalist forecasters of the end of infectious diseases in developed countries recognized that the job was far from done in developing countries. Despite many successes, such as the eradication of smallpox in the late 1970s and the recent increase in rates of vaccination among children, infectious diseases are still responsible for approximately 19% of deaths worldwide, with much higher proportions among infants and children leading to a much higher proportion of years of life lost. Although some infectious disease causes of death decreased between 1990 and 2010, AIDS deaths increased about fivefold, and deaths due to malaria were estimated to have increased by about 20%.

In this section, Fauci and Morens open with a review of milestones in infectious diseases over 200 years (their review appeared as part of the *New England Journal of Medicine's* 200th anniversary series). Although Piot and Quinn emphasize the multisectoral aspects of the global response to HIV/AIDS that make it a "model" for attacking other diseases, they still acknowledge the fragility of the progress made and the fact that less than 25% of all persons with HIV were receiving antiretroviral therapy or were on therapy with successful viral suppression. Fineberg discusses the response to the 2009 H1N1 influenza epidemic, marking the first time that the World Health Organization activated new provisions of the 2005 International Health Regulations, which went into effect in 2007. He also and draws lessons regarding the world's ability to respond to any global public health emergency.

In 2013, the emergence of Ebola virus disease (EVD) in West Africa was a vivid reminder of the ability of infectious diseases to devastate whole societies. It exposed frailties in weak health systems nationally as well as the

international ability to respond. Twenty-four prior documented outbreaks of this disease with a high rate of fatalities had occurred in rural areas, often centered on hospitals, and had been either self-limiting after infected people recovered or died or had been contained by public health interventions that included the isolation of patients, contact tracing, and the disposal of infectious cadavers. The current epidemic is radically different because it spread across borders and into cities. The numbers of infected patients soon overwhelmed inadequate health facilities, leading to an inability to isolate and treat those who were infectious. The international response is acknowledged to have been far too slow. Kanapathipillai, Baden, and Sprecher review the history of this epidemic and the progress made by mid-2015.

Critical to the response to and control of many infectious diseases is the manufacture and distribution of effective vaccines. The AIDS pandemic is a reminder of the limits of our ability to produce vaccines against some infectious organisms; 30 years after the isolation of the virus, no highly effective vaccine has been successfully tested. Nabel reviews the successes and failures of "traditional" approaches to vaccine design as well as some of the newer techniques that may help develop new vaccines and shorten the development time for vaccines that need to be redesigned annually, such as the influenza vaccine. Finally, eradicating a disease once and for all removes the threat of that disease along with the associated costs of controlling it. Although only a single human disease (smallpox) has been successfully eradicated, the eradication of dracunculiasis (Guinea worm) is tantalizingly close. Hopkins discusses the epidemiological criteria necessary to set a goal of eradicating a disease along with the array of logistical, sociocultural, and political forces that must be aligned in order to achieve this goal.

References

1. Fairchild AL, Oppenheimer GM (1998). Public health nihilism vs. pragmatism: history, politics, and the control of tuberculosis. *Am J Public Health* 88(7):1105–1117. PMCID: PMC1508245.
2. Spellberg B, Taylor-Blake B (2013). On the exoneration of Dr. William H. Stewart: debunking an urban legend. *Infect Dis Poverty* 2(1):3. PMCID: PMC3707092.
3. Fauci AS (2001). Infectious diseases: considerations for the 21st century. *Clin Infect Dis* 32(5):675–685.
4. Brandt AM (2013). How AIDS invented global health. *N Engl J Med* 368(23):2149–2152.

The Perpetual Challenge of Infectious Disease*
Anthony S. Fauci and David M. Morens

Among the many challenges to health, infectious diseases stand out for their ability to have a profound impact on the human species. Great pandemics and local epidemics alike have influenced the course of wars, determined the fates of nations and empires, and affected the progress of civilization, making infections compelling actors in the drama of human history.[1-11]

The Uniqueness of Infectious Diseases

Infections have distinct characteristics that, when considered together, set them apart from other diseases (Box 4.1). Paramount among these characteristics is their unpredictability and their potential for explosive global effect, as exemplified by the bubonic–pneumonic plague pandemic in the 14th century,[1-12] the 1918 influenza pandemic,[13,14] and the current pandemic of human immunodeficiency virus (HIV) infection and the acquired immunodeficiency syndrome (AIDS),[15] among others. Infectious diseases are usually acute and unambiguous in their nature. The onset of an infectious illness, unlike the onset of many other types of disease, in an otherwise healthy host can be abrupt and unmistakable. Moreover, in the absence of therapy, acute infectious diseases often pose an all-or-nothing situation, with the host either quickly dying or recovering spontaneously, and usually relatively promptly, often with lifelong immunity to the specific infecting pathogen.

Not only are some infectious diseases transmissible to others, a unique characteristic among human diseases, but their transmission mechanisms are relatively few (including inoculation and airborne and waterborne transmission), well understood, and comparatively easy to study, both experimentally and in the

---

*This article is modified from an article that appeared as part of the NEJM 200th Anniversary Series

BOX 4.1 Characteristics of Infectious Diseases That Set Them Apart from Other
         Human Diseases

Potential for unpredictable and explosive global impact

Frequent acquisition by host of durable immunity against reinfection after recovery

Reliance of disease on a single agent without requirement for multiple cofactors

Transmissibility

Potential for becoming preventable

Potential for eradication

Evolutionary advantage over human host because of replicative and mutational
capacities of pathogens that render them highly adaptable

Close dependence on the nature and complexity of human behavior

Frequent derivation from or coevolution in other animal species

Possibility of treatment for having multiplying effects on preventing infection in
contacts and the community and on microbial and animal ecosystems

---

field. In addition, such transmission is generally amenable to medical and public health interventions. Unlike many chronic and lifestyle-associated diseases
resulting from multiple, interacting risk cofactors, most infectious diseases are
caused by a single agent, the identification of which typically points the way not
only to general disease-control measures (e.g., sanitation, chemical disinfection,
hand washing, or vector control) but also to specific medical measures (e.g., vaccination or antimicrobial treatment).

Given their nature, infectious diseases are potentially preventable with personal
protection, general public health measures, or immunologic approaches such as
vaccination. As preventive measures have become more effective and efficient, history has shown that certain infectious diseases, particularly those with a broad
global health impact and for which there is no nonhuman host or major reservoir,
can be eliminated. Such diseases include poliomyelitis, which has been eliminated
in the Western Hemisphere,[16] and smallpox, which has been eradicated globally.[9]

Another unique aspect is that the extraordinary adaptability of infectious
pathogens (i.e., their replicative and mutational capacities) provides them with
a temporary evolutionary advantage against pressures aimed at their destruction. These pressures include environmental factors and antimicrobial drugs, as
well as the human immune response. At the same time, such adaptations provide us with opportunities to respond with new vaccine antigens, such as annually updated influenza vaccines,[17] or new or different anti-infective agents. This
back-and-forth struggle between human ingenuity and microbial adaptation
reflects a perpetual challenge.[12,18,19]

Infectious diseases are closely dependent on the nature and complexity of
human behavior, since they directly reflect who we are, what we do, and how we
live and interact with other people, animals, and the environment.[19-30] Infectious
diseases are acquired specifically and directly as a result of our behaviors and

lifestyles, from social gatherings, to travel and transportation, to sexual activity, to occupational exposures, to sports and recreational activities, to what we eat and drink, to our pets, to the environment—even to the way we care for the ill in hospitals and other health care environments. Moreover, microbial colonizing infections that lead to long-term carriage without disease (e.g., within the endogenous human microbiome) may influence the development of infections with exogenous microbes[31,32] and also have an effect on general immunologic and physiologic homeostasis,[33,34] including effects on nutritional status. Human microbiomes seem to reflect, and may even have helped to drive, human evolution.[35]

In this struggle, infectious diseases are intimately and uniquely related to us through our immune systems. The human immune system, including the primitive innate system and the specific adaptive system,[36] has evolved over millions of years from both invertebrate and vertebrate organisms, developing sophisticated defense mechanisms to protect the host from microbes.[37] In effect, the human immune system evolved as a response to the challenge of invading pathogens. Thus, it is not by accident that the fields of microbiology and immunology arose and developed in close association long before they came to be considered distinct disciplines.

Disease Emergence and Reemergence

Because infectious pathogens are evolutionarily dynamic, the list of diseases they cause is ever-changing and continually growing. Since newly emerging infectious agents do not arise spontaneously, they must recently have come from somewhere else, usually from animal infections, as occurred with HIV infection, influenza, and the severe acute respiratory syndrome. This interspecies transmission underscores the importance of interdigitating the study of human and animal diseases[19,23,38-40] and recognizing the central role that microbial reservoirs, including those in animals, vectors, and the environment, play in human infectious diseases.[19,38] Preexisting or established infectious diseases also may reemerge in different forms, as in extensively drug-resistant tuberculosis,[41] or in different locations, as in West Nile virus infection in the United States,[42] to cause new epidemics (Table 4.1). Indeed, many human infectious diseases seem to have patterns of evolution, sometimes played out over thousands of years, in which they first emerge and cause epidemics or pandemics, become unstably adapted to human populations, undergo periodic resurgences, and eventually become endemic with the potential for future outbreaks (Fig. 4.1).[12,19,43,44]

Historical Perspectives and Current Status

Just over a decade before the publication of the first issue of the *Journal*, President George Washington died of an acute infectious disease believed to have been bacterial epiglottitis.[45] Washington's life reflects the history of his era and provides

TABLE 4.1 Broad Categories of Infectious Diseases*

Type of Disease	Description
Established infectious diseases	Endemic diseases that have been prevalent for a sufficient period of time to allow for a relatively stable and predictable level of morbidity and mortality (e.g., viral and bacterial respiratory and diarrheal diseases, drug-susceptible malaria and tuberculosis, tropical diseases such as helminthic and other parasitic diseases, nosocomial infections)
Newly emerging infectious diseases	Diseases that are recognized in the human host for the first time (e.g., HIV/AIDS, Nipah virus, severe acute respiratory syndrome, ebola virus disease)
Reemerging infectious diseases	Diseases that historically have infected humans but continue to reappear either in new locations (e.g., West Nile virus in the United States) or in resistant forms (e.g., influenza, methicillin-resistant *Staphylococcus aureus,* drug-resistant malaria) or reappear after apparent control or elimination (e.g., polio in parts of Africa, cholera in Haiti, dengue in Florida) or under unusual circumstances (e.g., deliberately released agents, including the anthrax release in 2001)

*Categories of infectious diseases include those that are newly emerging, those that have become established and may periodically reemerge, and those that have become stably endemic.[19] Modern concepts that relate to emerging infections are more fully described in an influential 1992 report by the Institute of Medicine.[20]

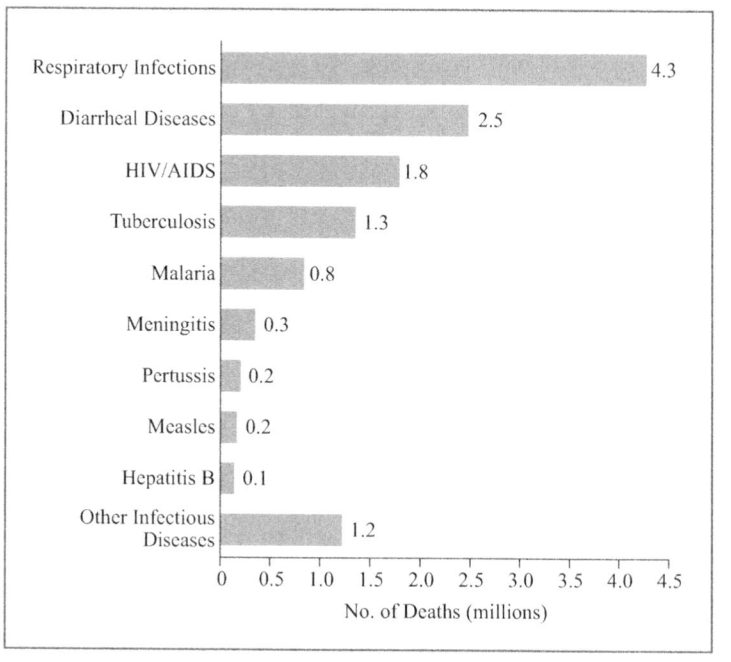

FIGURE 4.1 **Leading Causes of Global Deaths from Infectious Diseases** *Of an estimated 58.8 million annual deaths worldwide, approximately 15.0 million (25.5%) are believed to be caused by infectious diseases. Cause-specific mortality estimates are provided by the World Health Organization.[43,44] The data do not include deaths from secondary infectious causes, such as rheumatic fever and rheumatic heart disease, liver cancer and cirrhosis, or other chronic diseases.*

both a window into infectious diseases two centuries ago and a benchmark for measuring our remarkable progress since then. Washington was born in 1732, just before the deadliest diphtheria epidemic on the North American continent. He was scarred by smallpox, survived multiple debilitating bouts of malaria, suffered wound infections and abscesses, nursed his brother on a tropical island as he died of tuberculosis, and even had an influenza pandemic named after him (the Washington influenza of 1789–1790). During his presidency, he stayed in the then-capital city of Philadelphia while most of the government fled during the nation's deadliest yellow fever epidemic.[5,12] At the time of Washington's birth, there was no well-defined concept of infection or immunity, no vaccines, almost no specific or effective treatments for infectious diseases,[3,46] and little idea that any treatment or public health measure could reliably control epidemic diseases.

During Washington's lifetime, infectious diseases were the defining challenges of human existence. No one alive then could have imagined the astonishing breakthroughs that lay ahead. In this regard, it is noteworthy that almost all the major advances in understanding and controlling infectious diseases have occurred in the past two centuries (Table 4.2, and interactive timeline available at NEJM.org). Experimental animal-transmission studies that were conducted soon after the War of 1812 were followed by the development of better microscopes, which linked fungi to skin diseases and protozoa to mucosal diseases—for example, Alfred Donné's 1836 work with *Trichomonas vaginalis* and David Gruby's studies of *Candida albicans* in the early 1840s. The breakthroughs in the late 1800s, which taken together provided the compelling unifying principle of infectious diseases and must surely rank among the most important advances in the medical sciences, were the characterization of specific cultivatable microorganisms and proof of their association with specific diseases. This triumph was led by the work of Davaine and Koch in establishing anthrax as the first fully characterized infectious disease.[47,48] This seminal process was facilitated by the development of defined criteria for establishing causality (Koch's postulates).

Additional breakthroughs followed quickly, including the discovery and characterization of pathogen-specific immune responses; the demonstration that when inactivated by heat or chemicals or grown under limiting conditions that changed certain biologic properties (e.g., attenuation), organisms or their products could safely stimulate protective responses in a host; and development of anti-infective serums and chemicals to destroy pathogens. Over the next 135 years, a wide array of vaccines and antibiotics and, more recently, antiviral agents have saved hundreds of millions of lives, greatly extended the human life span, and reduced untold suffering. Undeniably, these countermeasures against infectious disease rank among the greatest achievements in public health and medicine.

History reminds us that new challenges in infectious diseases will continue to emerge and reemerge. We must be prompt in identifying them and devising new countermeasures. In this effort, we still follow the familiar pathway that was set down in the late 1800s for the identification and characterization, both clinical and epidemiologic, of the causative agent; the characterization of the human immune

TABLE 4.2 Selected Infectious Diseases of Importance from 1812 to the Present

Disease	1812	1912	2012
Malaria	Cause unknown; wealthy persons flee to higher elevations in malaria season; "Jesuit's bark" (containing quinine) used to treat symptoms	Causative organism identified in 1880 (Laveran; Nobel Prize awarded 1907); anopheles mosquito identified as principle vector (Sir Ronald Ross; Nobel Prize awarded 1902); vector-control attempts under way	Genomes of the host (human), two of the principal parasites (*Plasmodium falciparum* and *vivax*), and the principal vector (*Anopheles gambiae*) sequenced; drugs for treatment and prophylaxis; vaccines under development; successes with public health control, but malaria still causes >800,000 annual deaths
Variola (smallpox)	Cause unknown; control begins in the developed world with Jenner's 1798 publication on vaccination	Variola greatly controlled by vaccination in the developed world; developing world still has deadly epidemics	Variola eradicated in 1980 through aggressive global vaccination campaign
Plague	Cause and mode of transmission unknown; frightening disease for millennia; no good control measures; global quarantine systems not completely effective	1890s pandemic brings plague to the U.S. for the first time (1900); disease becomes enzootic and endemic, but fears of Black Death pandemic begin to subside	Plague a minor disease in U.S.; sporadic outbreaks still occur in the developing world, but fear of pandemics has subsided
Yellow fever	Cause and mode of transmission unknown; the "American Plague" is most frightening U.S. disease after deadly epidemics in 1793–1798, which led to forerunner of the U.S. Public Health Service (1798)	U.S. Public Health Service forerunner sets up Hygienic Laboratory (1887) to study the microbiology of infectious diseases, eventually becoming the National Institutes of Health; transmission by *Aedes aegypti* shown by Walter Reed team (1900); vector control efforts by Gorgas in Cuba and Panama soon lead to substantial control	Effective live attenuated vaccine developed in 1936; yellow fever is largely gone from the developed world and greatly reduced in the developing world
Tuberculosis	Cause unknown; consumption an old and feared disease; on the rise in the industrial age	Recognized as the deadliest infectious disease of the 19th century; organism discovered by Robert Koch in 1882; beginning to be controlled by public health measures and sanatorium movement	Bacille Calmette–Guérin vaccine (marginally effective against transmission of pulmonary tuberculosis) in 1921; antituberculosis chemotherapy initiated in 1950s; control in the developed world upset by HIV pandemic and in the developing world is never achieved; 1.3 million still die annually; emergence of multidrug-resistant and extremely drug-resistant tuberculosis; better vaccines actively pursued

TABLE 4.2 Continued

Disease	1812	1912	2012
Wound infections and puerperal fever	Causes unknown; amputations without anesthesia are often ineffective; maternal postpartum deaths common	General anesthesia introduced in 1840s; puerperal streptococcal infections controlled by hand washing in mid-19th century; aseptic technique introduced in 1867; causative organisms isolated in late 1900s	Antibiotics, first used in the late 1930s, are common by the early 1950s in the developed world
Diphtheria	"Throat distemper" (caused by diphtheria and streptococci, sometimes in combination) is a major cause of childhood deaths	Causative organism discovered in 1884; diphtheria anti-toxin (1894) is the first passive immunotherapy	Vaccine produced in 1913; disease controlled in developed world
Poliomyelitis	Not well described but probably endemic	First U.S. epidemic in Vermont in 1894; recurring epidemics cause fear in the U.S. during next 60 years	Inactivated Salk and live Sabin vaccines introduced in 1955 and 1962, respectively; effective global control has led to near eradication
HIV/AIDS	Unknown	May have emerged in Africa but was not recognized	First reported in 1981; causative virus identified in 1983–1984 by Luc Montagnier and Robert Gallo; combination antiretroviral therapy greatly prolongs the lives of infected patients
Ebola Virus		May have been present in Africa but was not recognized	First reported in 1976; more than 20 subsequent outbreaks were contained with a cumulative total of fewer than 1600 deaths; major outbreak starting in 2014 in Guinea, Sierra Leone and Liberia causes more than 11,000 deaths by May, 2015

response to the pathogen; and the development of pathogen-specific diagnostic tests, treatment strategies, and public health prevention strategies such as vaccinations.[49]

Diagnosis and Characterization of Pathogens

In the late 1800s, the realization that identifiable microbes caused specific diseases led to pathogen-specific medical diagnosis. Although the time-honored techniques of growing bacteria in broth or solid cultures and staining and examining them under microscopes are still important today, newer technologies have transformed the field of microbial diagnosis. Among the first emerging epidemic diseases to be identified by one such method was the hantavirus pulmonary syndrome, a centuries-old disease caused by an unknown phlebovirus (Sin Nombre)

that was discovered unexpectedly in 1993[50] by the application of a then-novel molecular genetic technique, polymerase chain reaction (PCR). This followed quickly on the 1992 discovery of the previously unknown agent causing an infectious chronic condition, Whipple's disease.[51] Less than a year later, PCR-related subtraction techniques solved a century-old mystery of the cause of Kaposi's sarcoma, human herpesvirus 8.[52] Now, less than two decades later, sophisticated, high-throughput, rapid sequencing of the genomes of pathogens not only dramatically hastens initial identification but also detects individual genetic variants,[53] facilitating identification of the genetic basis of drug resistance. Additional gene-based diagnostic tools include microchips and other technologies that detect short sequences of many different genes or their proteins, allowing simultaneous diagnosis or diagnostic elimination of multiple pathogens. New serologic techniques such as enzyme-linked immunosorbent assay can be many times more sensitive than traditional techniques in detecting and measuring antibodies to pathogens. Furthermore, monoclonal antibody techniques, which involve the use of cellular clones to produce antibodies against specific pathogen epitopes, have been adapted for the purposes of diagnosis, identification of the molecular structures of pathogens, elucidation of the natural history and pathogenesis of infectious diseases, development of conformationally accurate immunogens to be used as vaccine candidates,[54] and even treatment.[55] Many of these data-rich approaches require sophisticated bioinformatics systems (e.g., phylogenetic comparisons and genome construction analyses).

Vaccine Development

Vaccines against infectious diseases such as anthrax and rabies have been produced since the late 1870s. Only in the past half century, however, have technological advances in vaccination led to dramatic changes in the field of disease prevention. The World Health Organization now estimates that each year more than 120 different types of vaccines save 2.5 million lives and with optimal uptake could save an additional 2 million.[56] Trivalent combined inactivated and live attenuated poliomyelitis vaccines were licensed in 1955 and 1962, respectively; a live attenuated trivalent vaccine against three unrelated diseases (measles, mumps, and rubella) was licensed in 1971; and a variety of vaccine approaches and platforms have been introduced since then. It is now possible to determine high-resolution crystallographic structures of pathogens and use this information to design vaccines directed at the most relevant epitopes in the microbe's complex structure, an approach known as structure-based vaccine design.[57]

Treatment

Successful treatment with pathogen-immune serum was another critical breakthrough of the late 19th century.[55] This approach to therapy also encouraged

scientists to develop chemicals to kill the specific pathogens that they were regularly identifying. Ehrlich succeeded first in 1910 with his magic bullet against syphilis (arsphenamine, or salvarsan[58]). Within two decades, a new generation of scientists was working on what would eventually be called antibiotics. As a result of these efforts, sulfa drugs were developed in 1936, and penicillin in 1943.[59,60] In the United States, tuberculosis had been only partially controlled by public health measures and incompletely effective vaccines.[61] It was not until the introduction of specific antituberculosis therapy in the 1950s[62] that sanatoriums were emptied and cases of active disease were substantially reduced. Antibiotics have revolutionized the treatment of many other important bacterial infections and have saved many millions of lives since their introduction.

When antiviral drugs were first developed in the 1960s, they did not seem to be particularly promising, with a few exceptions. In response to the HIV/AIDS pandemic, however, the development of antiretroviral drugs markedly expanded the arsenal of available antiviral agents and invigorated the research-and-development pathway for these important drugs. Effective combinations of powerful antiretroviral drugs have led to substantial prolongation of the lives of millions of persons with previously almost invariably fatal HIV infection, a true landmark in therapies for infectious diseases.[15,63]

All antibiotic and antiviral drugs, however, share an inherent weakness: the organisms against which they are directed almost invariably evolve mechanisms of resistance. Bacteria become resistant by a variety of mechanisms.[64] The evolution of antimicrobial resistance is enhanced by overuse of antibiotics in animals and by inappropriate use in humans. Many viruses, particularly RNA viruses such as influenza virus, rapidly develop mutations even in a single brief replication cycle. A number of approaches have been pursued to meet the ever-present challenge of antimicrobial resistance. The development of new classes of antibiotic, antiviral, and antiparasitic agents aimed at diverse microbial targets, often with the use of high-throughput screening of compounds,[65] is strengthening and broadening the therapeutic armamentarium. In addition, combination therapies (e.g., antiretroviral agents for HIV infection and multidrug approaches to tuberculosis) have proved to be successful in slowing the emergence of resistance.

Public Health Achievements

Breakthroughs in the field of infectious diseases have had far-reaching effects, including the realization of the critical importance of clean water and basic sanitation and hygiene for the prevention of a great number of infectious diseases. In addition, disease-specific approaches to prevention and treatment have led in many cases to the widespread control of diseases that historically have caused substantial morbidity and mortality.[66] The treatment of infectious diseases is in itself a prevention measure, limiting or preventing transmission to others. Eradication, the ultimate goal in facing the threat of an established or emerging infectious disease, is no longer unrealistic. Specifically, in addition to the millions

of lives saved by vaccines and antibiotics, certain infectious diseases have been eliminated from large regions of the world or even completely eradicated, an accomplishment rarely, if ever, seen in other medical disciplines. In 1980, smallpox became the first eradicated disease,[9] making this among the most momentous achievements in human disease control. In May 2011, the veterinary morbillivirus disease rinderpest was declared eradicated, and its presumed descendant, human measles virus, is now being targeted for eradication.[67] Poliomyelitis has been eliminated from several regions of the world, and it is hoped that within a reasonable period, it will be eradicated globally.[68] Dracunculiasis (guinea worm disease) is also almost completely eradicated.[69] These are just a few examples of what has been and can be accomplished by aggressive and concerted public health measures using the tools provided by basic and clinical research.

New Vistas

An unanticipated outcome of the explosion of information concerning the microbial world is the recognition that a growing number of chronic diseases that were once attributed to host, environmental, or lifestyle factors or to unknown causes are actually directly or indirectly caused by infectious agents that potentially can be controlled through prevention and treatment. For example, liver cancer and cirrhosis are complications of hepatitis B and C infections, cervical cancer is a complication of human papillomavirus (HPV) infection, and gastric and duodenal ulcers may result from *Helicobacter pylori* infection.[70–72] Vaccines against two of these agents, hepatitis B and HPV, are already in use, exemplifying the concept of cancer-preventing vaccines. *H. pylori* infection can be cured with antibiotics, and chronic hepatitis B and C infections are being treated by means of antiviral regimens with growing success rates. Certain autoimmune conditions have also been attributed to infections. For example, enteric microbes have been associated with inflammatory arthritides, and *Campylobacter jejuni* and certain viruses have been associated with the Guillain–Barré syndrome.[73] In addition, with new technologies and approaches, scientists are exploring new facets of microbiology, including the role of the human microbiome in maintaining homeostasis in the ecosystems of our bodies and its possible relationship to conditions such as obesity and inflammatory bowel disease.[74]

The Perpetual Challenge

We are living in a remarkable era. Almost all the major advances in understanding and controlling infectious diseases have occurred during the past two centuries, and momentous successes continue to accrue. These breakthroughs in the prevention, treatment, control, elimination, and potential eradication of infectious diseases are among the most important advances in the history of medicine.

Nevertheless, because of the evolutionary capacity of infectious pathogens to adapt to new ecologic niches created by human endeavor, as well as to pressures directed at their elimination, we will always confront new or reemerging infectious threats. The ongoing Ebola Virus outbreak in West Africa is the latest example of an emergent threat. Our successes in meeting these threats have come not just from isolated scientific triumphs but also from broad approaches that complement the battle against infectious diseases on many different fronts, including constant surveillance of the microbial landscape, clinical and public health efforts, and efficient translation of new discoveries into disease-control applications. These efforts are driven by the necessity of expecting the unexpected and being prepared to respond when the unexpected occurs. It is a battle that has been well fought for more than two centuries but that will almost certainly still be raging, in now-unimagined forms, two centuries from now. The challenges are truly perpetual. Our response to these challenges must be perpetual as well

References

1. Hecker JFC. Der schwarze Tod im vier-zehnten Jahrhundert. Berlin: Friedrich August Herbig, 1832.
2. Prinzing F. Epidemics resulting from wars. Oxford, England: Clarendon Press, 1916.
3. Winslow C-EA. The conquest of epidemic disease: a chapter in the history of ideas. Princeton, NJ: Princeton University Press, 1943.
4. Duffy J. Smallpox and the Indians in the American colonies. Bull Hist Med 1951;25:324–41.
5. Powell JH. Bring out your dead; the great plague of yellow fever in Philadelphia in 1793. Philadelphia: University of Pennsylvania Press, 1949.
6. Cartwright FF, Biddiss MD. The impact of infectious diseases. In: Cartwright FF, Biddiss MD. Disease and history. New York: Crowell, 1972:113–36.
7. Ampel NM. Plagues—what's past is present: thoughts on the origin and history of new infectious diseases. Rev Infect Dis 1991;13:658–65.
8. Krause RM. The origin of plagues: old and new. Science 1992;257:1073–78.
9. Fenner F. Smallpox: emergence, global spread, and eradication. Hist Philos Life Sci 1993;15:397–420.
10. McNeill WH. Plagues and peoples. Garden City, NY: Anchor Press/Doubleday, 1976.
11. Diamond JM. Guns, germs, and steel: the fates of human societies. New York: W.W. Norton, 1997.
12. Morens DM, Folkers GK, Fauci AS. Emerging infections: a perpetual challenge. Lancet Infect Dis 2008;8:710–19.
13. Jordan EO. Epidemic influenza: a survey. Chicago: American Medical Association, 1927.
14. Morens DM, Fauci AS. The 1918 influenza pandemic: insights for the 21st century. J Infect Dis 2007;195:1018–28.
15. De Cock KM, Jaffe HW, Curran JW. Reflections on 30 years of AIDS. Emerg Infect Dis 2011;17:1044–48.

16. de Quadros CA, Andrus JK, Olive JM, Guerra de Macedo C, Henderson DA. Polio eradication from the Western Hemisphere. Annu Rev Public Health 1992;13:239–52.

17. Morens DM, Taubenberger JK, Fauci AS. The persistent legacy of the 1918 influenza virus. N Engl J Med 2009;361:225–29. [Erratum, N Engl J Med 2009;361:1123.]

18. Lederberg J. Infectious history. Science 2000;288:287–93.

19. Morens DM, Folkers GK, Fauci AS. The challenge of emerging and re-emerging infectious diseases. Nature 2004;430:242–49. [Erratum, Nature 2010;463:122.]

20. Lederberg J, Shope RE, Oaks SC Jr, eds. Emerging infections: microbial threats to health in the United States. Washington, DC: National Academy Press, 1992.

21. Neu HC. The crisis in antibiotic resistance. Science 1992;257:1064–73.

22. Garrett L. The coming plague: newly emerging diseases in a world out of balance. New York: Farrar, Straus and Giroux, 1994.

23. Quinn TC. Population migration and the spread of types 1 and 2 human immunodeficiency viruses. Proc Natl Acad Sci U S A 1994;91:2407–14.

24. Morse SS. Factors in the emergence of infectious diseases. Emerg Infect Dis 1995;1:7–15.

25. Guerrant RL, Blackwood BL. Threats to global health and survival: the growing crises of tropical infectious diseases—our "unfinished" agenda. Clin Infect Dis 1999;28:966–86.

26. Butler JC, Crengle S, Cheek JE, et al. Emerging infectious diseases among indigenous peoples. Emerg Infect Dis 2001;7:Suppl:554–55.

27. Fauci AS. Infectious diseases: considerations for the 21st century. Clin Infect Dis 2001;32:675–85.

28. McMichael AJ. Human frontiers, environments and disease: past patterns, uncertain futures. Cambridge, England: Cambridge University Press, 2001.

29. Smolinski MS, Hamburg MA, Lederberg J, eds. Microbial threats to health: emergence, detection, and response. Washington, DC: National Academy Press, 2003.

30. Lee JH. Methicillin (oxacillin)-resistant Staphylococcus aureus strains isolated from major food animals and their potential transmission to humans. Appl Environ Microbiol 2003;69:6489–94.

31. Kane M, Case LK, Kopaskie K, et al. Successful transmission of a retrovirus depends on the commensal microbiota. Science 2011;334:245–49.

32. Kuss SK, Best GT, Etheredge CA, et al. Intestinal microbiota promote enteric virus replication and systemic pathogenesis. Science 2011;334:249–52.

33. Ichinohe T, Pang IK, Kumamoto Y, et al. Microbiota regulates immune defense against respiratory tract influenza A virus infection. Proc Natl Acad Sci U S A 2011;108:5354–59.

34. Relman DA. Microbial genomics and infectious diseases. N Engl J Med 2011;365:347–57.

35. Walter J, Ley R. The human gut microbiome: ecology and recent evolutionary changes. Annu Rev Microbiol 2011;65:411–29.

36. Medzhitov R. Recognition of microorganisms and activation of the immune response. Nature 2007;449:819–26.

37. Haynes BF, Soderberg KA, Fauci AS. Introduction to the immune system. In: Longo DL, Fauci AS, Kasper DL, Hauser SL, Jameson JL, Loscalzo J. Harrison's principles of internal medicine. 18th ed. Vol. 2. The immune system in health and disease. New York: McGraw-Hill Medical, 2012:2650–85.

38. Woolhouse M, Gaunt E. Ecological origins of novel human pathogens. Crit Rev Microbiol 2007;33:231–42.
39. Parrish CR, Holmes EC, Morens DM, et al. Cross-species virus transmission and the emergence of new epidemic diseases. Microbiol Mol Biol Rev 2008;72:457–70.
40. Keesing F, Belden LK, Daszak P, et al. Impacts of biodiversity on the emergence and transmission of infectious diseases. Nature 2010;468:647–52.
41. Dheda K, Warren RM, Zumla A, Grobusch MP. Extensively drug-resistant tuberculosis: epidemiology and management challenges. Infect Dis Clin North Am 2010;24:705–25.
42. Murray KO, Walker C, Gould E. The virology, epidemiology, and clinical impact of West Nile virus: a decade of advancements in research since its introduction into the Western Hemisphere. Epidemiol Infect 2011;139:807–17.
43. The global burden of disease: 2004 update. Geneva: World Health Organization, 2008.
44. World health statistics 2011. Geneva: World Health Organization, 2011.
45. Morens DM. Death of a president. N Engl J Med 1999;341:1845–49.
46. Jarcho S. The concept of contagion in medicine, literature, and religion. Malabar, FL: Krieger, 2000.
47. Morens DM. Characterizing a "new" disease: epizootic and epidemic anthrax, 1769-1780. Am J Public Health 2003;93:886–93.
48. Koch R. Die Aetiologie der Milzbrand-Krankheit, begründet auf die Entwicklungsgeschichte des Bacillus Anthracis. Beiträge zur Biologie der Pflanzen 1876;2:277–310.
49. Lipkin WI. Microbe hunting. Microbiol Mol Biol Rev 2010;74:363–77.
50. Hjelle B, Jenison S, Torrez-Martinez N, et al. A novel hantavirus associated with an outbreak of fatal respiratory disease in the southwestern United States: evolutionary relationships to known hantaviruses. J Virol 1994;68:592–96.
51. Relman DA, Schmidt TM, MacDermott RP, Falkow S. Identification of the uncultured bacillus of Whipple's disease. N Engl J Med 1992;327:293–301.
52. Chang Y, Cesarman E, Pessin MS, et al. Identification of herpes-like DNA sequences in AIDS-associated Kaposi's sarcoma. Science 1994;266:1865–69.
53. Pallen MJ, Loman NJ, Penn CW. High-throughput sequencing and clinical microbiology: progress, opportunities and challenges. Curr Opin Microbiol 2010;13:625–31.
54. Zhou T, Georgiev I, Wu X, et al. Structural basis for broad and potent neutralization of HIV-1 by antibody VRC01. Science 2010;329:811–17.
55. Krause RM, Dimmock NJ, Morens DM. Summary of antibody workshop: the role of humoral immunity in the treatment and prevention of emerging and extant infectious diseases. J Infect Dis 1997;176:549–59.
56. Maurice JM. State of the world's vaccines and immunization. 3rd ed. Geneva: World Health Organization, 2009.
57. Schief WR, Ban Y-EA, Stamatatos L. Challenges for structure-based HIV vaccine design. Curr Opin HIV AIDS 2009;4:431–40.
58. Parascandola J. From mercury to miracle drugs: syphilis therapy over the centuries. Pharm Hist 2009;51:14–23.
59. Feldman HA. The beginning of antimicrobial therapy: introduction of the sulfonamides and penicillins. J Infect Dis 1972;125:Suppl:22–46.
60. Spink WW. The drama of sulfanila-mide, penicillin and other antibiotics 1936-1972. Minn Med 1973;56:551–56.

61. Morens DM. At the deathbed of consumptive art. Emerg Infect Dis 2002;8:1353–58.
62. McDermott W. The story of INH. J Infect Dis 1969;119:678–83.
63. van Sighem AI, Gras LA, Reiss P, Brinkman K, de Wolf F. Life expectancy of recently diagnosed asymptomatic HIV-infected patients approaches that of uninfected individuals. AIDS 2010;24:1527–35.
64. Davies J, Davies D. Origins and evolution of antibiotic resistance. Microbiol Mol Biol Rev 2010;74:417–33.
65. Agarwal AK, Fishwick CW. Structure-based design of anti-infectives. Ann N Y Acad Sci 2010;1213:20–45. [Erratum, Ann N Y Acad Sci 2011;1228:175–78.]
66. Armstrong GL, Conn LA, Pinner RW. Trends in infectious disease mortality in the United States during the 20th century. JAMA 1999;281:61–66.
67. Morens DM, Holmes EC, Davis AS, Taubenberger JK. Global rinderpest eradication: lessons learned and why humans should celebrate too. J Infect Dis 2011;204:502–505.
68. Modlin JF. The bumpy road to polio eradication. N Engl J Med 2010;362:2346–49.
69. Hopkins DR, Ruiz-Tibén E, Downs P, Withers PC Jr, Roy S. Dracunculiasis eradication: neglected no longer. Am J Trop Med Hyg 2008;79:474–79.
70. Fredricks DN, Relman DA. Infectious agents and the etiology of chronic idiopathic diseases. Curr Clin Top Infect Dis 1998;18:180–200.
71. Parsonnet J, ed. Microbes and malignancy: infection as a cause of human cancers. New York: Oxford University Press, 1999.
72. Sanders MK, Peura DA. Helicobacter pylori-associated diseases. Curr Gastroenterol Rep 2002;4:448–54.
73. Vucic S, Kiernan MC, Cornblath DR. Guillain-Barré syndrome: an update. J Clin Neurosci 2009;16:733–41.
74. Kinross JM, Darzi AW, Nicholson JK. Gut microbiome-host interactions in health and disease. Genome Med 2011;3:14.

{ 5 }

Response to the AIDS Pandemic

A GLOBAL HEALTH MODEL

Peter Piot and Thomas C. Quinn

Just over three decades ago, a new outbreak of opportunistic infections and Kaposi's sarcoma was reported in a small number of homosexual men in California and New York.[1,2] This universally fatal disease, which was eventually called the acquired immunodeficiency syndrome (AIDS), was associated with a complete loss of CD4+ T cells. Within the first year of its description, the disease was also identified in patients with hemophilia, users of injection drugs, blood-transfusion recipients, and infants born to affected mothers. Soon thereafter, a heterosexual epidemic of AIDS was reported in Central Africa, preferentially affecting women.[3,4] Little did we know at the time that this small number of cases would eventually mushroom into tens of millions of cases, becoming one of the greatest pandemics of modern times.

Within 2 years after the initial reports of AIDS, a retrovirus, later called the human immunodeficiency virus (HIV), was identified as the cause of AIDS.[5] Diagnostic tests were developed to protect the blood supply and to identify those infected. Additional prevention measures were implemented, including risk-reduction programs, counseling and testing, condom distribution, and needle-exchange programs. However, HIV continued to spread, infecting 10 million persons within the first decade after its identification.

The second decade of AIDS was marked by further intensification of the epidemic in other areas of the world, including the southern cone of Africa, which saw an explosive HIV epidemic. Asia and the countries of the former Soviet Union also reported a marked increase in the spread of HIV. However, by the mid-1990s, with the discovery of highly active antiretroviral therapy, rates of death in developed countries started to decline. The use of antiretroviral drugs during pregnancy also resulted in a substantial decline in mother-to-child transmission of HIV in high-income countries. However, without access to antiretroviral drugs in low- and middle-income countries, rates of death and mother-to-child transmission continued to increase, with 2.4 million deaths and more than 3 million new infections reported in 2001. Of these new infections, two thirds occurred in sub-Saharan Africa.[6]

International Response to AIDS—a Global Health Model

It was not until the third decade of the epidemic that the world's public health officials, community leaders, and politicians united to combat AIDS. In 2001, the United Nations General Assembly endorsed a historic Declaration of Commitment on HIV/AIDS, a commitment that was renewed in 2011.[7] These actions resulted in the formation of the Global Fund to Fight AIDS, Tuberculosis, and Malaria, which was established to finance anti-AIDS activities in developing countries. In 2003, President George W. Bush announced the President's Emergency Plan for AIDS Relief (PEPFAR), which allocated billions of dollars to the countries hardest hit by AIDS.

This unprecedented global response to the AIDS pandemic can serve as a model for the response to other global health threats. For example, the global AIDS response incorporated a multisectoral approach that involved public health officials, clinicians, politicians, and leaders in civil society, business and labor, the armed forces, and the law, working in concert and with financial resources in excess of $15 billion per year[8] to reduce the incidence of HIV infection and associated mortality. The response to the pandemic required a coordinated global effort, which has been led by the Joint United Nations Program on HIV/AIDS (UNAIDS) since 1996. This transformational response helped redefine what is meant by health diplomacy and led to a new culture of accountability in international development. Tiered pricing of medicines became commonplace, and renewed optimism provided a boost for research on other neglected global health issues. This response to the AIDS pandemic highlighted the shortage of health care workers, inadequate availability of essential medications, and weaknesses in primary health care and public health systems. The stigma of HIV infection and inequities in the care of those infected focused attention on social and medical equity and human rights.

Although it has been argued that the provision of health care for patients with other conditions may have suffered from "vertical" AIDS programs (i.e., programs focused exclusively on AIDS), especially because of their recruitment of scarce health care workers,[9] there is also evidence that the AIDS response has had multiple collateral benefits, including a major increase in attention to and funding for global health issues, particularly malaria and tuberculosis, and a strengthening of services for maternal and child health in some countries.[10-12] The unified and integrated response to AIDS, although far from perfect, can serve as a model for society's future response to the growing epidemic of chronic diseases, obesity, and injuries, along with maternal and child health.[13]

The Fourth Decade of AIDS

UNAIDS estimates that in 2011, a total of 34.2 million persons were living with HIV infection, as compared with 29.1 million in 2001; 2.5 million persons were newly infected in 2011, a 22% decline from the number in 2001, and 1.7 million

died, a decline of 26% from 2005, when the number of AIDS deaths peaked at 2.3 million.[8,14] Similarly, the number of new infections among neonates and infants decreased from a peak of 570,000 in 2003 to 330,000 in 2011 as a result of interventions to prevent mother-to-child transmission.

However, these global figures hide a wide diversity. Figure 5.1 shows the prevalence of HIV infection among adults according to country, with sub-Saharan Africa continuing to be the most affected continent, followed by Eastern Europe and the Caribbean.[15] A special case is southern Africa, where HIV infection has become hyperendemic, with an overall prevalence among adults of up to 31% in Swaziland, 25% in Botswana, and 17% in South Africa. In Swaziland, the prevalence among women between the ages of 30 and 34 years is an astonishing 54%.[7] Even within a country, the prevalence of HIV infection varies widely according to region and risk group. In 2010, the prevalence of antenatal HIV infection in South Africa ranged from 18.4% in the Northern Cape province to 39.5% in KwaZulu Natal.[16] Men who have sex with men, female sex workers, users of injection drugs, truck drivers, fishermen, and military personnel are disproportionately affected around the world.[17-22]

There is also heterogeneity in epidemiologic trends. Whereas the spread of HIV infection is slowing in most regions, the incidence of infection continues to increase in Eastern Europe and several Asian countries.[14] There is also a resurgence of HIV infection caused by increased risk behavior among men who have sex with men in several European cities—for example, a reported 68% increase in sexual risk behavior among such men in Amsterdam[23]—in spite of high rates of HIV testing and access to antiretroviral therapy. At the same time, HIV infection is spreading to previously unaffected populations, such as injection-drug users in parts of Africa and men who have sex with men across Asia and Africa, where widespread homophobia drives these men underground.

Progress in Treatment of HIV Infection

Twenty-six antiretroviral drugs have been licensed for the treatment of HIV infection. The availability of these drugs led to reductions in mortality starting in the late 1990s in the United States and Europe. Subsequent reductions in the cost of antiretroviral therapy, the availability of generic antiretroviral drugs, and increases in international financial aid led to a marked expansion in drug availability. As a result, the number of persons receiving antiretroviral therapy in low- and middle-income countries rose from less than 200,000 persons in 2001 to 8 million persons in 2011[14] (Fig. 5.2). In addition, the death rates in some of the hardest-hit countries have started to decline.[24]

With the life expectancy of a patient with HIV infection receiving treatment approaching that of a person without HIV infection,[25,26] there has been an increased emphasis on starting antiretroviral therapy as early as possible in the course of infection. The revised 2012 guidelines of the U.S. Department of Health and Human Services recommend the initiation of antiretroviral therapy in all

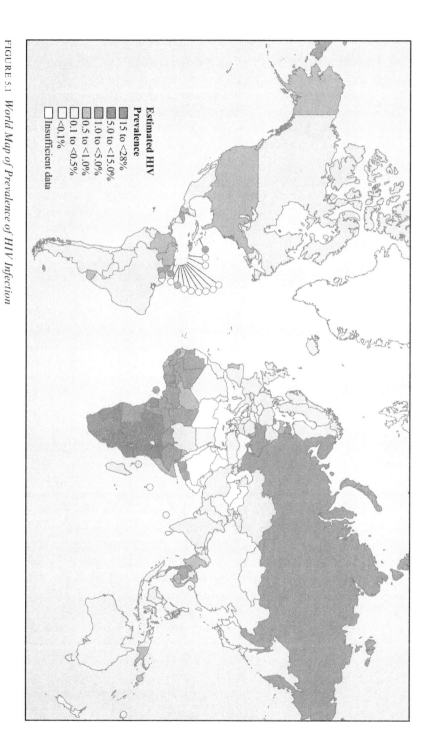

FIGURE 5.1 *World Map of Prevalence of HIV Infection*

Data are from UNAIDS,[15] UNICEF (www.unicef.org), and the World Bank (www.worldbank.org). An interactive version of this map is available at NEJM.org.

Estimated HIV Prevalence

- 15 to <28%
- 5.0 to <15.0%
- 1.0 to <5.0%
- 0.5 to <1.0%
- 0.1 to <0.5%
- <0.1%
- Insufficient data

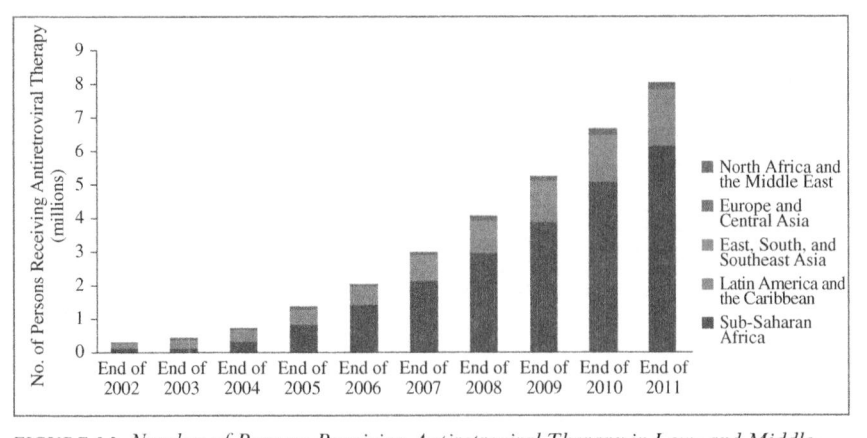

FIGURE 5.2 *Number of Persons Receiving Antiretroviral Therapy in Low- and Middle-Income Countries, According to Region (2002–2011)*

Data are from UNAIDS.[14]

persons with HIV infection.[27] These recommendations are based on evidence regarding the association between ongoing HIV replication and disease progression. In addition, because the use of antiretroviral therapy prevents the transmission of HIV in discordant couples (i.e., in which one person is infected and the other is not),[28] the guidelines recommend that such therapy be offered to all patients with HIV infection in order to reduce the risk for their sexual partners.

At variance with the U.S. and European guidelines,[29] World Health Organization guidelines continue to recommend the initiation of antiretroviral therapy in all persons with CD4 counts of 350 per cubic millimeter or less, with recognition of the limitations of cost and availability in many countries.[30] However, all guidelines strongly recommend antiretroviral therapy for all infected persons (regardless of the CD4 count) who are pregnant or who have a history of an AIDS-defining illness, tuberculosis, or coinfection with hepatitis B virus. The guidelines were recently updated to recommend antiretroviral therapy for HIV-discordant couples[31] (Table 5.1).

Despite advances in the accessibility of antiretroviral therapy, many challenges remain in the provision of care for persons with HIV infection. In the United States, the Centers for Disease Control and Prevention estimates that 1.2 million persons were living with HIV infection in 2008; of these persons, only 28% ultimately had suppressed viral levels, meaning that a majority were infectious owing to an insufficient uptake of testing, access to antiretroviral therapy, and adherence to therapy.[32–34] In one study in Mozambique involving 7005 persons with HIV infection, only half were enrolled in programs providing care, and only a small proportion ultimately started antiretroviral therapy and maintained adherence to the regimen at a rate of more than 90% for more than 180 days[35] (Fig. 5.3). These numbers reflect insufficient access and adherence to treatment that are mostly due to an inconsistent pattern of diagnosis, linkage to care, use of the CD4 count as a threshold for the initiation of therapy, and retention in care. In sub-Saharan Africa, the proportion of the population that

TABLE 5.1 Guidelines for the Initiation of Antiretroviral Drugs in Adults with HIV Infection*

Clinical Condition or CD4 Count	Recommendations to Start Treatment		
	DHHS 2013[27]	EACS 2012[29]	WHO 2010[30,31]†
CD4 count			
≤350 cells/mm³	Yes (AI)	Yes	Yes
>350–500 cells/mm³	Yes (AII)	Asymptomatic patients, consider therapy: symptomatic patients, yes	Stage 1 or 2, defer therapy; stage 3 or 4, yes
>500 cells/mm³	Yes (BIII)	Asymptomatic patients, defer therapy: symptomatic patients, yes	Stage 1 or 2, defer therapy; stage 3 or 4, yes
Pregnancy	Yes (AI)	Yes	Yes
History of AIDS-defining illness	Yes (AI)	Yes	Yes
HIV-associated nephropathy	Yes (AII)	Yes	Yes
Coinfection with tuberculosis	Yes (AII)	Yes	Yes
Coinfection with HBV	Yes (AII)	Yes, when treatment is indicated for HBV; defer therapy if HBV infection does not require treatment and CD4 count is >500 cells/mm³; consider therapy if CD4 count is 350–500 cells/mm³	Yes, when treatment is indicated for HBV infection
Coinfection with hepatitis C virus	Yes (BII)	Yes, if CD4 count is <500 cells/mm³; defer or consider therapy if CD4 count is ≥500 cells/mm³	Not specified
Risk of transmission			
Perinatal transmission	Yes (AI)	Yes	Yes
Heterosexual transmission	Yes (AI)	Strongly consider	Yes
Other sexual-transmission risk groups	Yes (AIII)	Strongly consider	Not specified

Preferred combination regimens

Patients receiving first-time therapy	Tenofovir and emtricitabine‡ plus one of the following: efavirenz (AI), ritonavir-boosted atazanavir (AI), ritonavir-boosted darunavir (AI), or raltegravir (AI)	Tenofovir and emtricitabine‡ or abacavir and lamivudine, plus one of the following: nevirapine, efavirenz, rilpivirine; ritonavir-boosted atazanavir, darunavir, or lopinavir; or raltegravir	Zidovudine or tenofovir, plus lamivudine or emtricitabine, plus efavirenz or nevirapine
Coinfection with tuberculosis§	Regimens listed above	Tenofovir and emtricitabine‡ plus either efavirenz or ritonavir-boosted protease inhibitor, plus rifabutin	Zidovudine or tenofovir, plus lamivudine or emtricitabine, plus efavirenz
Coinfection with HBV	Tenofovir and emtricitabine‡ plus efavirenz (AI) or regimens listed above	Tenofovir plus emtricitabine‡ plus efavirenz or same regimens as those for all patients	Tenofovir and emtricitabine‡ plus efavirenz
Pregnancy	Zidovudine and lamivudine, plus ritonavir-boosted atazanavir or lopinavir (AI)	Zidovudine and lamivudine, plus ritonavir-boosted lopinavir, saquinavir, or atazanavir	Zidovudine and lamivudine plus nevirapine

Note: These recommendations have been updated by the WHO, see their website for details. www.who.int/hiv/pub/guidelines/en/

*Recommendations are rated as follows: A, strong; B, moderate; and C, optional. Evidence is rated as follows: I, data from randomized, controlled trials; II, data from well-designed, nonrandomized trials or observational cohort studies with long-term clinical outcomes; and III, expert opinion. DHHS denotes Department of Health and Human Services, EACS European AIDS Clinical Society, HBV hepatitis B virus, and WHO World Health Organization.

†WHO stages include the following symptoms: stage 1, asymptomatic with generalized lymphadenopathy; stage 2, moderate weight loss, recurrent respiratory and oral infections, and herpes zoster; stage 3, severe weight loss, chronic diarrhea, thrush, severe bacterial infections, and tuberculosis within the past 2 years; stage 4, opportunistic infections, HIV wasting syndrome, and HIV encephalopathy.

‡Lamivudine can be used instead of emtricitabine and vice versa.

§In patients with HIV infection and tuberculosis, antiretroviral therapy should be started within 2 weeks after the initiation of treatment for tuberculosis if the CD4 count is less than 50 cells per cubic millimeter (AI). For patients with a CD4 count of 50 cells or more per cubic millimeter, therapy can be delayed beyond 2 weeks. The dose of antiretroviral therapy should be adjusted when used in combination with rifampin or rifabutin.

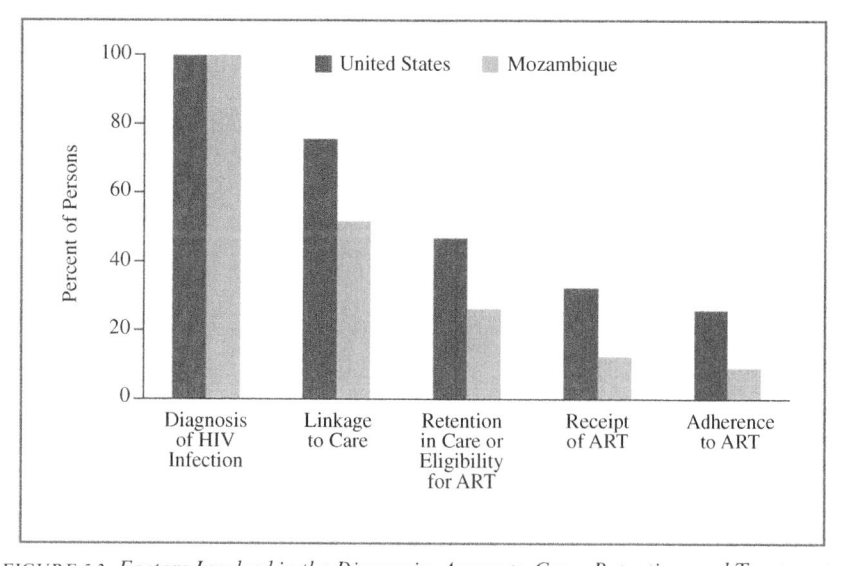

FIGURE 5.3 *Factors Involved in the Diagnosis, Access to Care, Retention, and Treatment of HIV Infection in the United States and Mozambique*

Data for the United States are derived from Gardner et al.,[33] and data for Mozambique are derived from Micek et al.[35] Data for adherence to antiretroviral therapy for the United States represent the proportion of persons with viral suppression, whereas for Mozambique, the data represent the proportion of persons with adherence to antiretroviral therapy, according to responses on questionnaires and pill counts among persons who were retained in care for more than 1 year (since viral levels were not obtained).

is being tested for HIV remains low. In low- and middle-income countries, the average CD4 count at the time of initiation of antiretroviral therapy remains low, with a median of 124 cells per cubic millimeter.[36] Intensified efforts are needed to identify persons who are infected, initiate therapy with standardized effective regimens, and encourage adherence to the regimen and retention in the program of care. Only with success at each stage in the continuum of care can the ultimate goals of improving health, extending lives, and preventing further HIV transmission be achieved.

Evolution of Prevention Strategies

A reduction in the incidence of HIV infection has been a top priority for AIDS control. The initial prevention strategy was based on behavioral change: abstinence, fidelity to a single partner, and use of a condom. This strategy met with only limited success, with Thailand's 100% condom campaign and Uganda's initial AIDS response being exceptions.[37,38] There is growing evidence that the relative decline of more than 25% in the incidence of HIV infection from 2000 through 2010 in several African countries is the result of behavioral change.[39] The rate of condom use continues to increase, with several countries (including South Africa, India, and Botswana) reporting a rate of condom use of more than 75%

during high-risk sexual intercourse.[6] However, condom use is still low in many other countries. A cause for concern is the finding that in several African countries (e.g., Uganda, Rwanda, and Zimbabwe), the number of men and women reporting multiple partners was higher in 2011 than the number 5 to 10 years earlier.[14]

Among injection-drug users, access to sterile injection equipment and drug-substitution therapy (referred to as harm reduction) is highly effective in reducing the spread of HIV infection.[40] Yet several countries in Eastern Europe and Asia in which HIV epidemics are driven by injection-drug use continue to use ineffective, punitive approaches. The result is a sustained high incidence of HIV infection, which also feeds the sexual spread of HIV.[41] Structural approaches,[42] such as programs to reduce violence against women[43] and the use of cash transfers (i.e., cash payments that can be used for food purchases, transportation, education, health care, or other expenses) among adolescent school girls in Malawi,[44] should be integrated more widely into HIV-prevention agendas. In addition, laws that drive men with same-sex partners underground or prohibit harm reduction for injection-drug users can be major obstacles to effective HIV prevention.[17] That such laws can be reversed was illustrated in India, where same-sex relations were decriminalized in 2009.

Biomedical Advances in Prevention

MALE CIRCUMCISION

The first major biomedical breakthrough in prevention was the finding of reduced susceptibility to HIV infection among circumcised men, with an efficacy rate of 50 to 60% shown in three clinical trials.[45-47] Three years after the completion of the circumcision trial in Rakai, Uganda, high rates of community effectiveness (73%) in decreasing the incidence of HIV infection have been reported.[48] With an estimated cost per infection averted in the range of $150 to $900 over a 10-year period (depending on the local incidence of HIV infection), male circumcision appears to be one of the most cost-effective preventive approaches, requiring only a one-time intervention.[49]

PREEXPOSURE PROPHYLAXIS

Preexposure prophylaxis (i.e., the use of antiretroviral therapy before sex) with 1% tenofovir gel was reported to reduce HIV acquisition by 39% in women.[50] Daily use of oral combination prophylaxis with tenofovir and emtricitabine among HIV-negative homosexual men who had multiple partners reduced HIV acquisition by 44%.[51] In both studies, greater efficacy was observed among persons who had high levels of adherence to the medication regimen. Daily use of tenofovir or tenofovir plus emtricitabine reduced HIV acquisition by 66% and 73%, respectively, among unaffected partners in HIV-discordant couples[52] and

among young heterosexuals in Botswana.[53] Although these findings are encouraging, two studies had conflicting results, with findings of no efficacy for either oral or gel tenofovir.[54,55] Such discrepancies in results may be due to low adherence to the drug regimens or differences in mucosal penetration. Recently, the Food and Drug Administration approved the daily use of oral emtricitabine and tenofovir disoproxil fumarate (Truvada, Gilead Sciences) for preexposure prophylaxis in combination with safer sex practices to reduce the risk of sexually acquired HIV infection among adults at high risk.

TREATMENT AS PREVENTION

Viral load is the single greatest risk factor for all modes of HIV transmission,[56] and treatment as prevention is based on the fact that antiretroviral therapy can reduce plasma and genital viral loads to undetectable levels, thereby reducing infectiousness.[28] This principle was first proved for the prevention of mother-to-child transmission[57] and was subsequently proved for the prevention of sexual transmission among discordant couples, with a reduction of 96% in the transmission rate.[28] This shift in focus from the use of antiretroviral agents for the treatment of HIV infection to their prophylactic use for the elimination of viral transmission has inspired optimism for achieving the goal of an AIDS-free generation.

COMBINATION PREVENTION

There is consensus that no single intervention can stop the spread of HIV and that combination prevention is the best approach.[58] Effective biomedical interventions coupled with behavioral and structural approaches may now successfully reduce the incidence of HIV infection to very low levels and ultimately control the epidemic. There is also a need to test in randomized trials the efficacy of treatment as prevention at the population level and to determine the optimal program design (in combination with specific preventive interventions), as well as ensuring good treatment coverage for persons in immediate need of clinical treatment.

From the perspectives of both efficacy and cost-effectiveness, HIV prevention should focus on populations at highest risk for transmission and should be customized to a wider range of realities than is currently the case. All components of combination prevention require some form of behavioral intervention, including adherence to condom use, antiretroviral-based prevention, and prevention of behaviors associated with an increased risk of infection. However, even when the most effective HIV interventions are used, most mathematical models suggest that by 2031—50 years after the identification of AIDS—there may still be as many as 1 million new infections globally every year.[59,60] Although a vaccination trial in Thailand showed an efficacy of 31%, providing a much-needed boost to vaccine research,[61] the search for such effective prophylaxis still eludes investigators.

The Challenges Ahead

After 30 years of the AIDS epidemic, more than 34 million persons are still living with HIV infection worldwide, and the global response will clearly have to be sustained for at least several decades. An impressive array of evidence-based interventions can be implemented to treat established infections and prevent new ones. Studies of high-risk populations have shown that HIV infection can be prevented even in the most challenging settings. Nevertheless, UNAIDS reports that only 60% of sex workers, 46% of injection-drug users, and 40% of men who have sex with men were reached by HIV-prevention programs in 2008, and the incidence of HIV infection is rising again in several countries, including Uganda.[8,14]

In 2011, less than 25% of all persons with HIV infection had access to antiretroviral therapy or had virologic suppression from receipt of such therapy.[14] To ensure access to antiretroviral drugs, many lower-income countries are still almost entirely dependent on international aid, which has declined in recent years. As a result of successful therapy and increased life expectancy, we are witnessing an increase in the need for care for chronic diseases among persons with HIV infection. Thus, we need to develop innovative solutions for care delivery, including shifting specific tasks to health workers aside from clinicians and integrated service delivery in the community.

In conclusion, great progress has been made in the global response to the AIDS epidemic, but these achievements are fragile because of the enormous challenge of sustaining political, programmatic, and technical commitment, along with national and international funding. A certain level of AIDS fatigue on the part of funders and public health and political leaders coincides with the unprecedented opportunities for using new tools to control AIDS. Prevention and care now need to be targeted strategically, and creative combinations of behavioral, biomedical, and structural interventions need to be widely implemented.[59,60] These programs will require universal access, large-scale implementation, careful monitoring and evaluation, financial and technical resources, and robust commitment. Only then may we begin to see a substantial effect on the global spread of HIV infection.

References

1. Pneumocystis pneumonia—Los Angeles. MMWR Morb Mortal Wkly Rep 1981;30:250–52.
2. Kaposi's sarcoma and Pneumocystis pneumonia among homosexual men—New York City and California. MMWR Morb Mortal Wkly Rep 1981;30:305–308.
3. Piot P, Quinn TC, Taelman H, et al. Acquired immunodeficiency syndrome in a heterosexual population in Zaire. Lancet 1984;2:65–69.
4. Quinn TC, Mann JM, Curran JW, Piot P. AIDS in Africa: an epidemiologic paradigm. Science 1986;234:955–63.

5. Gallo RC, Montagnier L. The discovery of HIV as the cause of AIDS. N Engl J Med 2003;349:2283–85.

6. Piot P, Bartos M, Ghys PD, Walker N, Schwartländer B. The global impact of HIV/AIDS. Nature 2001;410:968–73.

7. World AIDS Day report 2011—how to get to zero: Faster. Smarter. Better. Geneva: Joint United Nations Programme on HIV/AIDS (UNAIDS), 2011.

8. Global AIDS response progress reporting 2012. Geneva: Joint United Nations Programme on HIV/AIDS (UNAIDS), 2012.

9. Shiffman J. Has donor prioritization of HIV/AIDS displaced aid for other health issues? Health Policy Plan 2008;23:95–100.

10. El-Sadr WM, Abrams EJ. Scale-up of HIV care and treatment: can it transform healthcare services in resource-limited settings? AIDS 2007;21:Suppl 5:S65-S70.

11. Rasschaert F, Pirard M, Philips MP, et al. Positive spill-over effects of ART scale up on wider health systems development: evidence from Ethiopia and Malawi. J Int AIDS Soc 2011;14:Suppl 1:S3.

12. Harries AD, Zachariah R, Jahn A, Schouten EJ, Kamoto K. Scaling up antiretroviral therapy in Malawi—implications for managing other chronic diseases in resource-limited countries. J Acquir Immune Defic Syndr 2009;52:Suppl 1:S14-S16.

13. Lamptey P, Merson M, Piot P, Reddy KS, Dirks R. Informing the 2011 UN Session on Noncommunicable Diseases: applying lessons from the AIDS response. PLoS Med 2011;8(9):e1001086.

14. Global report: UNAIDS report on the global AIDS epidemic 2012. Geneva: Joint United Nations Programme on HIV/AIDS (UNAIDS), 2012.

15. AIDSinfo: epidemiological status. Geneva: Joint United Nations Programme on HIV/AIDS (UNAIDS), 2012 (http://www.unaids.org/en/dataanalysis/datatools/aidsinfo/).

16. The 2010 national antenatal HIV and syphilis prevalence survey in South Africa. Pretoria: South Africa National Department of Health, 2011.

17. Beyrer C, Baral SD, van Griensven F. The global epidemiology of HIV infection among men who have sex with men. Lancet 2012;380:367–77.

18. Baral S, Beyrer C, Muessig K, et al. Burden of HIV among female sex workers in low-income and middle-income countries: a systematic review and meta-analysis. Lancet Infect Dis 2012;12:538–49.

19. Mathers BM, Degenhardt L, Phillips B, et al. Global epidemiology of injecting drug use and HIV among people who inject drugs: a systematic review. Lancet 2008;372:1733–45.

20. MacPherson EE, Sadalaki J, Njoloma M, et al. Transactional sex and HIV: understanding the gendered structural drivers of HIV in fishing communities in Southern Malawi. J Int AIDS Soc 2012;15:Suppl 1:1–9.

21. Pandey A, Benara SK, Roy N, et al. Risk behaviour, sexually transmitted infections and HIV among long-distance truck drivers: a cross-sectional survey along national highways in India. AIDS 2008;22:Suppl 5:S81-S90.

22. Abebe Y, Schaap A, Mamo G, et al. HIV prevalence in 72,000 urban and rural male army recruits, Ethiopia, 1999-2000. Ethiop Med J 2003;41:Suppl 1:25–30.

23. Bezemer D, de Wolf F, Boerlijst MC, et al. A resurgent HIV-1 epidemic among men who have sex with men in the era of potent antiretroviral therapy. AIDS 2008;22:1071–77.

24. Bendavid E, Holmes C, Bhattacharya J, Miller G. HIV development assistance and adult mortality in Africa. JAMA 2012;307:2060–67.

25. Antiretroviral Therapy Cohort Collaboration. Life expectancy of individuals on combination antiretroviral therapy in high-income countries: a collaborative analysis of 14 cohort studies. Lancet 2008;372:293–99.

26. Mills EJ, Barnighausen T, Negin J. HIV and aging—preparing for the challenges ahead. N Engl J Med 2012;366:1270–73.

27. Panel on Antiretroviral Guidelines for Adults and Adolescents. Guidelines for the use of antiretroviral agents in HIV-1-infected adults and adolescents. Updated 2013. Washington, DC: Department of Health and Human Services, 2012 (http://aidsinfo. nih.gov/contentfiles/lvguidelines/adultandadolescentgl.pdf).

28. Cohen MS, Chen YQ, McCauley M, et al. Prevention of HIV-1 infection with early antiretroviral therapy. N Engl J Med 2011;365:493–505.

29. European guidelines for treatment of HIV infected adults in Europe: version 6.1. Paris: European AIDS Clinical Society, 2012 (http://www.europeanaidsclinicalsociety.org/images/stories/EACSPdf/EacsGuidelines-v6.1-2edition.pdf).

30. Antiretroviral therapy for HIV infection in adults and adolescents: recommendations for a public health approach (2010 revision). Geneva: World Health Organization (http://whqlibdoc.who.int/publications/2010/9789241599764_eng.pdf).

31. Guidance on couples HIV testing and counselling including antiretroviral therapy for treatment and prevention in serodiscordant couples. Geneva: Joint United Nations Programme on HIV/AIDS (UNAIDS), 2012.

32. HIV surveillance—United States, 1981–2008. MMWR Morb Mortal Wkly Rep 2011;60:689–93. [Erratum, MMWR Morb Mortal Wkly Rep 2011;60:852.]

33. Gardner EM, McLees MP, Steiner JF, Del Rio C, Burman WJ. The spectrum of engagement in HIV care and its relevance to test-and-treat strategies for prevention of HIV infection. Clin Infect Dis 2011;52:793–800.

34. Vital signs: HIV prevention through care and treatment—United States. MMWR Mortal Wkly Rep 2011;60:1618–23.

35. Micek MA, Gimbel-Sherr K, Baptista AJ, et al. Loss to follow-up of adults in public HIV care systems in central Mozambique: identifying obstacles to treatment. J Acquir Immune Defic Syndr 2009;52:397–405.

36. Gupta A, Nadkarni G, Yang WT, et al. Early mortality in adults initiating antiretroviral therapy (ART) in low- and middle-income countries (LMIC): a systematic review and meta-analysis. PLoS One 2011;6(12):e28691.

37. Stoneburner RL, Low-Beer D. Population-level HIV declines and behavioral risk avoidance in Uganda. Science 2004;304:714–18.[Erratum, Science 2004; 306:1477.]

38. Evaluation of the 100% condom programme in Thailand: case study. Geneva: Joint United Nations Programme on HIV/AIDS (UNAIDS), 2000.

39. The International Group on Analysis of Trends in HIV Prevalence and Behaviours in Young People in Countries Most Affected by HIV. Trends in HIV prevalence and sexual behaviour among young people aged 15-24 years in countries most affected by HIV. Sex Transm Infect 2010;86:Suppl 2:ii72–83. [Erratum, Sex Transm Infect 2011;87:8.]

40. Beasley R. Reducing harm: brief report. Washington, DC: Institute of Medicine of the National Academies, January 2010.

41. Beyrer C, Malinowska-Sempruch K, Kamarulzaman A, Kazatchkine M, Sidibe M, Strathdee SA. Time to act: a call for comprehensive responses to HIV in people who use drugs. Lancet 2010;376:551–63.

42. Gupta GR, Parkhurst JO, Ogden JA, Aggleton P, Mahal A. Structural approaches to HIV prevention. Lancet 2008;372:764–75.

43. Jan S, Ferrari G, Watts CH, et al. Economic evaluation of a combined micro-finance and gender training intervention for the prevention of intimate partner violence in rural South Africa. Health Policy Plan 2011;26:366–72.

44. Baird SJ, Garfein RS, McIntosh CT, Ozler B. Effect of a cash transfer programme for schooling on prevalence of HIV and herpes simplex type 2 in Malawi: a cluster randomised trial. Lancet 2012;379:1320–29.

45. Gray RH, Li X, Kigozi G, et al. The impact of male circumcision on HIV incidence and cost per infection prevented: a stochastic simulation model from Rakai, Uganda. AIDS 2007;21:845–50.

46. Auvert B, Taljaard D, Lagarde E, Sobngwi-Tambekou J, Sitta R, Puren A. Randomized, controlled intervention trial of male circumcision for reduction of HIV infection risk: the ANRS 1265 Trial. PLoS Med 2005;2(11):e298.

47. Bailey RC, Moses S, Parker CB, et al. Male circumcision for HIV prevention in young men in Kisumu, Kenya: a randomised controlled trial. Lancet 2007;369:643–56.

48. Gray R, Kigozi G, Kong X, et al. The effectiveness of male circumcision for HIV prevention and effects on risk behaviors in a posttrial follow-up study. AIDS 2012;26:609–615.

49. Tobian AA, Serwadda D, Quinn TC, et al. Male circumcision for the prevention of HSV-2 and HPV infections and syphilis. N Engl J Med 2009;360:1298–309.

50. Abdool Karim Q, Abdool Karim SS, Frohlich JA, et al. Effectiveness and safety of tenofovir gel, an antiretroviral microbicide, for the prevention of HIV infection in women. Science 2010;329:1168–74. [Erratum, Science 2011;333:524.]

51. Grant RM, Lama JR, Anderson PL, et al. Preexposure chemoprophylaxis for HIV prevention in men who have sex with men. N Engl J Med 2010;363:2587–99.

52. Baeten JM, Donnell D, Ndase P, et al. Antiretroviral prophylaxis for HIV-1 prevention in heterosexual men and women. N Engl J Med 2012;367:399–410.

53. Thigpen MC, Kebaabetswe PM, Paxton LA, et al. Antiretroviral preexposure prophylaxis for heterosexual HIV transmission in Botswana. N Engl J Med 2012;367:423–34.

54. Van Damme L, Corneli A, Ahmed K, et al. Preexposure prophylaxis for HIV infection among African women. N Engl J Med 2012;367:411–22.

55. Marrazzo J, Ramjee G, Nair G, et al. Pre-exposure prophylaxis for HIV in women: daily oral tenofovir, oral tenofovir/emtricitabine, or vaginal tenofovir gel in the VOICE Study (MTN 003). Presented at the 20th Conference on Retroviruses and Opportunistic Infections, Atlanta, March 3–6, 2013. abstract.

56. Quinn TC, Wawer MJ, Sewankambo N, et al. Viral load and heterosexual transmission of human immunodeficiency virus type 1. N Engl J Med 2000;342:921–29.

57. Garcia PM, Kalish LA, Pitt J, et al. Maternal levels of plasma human immunodeficiency virus type 1 RNA and the risk of perinatal transmission. N Engl J Med 1999;341:394–402.

58. Piot P, Bartos M, Larson H, Zewdie D, Mane P. Coming to terms with complexity: a call to action for HIV prevention. Lancet 2008;372:845–59.

59. Quinn T, Serwadda D. Preparing for the future of HIV/AIDS in Africa—a shared responsibility: brief report. Washington, DC: Institute of Medicine of the National Academies, November 2010.

60. The aids2031 Consortium. AIDS: taking a long-term view. Upper Saddle River, NJ: FT Press, 2010.

61. Rerks-Ngarm S, Pitisuttithum P, Nitayaphan S, et al. Vaccination with ALVAC and AIDSVAX to prevent HIV-1 infection in Thailand. N Engl J Med 2009;361:2209–20.

Pandemic Preparedness and Response
LESSONS FROM THE H1N1 INFLUENZA OF 2009
Harvey V. Fineberg

A number of viruses have pandemic potential. For example, the coronavirus responsible for the severe acute respiratory syndrome (SARS), which first appeared in southern China in November 2002, caused 8096 cases and 774 deaths in 26 countries before coming to a halt by July 2003 mainly owing to isolation and quarantine.[1] In terms of persistence, versatility, potential severity, and speed of spread, however, few viruses rival influenza virus. Endemic in a number of species, including humans, birds, and pigs, influenza virus causes annual outbreaks punctuated by occasional worldwide pandemics, which are characterized by sustained community spread in multiple regions of the world.

Beyond spread, the degree to which a pandemic is defined according to the severity of the disease, or whether it may be simply described as often producing many illnesses and deaths, remains ambiguous.[2] At its worst, pandemic influenza can be catastrophic: the great influenza pandemic of 1918–1919 is estimated to have infected 500 million persons worldwide and to have killed 50 to 100 million persons.[3] In a typical year of seasonal outbreaks in the Northern and Southern Hemispheres, influenza virus causes as many as 5 million cases of severe illness in humans and 500,000 deaths.[4]

Over the past decade, sporadic cases of severe influenza and deaths in humans have been caused by a number of avian influenza A viruses, including the H5N1 virus, first detected in 1997, and the H7N9 and H10N8 viruses, first reported in 2013. Such sporadic cases may be harbingers of a gathering pandemic, but the likelihood is difficult to judge because it is not known how frequently similar zoonotic episodes occurred silently in the past, when surveillance was more limited, and did not cause pandemics.

The most recent global pandemic was caused by the influenza A (H1N1) strain, which was first detected in North America in 2009 (influenza A[H1N1]pdm09). This event prompted the first activation of provisions under the 2005 International

Health Regulations (IHR), which went into effect in 2007.[5] Deliberations that led
to the 2005 IHR revisions were shaped by experience in the SARS outbreak of
2003. The regulations delineate the responsibilities of individual countries and
the leadership role of the World Health Organization (WHO) in declaring and
managing a public health emergency of international concern.

The 2009 H1N1 pandemic presented a public health emergency of uncertain
scope, duration, and effect. The experience exposed strengths of the newly implemented IHR as well as a number of deficiencies and defects, including vulnerabilities in global, national, and local public health capacities; limitations of scientific
knowledge; difficulties in decision making under conditions of uncertainty; complexities in international cooperation; and challenges in communication among
experts, policymakers, and the public.

At the request of the WHO, an international committee, which I chaired,
reviewed the experience of the pandemic, with special attention given to the function of the 2005 IHR and the performance of the WHO.[6] Since this was the first
time that the 2005 IHR was tested in a real-world situation, it was inevitable
that aspects of the response to the series of outbreaks and subsequent pandemic
could have been improved. Even though there were areas of outstanding performance, such as the timely identification of the pathogen, the development of
sensitive and specific diagnostics, and the creation of highly interactive networks
of public health officials, the most fundamental conclusion of the committee,
which applies today, is not reassuring: "The world is ill prepared to respond to a
severe influenza pandemic or to any similarly global, sustained and threatening
public-health emergency."[6]

In this article, I focus on lessons from the global response to the 2009 H1N1
pandemic. I identify some of the key successes and shortcomings in the global
response, on the basis of the findings and conclusions of the review committee.
The article concludes by pointing to steps that can improve global readiness to
deal with future pandemics.

Time Course of the 2009 H1N1 Pandemic

The first laboratory-confirmed cases of H1N1 influenza appeared in Mexico
in February and March of 2009. Cases that were detected in California in late
March were laboratory-confirmed by mid-April. By the end of April, cases had
been reported in a number of U.S. states and in countries on various continents, including Canada, Spain, the United Kingdom, New Zealand, Israel, and
Germany. On April 25, invoking its authority under the 2005 IHR, the WHO
declared a public health emergency of international concern and convened the
emergency committee called for in the regulations. The WHO also established
a dedicated internal group to coordinate the response to the widening outbreaks. As of June 9, 2009, a total of 73 countries had reported more than 26,000
laboratory-confirmed cases, and the WHO declared on June 11 that the situation met the criteria for phase 6—that is, a full-fledged pandemic (Table 6.1). By

TABLE 6.1 World Health Organization (WHO) Pandemic-Phase Descriptions and Main
Actions According to Phase

Phase	Estimated Probability of Pandemic	Description	Main Actions in Affected Countries	Main Actions in Nonaffected Countries
1	Uncertain	No animal influenza virus circulating among animals has been reported to cause infection in humans	Developing and implementing national pandemic-influenza preparedness and response plans and harmonizing them with national emergency preparedness and response plans	Same as in affected countries
2	Uncertain	An animal influenza virus circulating in domesticated or wild animals is known to have caused infection in humans and is therefore considered a specific potential pandemic threat	Same as phase 1	Same as phase 1
3	Uncertain	An animal or human–animal influenza reassortant virus has caused sporadic cases or small clusters of disease in people but has not resulted in a level of human-to-human transmission sufficient to sustain community-level outbreaks	Same as phase 1	Same as phase 1
4	Medium to high	Human-to-human transmission of an animal or human–animal influenza reassortant virus that is able to sustain community-level outbreaks has been verified	Rapid containment	Readiness for pandemic response

(*continued*)

TABLE 6.1 Continued

Phase	Estimated Probability of Pandemic	Description	Main Actions in Affected Countries	Main Actions in Nonaffected Countries
5	High to certain	The same identified virus has caused sustained community-level outbreaks in at least two countries in one WHO region	Pandemic response: each country implements the actions called for in its national plans	Readiness for imminent pandemic response
6	Pandemic in progress	In addition to the criteria for phase 5, the same virus has caused sustained community-level outbreaks in at least one other country in another WHO region	Same as phase 5	Same as phase 5

the time the pandemic had waned, in August 2010, virtually all countries had reported laboratory-confirmed cases (Fig. 6.1). An interactive graphic showing the timeline of the 2009 H1N1 pandemic is available at NEJM.org.

Evidence from the first outbreak in Mexico was alarming. An observational study of 899 hospitalized patients showed that 58 (6.5%) became critically ill, and of those, 41% died.[7] During the course of the pandemic, mortality among children, young adults, and pregnant women was much higher than in a typical influenza season, and there was substantial variation in severity among different regions of the world.[8] In general, older adults fared relatively well, and the total number of influenza-related deaths worldwide (estimated ranges of 123,000 to 203,000 deaths[8] and 105,700 to 395,600 deaths[9]) proved similar to the number in a relatively mild year of seasonal influenza. However, because of the proportionately higher mortality among children and young adults, the severity in terms of years of life lost was greater than in a typical year of seasonal influenza.[10]

2005 INTERNATIONAL HEALTH REGULATIONS

A number of provisions of the 2005 IHR proved helpful in dealing with the 2009 H1N1 pandemic. For example, the 2005 IHR established systematic approaches to surveillance, early-warning systems, and response in member states and promoted technical cooperation and sharing of logistic support. Communication among countries and the WHO was strengthened by the establishment in each member state of National Focal Points—national offices that would be responsible for rapid collection and dissemination of emerging data and guidance.

A static and potentially outdated list of notifiable diseases in previous regulations was replaced by a more flexible flow diagram and decision tool that

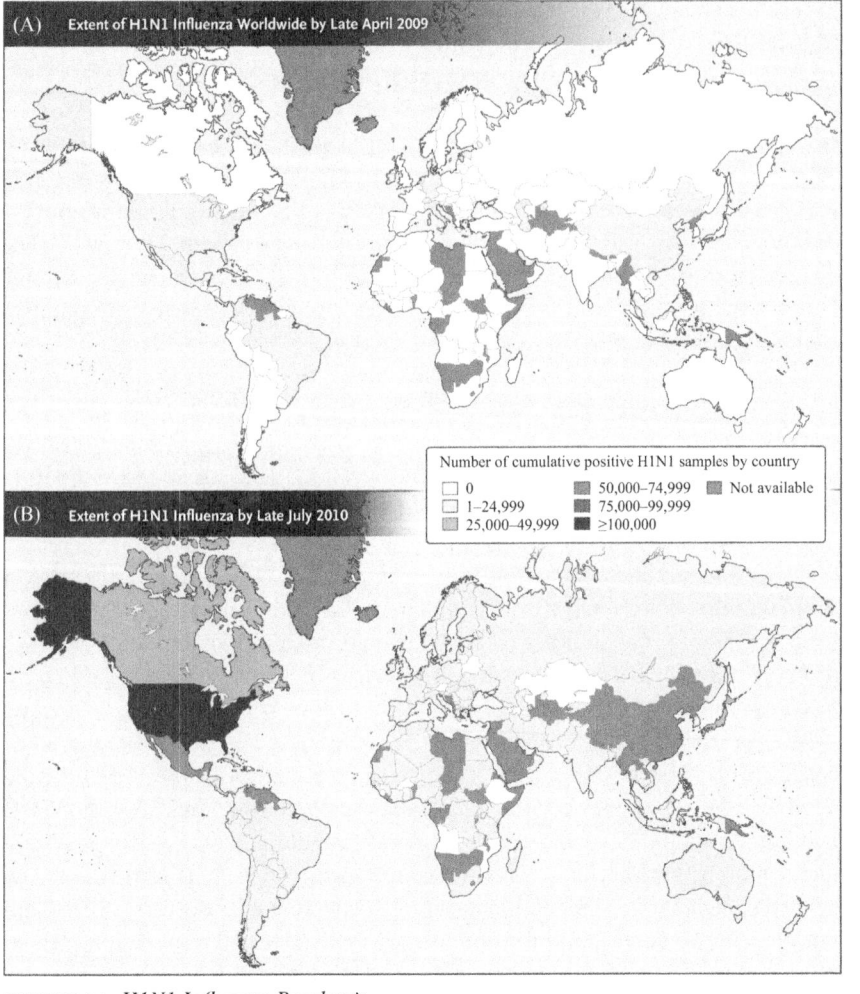

FIGURE 6.1 *H1N1 Influenza Pandemic*
Data are from the World Health Organization and http://fluNet.org.

identified conditions warranting public health action. The 2005 IHR required, for the first time, that member states implementing unilateral measures that interfere with international traffic and trade inform the WHO and that they also provide a public health rationale and scientific justification for those measures. Most important, the 2005 IHR formally assigned to the WHO the authority to declare a public health emergency of international concern and take a leading role in the global response.

Despite these positive features, many member states did not have in place the capacities called for in the IHR, nor were they on a path to meet their obligations by the 2012 deadline specified in the document. Of the 194 eligible states, 128 (66%) responded to a WHO questionnaire on their state of progress in 2011. Only

58% of the responding member states reported having developed national plans to meet their core capacity requirements, and only 10% claimed to have fully established the capacities called for in the IHR.[6]

The IHR fails to specify a basis for virus sharing and vaccine sharing. This has been partially ameliorated in a framework for pandemic-influenza preparedness, adopted in 2011, that calls on member states to encourage vaccine manufacturers to set aside a fraction of their pandemic-vaccine production for donation and for discounted pricing in developing countries.[11] A glaring gap in the IHR, which has not been remedied, is its lack of enforceable sanctions. For example, if a country fails to explain why it restricted trade or travel, no financial penalties or punitive trade sanctions are called for under the 2005 IHR.

WORLD HEALTH ORGANIZATION

The WHO is an indispensable global resource for leading and coordinating the response to a pandemic. In the 2009 H1N1 pandemic, the WHO had many notable achievements. The organization provided guidance to inform national influenza-preparedness plans, which were in place in 74 countries at the time of the first outbreak in North America, and helped countries monitor their development of IHR core capacities. The WHO Global Influenza Surveillance Network detected, identified, and characterized the virus in a timely manner and monitored the course of the pandemic.

Within 48 hours after the activation of provisions in the 2005 IHR, the WHO convened the first meeting of the emergency committee of experts who would advise the WHO on the status of the pandemic. Within 32 days after the WHO had declared a public health emergency of international concern, the first candidate reassortant vaccine viruses were developed, and vaccine seed strains and control reagents were made available within a few weeks. The Strategic Advisory Group of Experts on immunization at the WHO provided early recommendations on vaccine target groups and dose. The WHO provided prompt and valuable field assistance to affected countries and efficiently distributed more than 3 million courses of antiviral drugs to 72 countries.

Against this backdrop of accomplishment, the WHO confronted systemic difficulties and made a number of missteps in the course of coping with the unfolding pandemic. Although the WHO is the only global agency with legitimate authority to lead the response to a pandemic, it is burdened by a number of structural impediments. First, the WHO is simultaneously the moral voice for health in the world and the servant of its member states, which authorize the overall program and budget. National interests may conflict with a mandate to equitably protect the health of every person on the planet. Second, the budget of the WHO is incommensurate with the scope of its responsibilities. Only approximately one quarter of the budget comes from member-state assessments, and the rest depends on specific project support from countries and foundations. These budget realities and the personnel-management requirements inherent in being a United Nations agency constrain flexibility.

Third, the WHO is better designed to respond to focal, short-term emergencies, such as investigating an isolated outbreak of hemorrhagic fever in rural sub-Saharan Africa, or to manage a multiyear, steady-state disease-control program than to mount and sustain the kind of intensive, global response that is required to deal with a rapidly unfolding pandemic. Finally, the regional WHO offices are autonomous, with member states of the region responsible for the election of the regional director, budget, and program. Although this system allows for regional variation to suit local conditions, the arrangement limits the ability of the WHO to direct a globally coherent and coordinated response during a global health emergency.

In anticipation of a possible pandemic before 2009, public health authorities had focused on the threat of avian H5N1 influenza, and a signal feature among recognized cases of H5N1 influenza in humans was mortality exceeding 50%.[12] Hence, it was expected that a newly emerging pandemic virus would cause many deaths as well as widespread disease, and the WHO said as much on its website on pandemic preparedness in advance of the 2009 H1N1 pandemic.

The prospects of a pandemic depend on the transmissibility and virulence of the virus and on the susceptibility of the population, which may vary according to age and past exposure to influenza viruses. Although a catastrophic pandemic probably depends on the emergence of a new antigenic type of influenza virus, it does not follow that every newly emerging influenza virus will produce an especially severe burden of influenza. For example, in the 40 years between the mid-1930s and mid-1970s, the 5 years of greatest excess mortality from influenza in the United States were 1937, 1943, 1953, 1957, and 1960, but among these years, only 1957 was marked by a new antigenic type (H2N2), and 1968 (the year when H3N2 appeared) did not rank in the top five for severity.[13] The expectation of a very severe pandemic was understandable in the context of H5N1 but not necessarily for every new antigenic type.

Since the formal criteria for advancing from one phase to the next higher phase in an emerging pandemic were based entirely on the extent of spread and not on severity, this led to public confusion about exactly what the WHO meant by a pandemic. The WHO lacked a consistent, measurable, and understandable depiction of the severity of a pandemic. This situation was problematic because, regardless of the definition of a pandemic, the decisions about response logically depend on both spread and severity. In addition, the defining phase structure that was based on spread was needlessly complex in that it defined more stages than there were differentiated responses, and the structure that seemed suitable for planning proved less suited to operational management.

The weekly requests by the WHO for data were overwhelming for some countries, particularly those with limited epidemiologic and laboratory capacity. As the epidemic progressed, it was not always evident to country officials that the data they submitted were being analyzed and used. Rather than focus on laboratory-confirmed cases, a surveillance model that relied on syndromic surveillance and selective, systematic virologic testing might have been more revealing.[14] Public health officials in some countries, such as the U.K. Health Protection

Agency, produced weekly summaries that tracked domestic indicators of influenza spread and severity while noting pertinent global influenza activity, and this approach could hold lessons for other countries as well as for the WHO.[15]

When the WHO convened an expert group, typically for a 1- or 2-day consultation, the practice of the organization was not to disclose the identities of the experts until the consultation was concluded. Similarly, the WHO kept confidential the identities of emergency-committee members convened under the provisions of the IHR, who would advise the WHO on the status of the emerging pandemic. Although the intent was to shield the experts from commercial or political influences, the effect was to stoke suspicions about the potential links between individual members of the emergency committee and industry.[16] Although the review committee uncovered no evidence of inappropriate influence on the emergency committee, the decision to keep the members' identities secret fostered suspicions about WHO decision making, which were exacerbated by the failure to apply systematic and open procedures for disclosing, recognizing, and managing conflicts of interest. A practice of confidentiality that was arguably fitting for a 1-day consultation was ill-suited to an advisory function that extended over a period of months.

The failure to acknowledge legitimate criticisms, such as inconsistent descriptions of the meaning of a pandemic and the lack of timely and open disclosure of potential conflicts of interest, undermined the ability of the WHO to respond effectively to unfounded criticisms. For example, the WHO was wrongly accused of rushing to declare phase 6, or a full-fledged pandemic, because such action would trigger vaccine orders sought by manufacturers. This kind of suspicion proved hard for the WHO to dispel, despite the fact that the declaration of phase 6 was delayed until the sustained community spread in multiple countries in multiple WHO regions was incontrovertible.

The WHO made a number of operational missteps, including conferring with only a subset of the emergency committee, rather than inviting input from the full group, at a crucial point of deciding to declare progression from phase 4 to phase 5. Throughout the pandemic period, the WHO generated an unmanageable number of documents from multiple technical units within the organization and lacked a cohesive, overarching set of procedures and priorities for producing consistent and timely technical guidance. In addition, after the declaration of phase 6, a time when public awareness of the evolving pandemic was especially important, the WHO chose to diminish proactive communication with the media by discontinuing routine press conferences on the pandemic.

The most serious operational shortcoming, however, was the failure to distribute enough influenza vaccine in a timely way. Ultimately, 78 million doses of vaccine were sent to 77 countries, but mainly long after they would have done the most good. At its root, this reflected a shortfall in global vaccine-production capacity and technical delays due to reliance on viral egg cultures for production, as well as distributional problems. Among the latter were variation among wealthier countries and manufacturers in their willingness to donate vaccine, concerns about liability, complex negotiations over legal agreements with both

manufacturers and recipient countries, a lack of procedures to bypass national regulatory requirements for imported vaccine, and limited national and local capacities to transport, store, and administer vaccines. Some recipient countries thought that the WHO did not adequately explain that the liability provisions included in their recipient agreements were the same as the provisions accepted by purchasing countries.

Looking Ahead

In light of these structural impediments and operational deficiencies, the world was very fortunate that the 2009 H1N1 influenza pandemic was not more severe. On the basis of its analysis, the review committee offered 15 recommendations to the WHO and the member states (Box 6.1). The report and recommendations were endorsed by the member states at the 64th World Health Assembly in May 2011, and the relevant WHO departments incorporated the recommendations into their biennial work plans.[17] Some recommendations, such as improved protocols for vaccine sharing, have been carried out, some are within the power of

BOX 6.1 Recommendations of the WHO Review Committee on the Functioning of the 2005 International Health Regulations (IHR) in Relation to the 2009 H1N1 Influenza Pandemic

---

Accelerate the implementation of the core capacities required by the IHR

Enhance the WHO Event Information Site*

Reinforce evidence-based decisions on international travel and trade

Ensure necessary authority and resources for all National Focal Points[†]

Strengthen the internal capacity of the WHO for sustained response

Improve practices for the appointment of an emergency committee

Revise pandemic-preparedness guidance

Develop and apply measures to assess the severity of a pandemic

Streamline the management of guidance documents

Develop and implement a strategic, organization-wide communications policy

Encourage advance agreements for vaccine distribution and delivery

Establish a more extensive public health reserve workforce globally

Create a contingency fund for public health emergencies

Reach an agreement on the sharing of viruses, access to vaccines, and other benefits

Pursue a comprehensive influenza research and evaluation program

*The Event Information Site is a WHO website that, in the event of a pandemic, would serve as an authoritative resource to disseminate reliable, up-to-date, and readily accessible information related to the pandemic.

[†]National Focal Points are national offices that are responsible for the rapid collection and dissemination of emerging data and guidance.

---

the WHO to implement, and others depend on the actions and resources of the member states, which have yet to be committed to this purpose.

Beyond institutional, political, and managerial difficulties, the most fundamental constraints on pandemic preparedness are the limits of scientific understanding and technical capacity. Perhaps because only three or four influenza pandemics tend to occur each century, at least in recent centuries, the annals of influenza are filled with overly confident predictions based on insufficient evidence.[18] Studies designed to select for avian-origin viruses that can be transmitted more readily than the original virus in mammalian species (gain-of-function studies) may arguably help predict the pandemic potential of naturally occurring viruses but have raised concerns about the possibilities of intentional misuse and unintended consequences.[19,20] In the current state of scientific knowledge, however, no one can predict with confidence which influenza virus will become dangerous to human health and to what degree. The only way, potentially, to reduce this uncertainty is through a deeper biologic and epidemiologic understanding.

Disease detection, surveillance, and laboratory capacity are improving in many countries. The new techniques of Web-based field reports and analysis of Web-based search patterns can yield valuable intelligence that can give the world a head start on the next emerging pandemic.[21]

In addition to superior surveillance and agreements on virus and vaccine sharing, the world needs better antiviral agents and more effective influenza vaccines, greater production capacity, and faster throughput. One comprehensive assessment showed that the effectiveness of current influenza vaccines in practice is lower than is typically asserted, especially among elderly persons.[22] The traditional methods of influenza-vaccine production, which rely on egg cultures, are often too slow to keep up with a first wave of pandemic spread, and in total, the annual capacity of influenza-vaccine production covers less than one third of the global population.

In early 2013, the Food and Drug Administration approved the first trivalent influenza vaccine produced with the use of recombinant technology,[23] and other production methods are under active research and development. At least four lower-income countries have their own influenza-vaccine manufacturing facilities, and more are on the way. Most important, if research could yield a universal (non–strain-specific), long-lasting, safe, and effective vaccine against influenza, the annual frenzy of action against influenza would be transformed into a proactive, long-term prevention program.[24,25]

In the meantime, influenza outbreaks and pandemics will continue to challenge policymakers and public health leaders to make decisions under conditions of stress and uncertainty. Pandemics will challenge national authorities and the WHO to function more efficiently and effectively with insufficient resources. Preparation beyond planning, with advance protocols and agreements, the commitment of ready reserves of public health experts and a financial line of credit, and the fulfillment of the IHR requirements can all help. Whenever the next influenza pandemic arises, many more lives may be at risk. By heeding the lessons from the 2009 H1N1 pandemic, the international community will be able to cope more successfully the next time.

The views expressed in this article are those of the author and do not necessarily represent the views of the Institute of Medicine.

Members of the World Health Organization committee for the review of the 2009 H1N1 pandemic and 2005 International Health Regulations, on whose work this article is largely based, include Preben Aavitsland (Norway), Tjandra Y. Aditama (Indonesia), Silvia Bino (Albania), Eduardo Hage Carmo (Brazil), Martin Cetron (United States), Omar El Menzhi (Morocco), Yuri Fedorov (Russia), Andrew Forsyth (New Zealand), Claudia Gonzalez (Chile), Mohammad Mehdi Gouya (Iran), Amr Mohamed Kandeel (Egypt), Arlene King (Canada), Abdulsalami Nasidi (Nigeria), Paul Odehouri-Koudou (Ivory Coast), Nobuhiko Okabe (Japan), Mahmudur Rahman (Bangladesh), Palliri Ravindran (India), José Ignacio Santos (Mexico), Palanitina Tupuimatagi Toelupe (Samoa), Patricia Ann Troop (United Kingdom), Kumnuan Ungchusak (Thailand), Kuku Voyi (South Africa), Yu Wang (China), and Sam Zaramba (Uganda). The committee secretariat was led by Nick Drager and included Dominique Metais, Faith McLellan, Mary Chamberland, Nadia Day, Alice Ghent, Sue Horsfall, Janet Kincaid, Phillip Lambach, Linda Larsson, Fabienne Maertens, Joan Ntabadde, Les Olson, Magdalena Rabini, Sarah Ramsay, Mick Reid, Chastine Rodriguez, Alexandra Rosado-Miguel, and Natasha Shapovalova.

References

1. World Health Organization. Summary of probable SARS cases with onset of illness from 1 November 2002 to 31 July 2003 (based on data as of the 31 December 2003) (http://www.who.int/csr/sars/country/table2004_04_21/en).
2. Doshi P. The elusive definition of pandemic influenza. Bull World Health Organ 2011;89:532–38.
3. Taubenberger JK, Morens DM. 1918 Influenza: the mother of all pandemics. Emerg Infect Dis 2006;12:15–22.
4. Lozano R, Naghavi M, Foreman K, et al. Global and regional mortality from 235 causes of death for 20 age groups in 1990 and 2010: a systematic analysis for the Global Burden of Disease Study 2010. Lancet 2012;380:2095–128.
5. International health regulations (2005). 2nd ed. Geneva: World Health Organization, 2008.
6. Implementation of the International Health Regulations (2005): report of the Review Committee on the Functioning of the International Health Regulations (2005) in relation to pandemic (H1N1) 2009. Geneva: World Health Organization, May 5, 2011 (http://apps.who.int/gb/ebwha/pdf_files/WHA64/A64_10-en.pdf).
7. Domínguez-Cherit G, Lapinsky SE, Macias AE, et al. Critically Ill patients with 2009 influenza A(H1N1) in Mexico. JAMA 2009;302:1880–87.
8. Simonsen L, Spreeuwenberg P, Lustig R, et al. Global mortality estimates for the 2009 influenza pandemic from the GLaMOR project: a modeling study. PLoS Med 2013;10(11):e1001558.

9. Dawood FS, Iuliano AD, Reed C, et al. Estimated global mortality associated with the first 12 months of 2009 pandemic influenza A H1N1 virus circulation: a modelling study. Lancet Infect Dis 2012;12:687–95. [Erratum, Lancet Infect Dis 2012;12:655.]

10. Viboud C, Miller M, Olson D, Osterholm M, Simonsen L. Preliminary estimates of mortality and years of life lost associated with the 2009 A/H1N1 pandemic in the US and comparison with past influenza seasons. PLoS Curr 2010;2:RRN1153.

11. Pandemic influenza preparedness framework for the sharing of influenza viruses and access to vaccines and other benefits (http://www.ip-watch.org/weblog/wp-content/uploads/2011/04/PIP-Framework-16-April_2011.pdf).

12. World Health Organization. Cumulative number of confirmed human cases for avian influenza A(H5N1) reported to WHO, 2003-2013 (http://www.who.int/influenza/human_animal_interface/EN_GIP_20131008CumulativeNumberH5N1cases.pdf).

13. Dowdle WR. Influenza: epidemic patterns and antigenic variation. In: Selby P, ed. Influenza: virus, vaccine and strategy. New York: Academic Press, 1976:17–21.

14. Lipsitch M, Hayden FG, Cowling BJ, Leung GM. How to maintain surveillance for novel influenza A H1N1 when there are too many cases to count. Lancet 2009;374:1209–211.

15. Weekly epidemiological updates archive-(http://www.hpa.org.uk/Topics/InfectiousDiseases/InfectionsAZ/PandemicInfluenza/H1N1PandemicArchive/SIEpidemiologicalData/SIEpidemiologicalReportsArchive/influswarchiveweeklyepireports).

16. Flynn P. The handling of the H1N1 pandemic: more transparency needed. Council of Europe Parliamentary Assembly, 2010 (http://assembly.coe.int/CommitteeDocs/2010/20100329_MemorandumPandemie_E.pdf).

17. Hardiman MC, World Health Organization Department of Global Capacities, Alert and Response. World Health Organization perspective on implementation of International Health Regulations. Emerg Infect Dis 2012;18:1041–46.

18. Neustadt RE, Fineberg HV. The epidemic that never was: policy-making and the swine flu scare. New York: Vintage Books, 1983.

19. Herfst S, Schrauwen EJA, Linster M, et al. Airborne transmission of influenza A/H5N1 virus between ferrets. Science 2012;336:1534–41.

20. Imai M, Watanabe T, Hatta M, et al. Experimental adaptation of an influenza H5 HA confers respiratory droplet transmission to a reassortant H5 HA/H1N1 virus in ferrets. Nature 2012;486:420–28.

21. Brownstein JS, Freifeld CC, Madoff LC. Digital disease detection—harnessing the Web for public health surveillance. N Engl J Med 2009;360:2153–55, 2157.

22. Osterholm MT, Kelley NS, Sommer A, Belongia EA. Efficacy and effectiveness of influenza vaccines: a systematic review and meta-analysis. Lancet Infect Dis 2012;12:36–44. [Erratum, Lancet Infect Dis 2012;12:655.]

23. FDA approves new seasonal influenza vaccine made using novel technology. Press release of the Food and Drug Administration, Bethesda, MD, January 16, 2013 (http://www.fda.gov/NewsEvents/Newsroom/PressAnnouncements/ucm335891.htm).

24. Treanor J. Influenza vaccine—outmaneuvering antigenic shift and drift. N Engl J Med 2004;350:218–20.

25. Kanekiyo M, Wei C-J, Yassine HM, et al. Self-assembling influenza nanoparticle vaccines elicit broadly neutralizing H1N1 antibodies. Nature 2013;499:102–106.

Ebola Virus Disease

PAST AND PRESENT

Rupa Kanapathipillai, Armand G. Sprecher,
and Lindsey R. Baden

History

From June to November 1976, two outbreaks of viral hemorrhagic fever occurred in South Sudan and neighboring Zaire (now the Democratic Republic of Congo (DRC)) (Table 7.1).[1,2] The causative filovirus was named Ebola, after a nearby river associated with these outbreaks, and is now recognized to comprise five separate species; *Zaire ebolavirus, Sudan ebolavirus, Bundibugyo ebolavirus, Tai Forest ebolavirus,* and *Reston ebolavirus.*[3] All but the last of these have been shown to cause disease in humans. Case fatality rates (CFRs) associated with the different species vary widely, ranging from less than 40% for *Bundibugyo* to approximately 50% for *Sudan* to 70% to 90% for *Zaire* (Table 7.1).[3] Since identification of the virus, prior to the current outbreak, more than 20 outbreaks of Ebola virus disease (EVD) occurred across 7 countries in sub-Saharan Africa. The majority of documented outbreaks, including the currentWest African epidemic, were caused by the *Zaire ebolavirus.*[4] Historically this species has been associated with CFRs of 70% to 90%.[3] Studies of symptomatic patients with non-Lassa fever febrile illnesses in West Africa have revealed the presence of Ebola antibodies, suggesting that Ebola may have been present in this region prior to the current outbreak.[5,6]

The Current Outbreak in West Africa

In December 2013, a 2-year-old child in the Meliandou Village in Gueckedou, Guinea, died from a febrile illness associated with black stool and vomiting (Figure 7.1). In the following weeks, several family members and health care workers also died following onset of fever, diarrhea, and vomiting. Chains of transmission then spread to the Macenta and Kissidougou prefectures of Guinea.[7]

TABLE 7.1 Overview of Non-Laboratory-Related Ebola Outbreaks in Sub-Saharan Africa Since 1976

Year(s)	Country	Ebola Species	Reported Number of Cases	Reported Number of Deaths Among Cases (%)
March 2014–Present	Multiple countries	Zaire virus	27,345*	11184*
August–November 2014	DRC	Zaire virus	66	49 (74%)
November 2012– January 2013	Uganda	Sudan virus	6	3 (50%)
June–November 2012	DRC	Bundibugyo virus	36	13 (36.1%)
June–October 2012	Uganda	Sudan virus	11	4 (36.4%)
May 2011	Uganda	Sudan virus	1	1 (100%)
December 2008– February 2009	DRC	Zaire virus	32	15 (47%)
December 2007– January 2008	Uganda	Bundibugyo virus	149	37 (25%)
2007	DRC	Zaire virus	264	187 (71%)
2004	Sudan (South Sudan)	Sudan virus	17	7 (41%)
November– December 2003	Republic of the Congo	Zaire virus	35	29 (83%)
December 2002–April 2003	Republic of the Congo	Zaire virus	143	128 (89%)
October 2001– March 2002	Republic of the Congo	Zaire virus	57	43 (75%)
October 2001– March 2002	Gabon	Zaire virus	65	53 (82%)
2000–2001	Uganda	Sudan virus	425	224 (53%)
1996	South Africa	Zaire virus	2	1 (50%)
1996–1997 (July–January)	Gabon	Zaire virus	60	45 (74%)
1996 (January– April)	Gabon	Zaire virus	37	21 (57%)
1995	Democratic Republic of Congo (formerly Zaire)	Zaire virus	315	250 (81%)
1994	Cote d'Ivoire (Ivory Coast)	Tai Forest virus	1	0
1994	Gabon	Zaire virus	52	31 (60%)
1979	Sudan (South Sudan)	Sudan virus	34	22 (65%)
1977	Zaire	Zaire virus	1	1 (100%)
1976	Sudan (South Sudan)	Sudan virus	284	151 (53%)
1976	Zaire (Democratic Republic of Congo—DRC)	Zaire virus	318	280 (88%)

*Updated June 17 2015

Source: http://www.cdc.gov/vhf/ebola/outbreaks/history/chronology.html

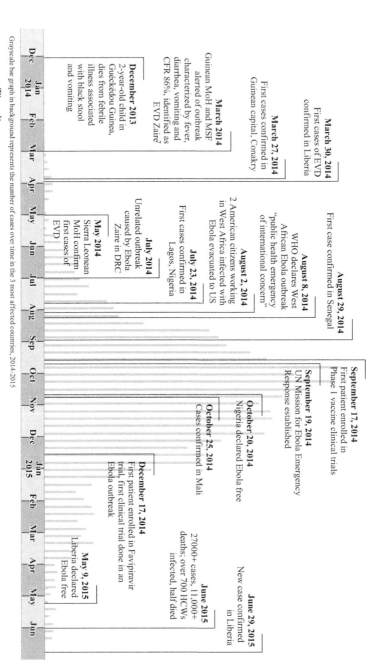

FIGURE 7.1 *Time line*

Grayscale bar graph in background represents the number of cases over time in the 3 most affected countries, 2014–2015

March 30, 2014
First cases of EVD
confirmed in Liberia

August 29, 2014
First case confirmed in Senegal

March 27, 2014
First cases confirmed in
Guinean capital, Conakry

March 2014
Guinean MoH and MSF
alerted of outbreak
characterized by fever,
diarrhea, vomiting and
CFR 86%, identified as
EVD Zaire[7]

December 2013
2-year-old child in
Guéckédou Guinea,
dies from febrile
illness associated
with black stool
and vomiting

July 2014
Unrelated outbreak
caused by Ebola
Zaire in DRC

May 2014
Sierra Leonean
MoH confirm
first cases of
EVD

August 2, 2014
2 American citizens working
in West Africa infected with
Ebola evacuated to US

July 23, 2014
First cases confirmed in
Lagos, Nigeria

August 8, 2014
WHO declares West
African Ebola outbreak
"public health emergency
of international concern"

September 17, 2014
First patient enrolled in
Phase 1 vaccine clinical trials

September 19, 2014
UN Mission for Ebola Emergency
Response established

October 20, 2014
Nigeria declared Ebola free

October 25, 2014
Cases confirmed in Mali
Ebola outbreak

December 17, 2014
First patient enrolled in Favipiravir
trial, first clinical trial done in an
Ebola outbreak

June 29, 2015
New case confirmed
in Liberia

June 2015
27000+ cases, 11,000+
deaths; over 700 HCWs
infected, half died

May 9, 2015
Liberia declared
Ebola free

Dec
Jan 2014
Feb
Mar
Apr
May
Jun
Jul
Aug
Sep
Oct
Nov
Dec
Jan 2015
Feb
Mar
Apr
May
Jun

In March 2014, hospitals and public health services in Gueckedou alerted the Guinean Ministry of Health and Médecins Sans Frontières (MSF) of an outbreak characterized by fever, severe diarrhea, and vomiting with a high CFR of 86%. Viral sequencing of blood specimens from affected patients identified the Ebola Zaire strain, distinct from strains identified in prior outbreaks from the DRC and Gabon.[7] Over a few weeks more cases occurred in Guinea Forestiere and the disease spread to Conakry, Liberia, with suspected cases in Sierra Leone. In the following 8 weeks, there was an encouraging decline in cases, the control and end of the initial Conakry transmission chains, and the apparent disappearance of cases in Sierra Leone and Liberia. However, from June to October, the number of cases increased exponentially in all three countries. Multiple factors are likely to have contributed to the initial spread of disease: with the exception of Tai Forest disease in Cote d'Ivoire, West African countries had never previously experienced an Ebola outbreak; thus health care workers (HCWs), laboratories, governments, and communities were unfamiliar with the disease's diagnosis and management. Liberia, Sierra Leone, and Guinea had severe shortages of HCWs prior to the outbreaks, with a ratio of about one or two doctors per 100,000 population; previous Ebola outbreaks were largely confined to rural areas, without the population density of urban settings and slums; the three most affected countries are among the world's poorest, with limited health care infrastructure. High population mobility within and across porous borders led to multiple independent responses in all three countries. Cultural beliefs and behavioral practices, particularly traditional burial and funeral practices involving the laying of hands on the body of the deceased, tended to spread the infection, as did the resistance of communities to control measures imposed by local governments. As in other Ebola-affected countries in the past, a significant distrust of the central government among rural populations interfered with the implementation of control measures, resulting in delayed responses among ambulances and burial teams. In short, unsafe burial practices, fear and stigma within communities, and the fact that many organizations and agencies were unfamiliar with the management of Ebola outbreaks—let alone an outbreak of such magnitude—fostered the spread of the epidemic.[8]

The necessary basic public health response measures far exceeded the human resource capabilities of any single governmental or nongovernmental organization to respond. The international response to this outbreak was slow.[9] Cases were identified in other countries in the region—Nigeria, Senegal and Mali—with successful containment in those countries.[10] An unrelated outbreak caused by Ebola (*Zaire*) began in the DRC on July 26, 2014—a country with substantial experience with Ebola; 69 cases were identified and the outbreak was successfully contained.[11] On August 2, 2 American citizens working in West Africa and infected with Ebola were evacuated back to the United States for medical care.[12] On August 8, the World Health Organization (WHO) declared the outbreak a "public health emergency of international concern."[13] At that time hundreds of confirmed and probable new cases were being identified each week in each of the three affected countries.[14]

In mid-September, the UN Security Council determined that the Ebola outbreak constituted a threat to international peace and security and unanimously passed a resolution asking member states to respond urgently to the crisis and refrain from isolating the affected countries.[15] UNMEER (UN Mission for Ebola Emergency Response) was established on September 19, 2014, as a temporary measure to help meet immediate financial, logistical, and human resource needs.

Epidemiological projections for the coming months predicted a range of incident cases from 20,000 infections by early November, to 1.4 million cases in Liberia and Sierra Leone by mid-January if additional interventions were not immediately put in place.[14,16] As international responses began to be mobilized, including military deployment, there remained insufficient deployment of qualified and trained medical staff to treat patients in the three worst-affected countries and insufficient mobilization of outbreak control operations with lack of contact tracing and health promotion.[9,17] An unprecedented number of HCWs were infected by Ebola during this outbreak, primarily in the three affected countries and in Nigeria: nearly 700 HCWs were infected by the end of 2014, half of whom died.[8] Several aid workers from outside the West African region were also infected and medically evacuated to Europe and North America. Secondary infection of three HCWs in total occurred in Spain and in the United States, leading to reevaluation of preparedness procedures and protocols, including quarantine of returning HCWs.[18–20]

Research into Ebola experimental therapies, vaccines, and diagnostics accelerated rapidly between August and December; with field studies commencing between December 2014 and February 2015.[21]

Control measures increased, including patient isolation and safe burial practices; by December over 2000 ETU beds were created and approximately 200 burial teams were carrying out safe burials, covering almost all districts in the three affected countries.[22] Increased international support, coordination, and logistics, including building and staffing of ETU units and collaboration with local communities, were met with a decline in incident cases by late 2014. By the time the ETU beds were made available, much of the inpatient infrastructure had become irrelevant. Multiple factors likely contributed to case decline, including changes in behavior in affected communities, increased availability of treatment beds, increased efforts to control infection including contact tracing, and safer burial practices.[9] As the number of Ebola cases decreased, an increased number of non-Ebola medical conditions began to come for care to ETUs. These encompassed a wide range of acute and chronic medical and surgical conditions including obstetric care, noncommunicable diseases, HIV, TB, malaria, and vaccine-preventable diseases such as measles due to widespread disruption of health services.[23] The usual background burden of illness that has largely gone untreated owing to hospital and clinic closings has likely resulted in major excess morbidity and mortality, probably dwarfing that due to EVD.

As of June 2015, over 27,000 cases and 11,000 deaths had resulted from the largest, most prolonged Ebola outbreak in history.[24] Incident cases continue to decrease in Guinea and Sierra Leone. Although Liberia was declared Ebola-free on May 9,

2015, further cases have emerged in the country.[24] Therefore the need for ongoing vigilance and an appropriate public health response cannot be underestimated, as no clear epidemiological links have been identified for a large number of cases confirmed in April to June.[24] Countries previously identified as Ebola endemic have experienced recurrent outbreaks every few years[4]; it stands to reason, therefore, that a long-term disease-management strategy for the West African region should be developed. An effort to improve the health care infrastructure and capacity in the region in order to manage not only ongoing case detection and management of Ebola but also of other medical conditions has yet to be prioritized.

Virology

Ebola virus, alongside Marburg virus, belongs to the Filoviridae family of viruses.[25] Filoviruses are negative-stranded, enveloped RNA viruses with a filamentous structure. Ebola virions have a diameter ranging from 80 nm to 14000 nm.[25] The Ebola virion contains an RNA genome encapsulated by a nucleoprotein, forming a ribonucleoprotein complex. The virus genome is 19 kb in length and comprises 7 genes in the order 3'-nucleoprotein-virion protein (VP) 35, VP40, glycoprotein, VP30, VP24, and RNA-dependent RNA polymerase-5'.[25,26] The glycoprotein is a transmembrane surface protein that forms trimeric spikes and is critical for viral attachment to host cells.[27] The ribonucleoprotein complex facilitates replication, transcription, evasion from interferon, and particle formation.[26] Further details are available at nejm.org.

Ecology

Ebola is thought to remain persistent in reservoir species in endemic areas; it is hypothesized that in the zoonotic reservoir species, the virus does not cause severe disease or death.[28] Humans, apes, and some other mammalian species develop severe disease and are therefore considered end hosts.[28] Viral antibodies and RNA have been identified in three species of fruit bats (*Hypsignathus monstrosus, Epomops franqueti,* and *Myonycteris torquata*) during previous outbreaks, although isolation of the virus from bats with serological and molecular evidence of infection has not occurred.[29,30] Rodents are also thought to be potential reservoirs.[31] Ebola has not been isolated from arthropod studies during previous epidemics.[32] Because the natural reservoir for Ebola has not been definitively identified, the mode of transmission to humans remains unknown. Hunting of fruit bats as a food source, with subsequent direct contact with an infected animal or its body fluids, is thought to be associated with transmission of virus from the zoonotic reservoir to the end host.[33] *Reston ebolavirus* has been identified in domestic pigs in the Phillipines.[34] It remains unclear whether other species are viral reservoirs.

Once humans are infected, viral transmission from person to person can occur following direct contact with body fluids or tissues of symptomatic patients.[35] Evidence from this outbreak and previous outbreaks suggests that asymptomatic infection can occur, although there is no evidence that this represents a significant source of disease transmission.[36–38]

Epidemiological studies of previous outbreaks have shown that exposure to body fluids, touching a deceased patient, and exposure during the late hospital phase of illness are associated with increased risk of transmission.[35]

Previous studies have demonstrated that viral antigen is detectable in increasing quantities from onset of clinical symptoms through about day 10 (approximate mean time of death in patients who do not survive) (Figure 7.2); in those who survive, antigen declines to undetectable levels by approximately day 14 or 15 after symptom onset.[39] IgM values have previously been shown to peak at approximately 18 days after onset, with mean IgG antibody titers reaching maximum levels slightly later (by approximately day 26).[39] Follow-up of few patients to 2 years suggests that IgG antibody persists.[39]

Studies of the *Sudan ebolavirus* outbreak in Uganda (2000) demonstrate that low viral RNA levels are detectable in blood at the time of onset of symptoms; however, these may not be reliably detectable in all patients during the first 72 hours of illness[40]—findings reinforced during the current Ebola outbreak.[41] RNA levels increase exponentially during acute illness and decrease to below the lower limit of RT-PCR detection in survivors.[12,40,42] RNA has been shown to peak at approximately day 6 to 8, with clearance of viremia at approximately day 16.[39] During acute infection, viral RNA has been detected by RT-PCR in a

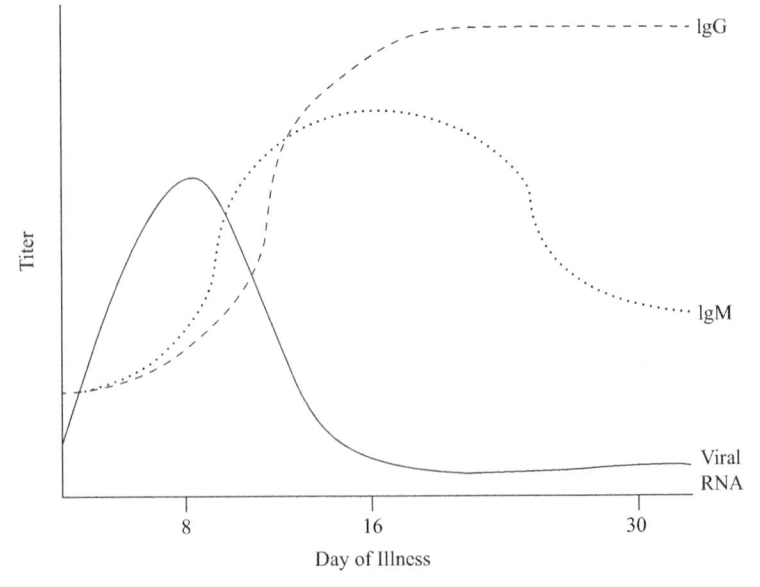

FIGURE 7.2 *Viral and antibody response to EBV infection*

Sources: Adapted from Ksiazek[39] and Kreuels.[42]

variety of body fluids including stool, vomit, saliva, breast milk, tears, semen, and amniotic fluid.[43,44] Infectious virus has been cultured from urine, semen, and aqueous humor 9 days, 6 months, and 14 weeks respectively after clearance of viremia.[42,45,46] Infectious virus has also been cultured from breast milk during convalescence.[43]

Indirect exposure to body fluids via fomites is thought to occur less commonly.[47] Although data are limited, laboratory studies of viral inactivation kinetics indicate that Ebola virus can remain viable on surfaces for days and maintains viability for a longer duration in liquid than in dried blood.[48,49]

Clinical Illness

Clinical descriptions of patients presenting to ETUs and those managed in well-resourced settings have found that early symptoms include fever (up to 40C/104F), fatigue, malaise, and body aches.[41] Some 95% of patients had symptom onset within 21 days after exposure, with a mean incubation of 11.4 days.[14] Gastrointestinal symptoms typically begins by day 3 to 5 of illness, with epigastric pain, nausea, vomiting, and diarrhea.[41,50] Watery diarrhea persists for up to 7 days; recurrent vomiting often results in inability to tolerate oral intake.[41] Diarrhea was reported in 50% to 65% of cases presenting to ETUs.[14,50,51] Quantification of diarrhea in this setting has been extremely difficult, although large-volume gastrointestinal loss occurs in a minority of cases. Associated symptoms include asthenia, headache, conjunctival injection, chest or abdominal pain, arthralgias, myalgias, and hiccups.[41] Clinical findings in the majority (60%) of patients—decreased conscious state, rapid thready pulse, oliguria, and tachypnea—are suggestive of metabolic acidosis, likely due to septic shock,[52] which may be complicated by hypovolemia in some cases. Hemorrhage has not been a major finding in this or any outbreak. Typically by day 10 of illness, symptom severity was noted to be improving in 40% of patients.[41]

Most deaths occurred between days 7 and 12 of illness; almost all patients who were alive on day 13 survived[41]; one study found that median time from symptom onset to admission, admission to death, and admission to survival was 5 days interquartile range (IQR)(IQR 3 to 7), 4 days (IQR 2 to 6), and 13 days (IQR 10 to 18) respectively.[53] Sudden death occurred in a few patients during the recovery phase of illness, possibly owing to fatal arrhythmias.[41] Significant risk factors for death include age equal to or greater than 45 years compared with younger ages[14,51] and the presence of a number of general symptoms—diarrhea,[14,51,53] weakness,[51] conjunctivitis,[14,53] difficulty breathing or swallowing,[14] confusion,[14,53] dizziness,[51] disorientation,[14] coma,[14] and hemorrhagic symptoms.[14] Higher viral load at time of presentation appeared to be associated with increased risk of death,[51] as were significant laboratory abnormalities at presentation, including elevated levels of blood urea nitrogen, creatinine, and aspartate aminotransferase.[51] Hepatic and renal dysfunction are consistent with findings during a previous outbreak of *Sudan ebolavirus*.[54] Pregnant women were found to be a particularly vulnerable

population, with high mortality in mothers and fetuses[41,55]; this is tragically compounded by significant transmission risk to birth attendants at delivery.[44]

Medical Management

Widely varying CFRs have been reported during the current epidemic.[14,50,51] CFRs within a single ETU in Sierra Leone varied between 24% and 85% by admission week over a 5-month study period between June and October 2014.[53] Notably only 5 of 24 (CFR 21.7%) patients managed in well-resourced settings died.[56] Conclusions about the efficacy of various uncontrolled medical interventions including experimental therapies and supportive care, particularly in the absence of systematic data about natural history of the illness, should be interpreted with caution.

Patient care in ETUs during this outbreak has been limited by the high volume of patients; at the peak of the outbreak, patients arrived moderately to severely ill and each clinician was often responsible for 30 to 50 patients.[41] Time spent with patients was limited to 60-minute intervals two to three times per day owing to the heat exposure and fluid loss associated with wearing personal protective equipment (PPE). Mainstays of treatment in ETUs include routine malaria treatment, antibiotics for intercurrent infections, analgesia, antiemetics, antidiarrheal medication, oral rehydration and—where safe and feasible—intravenous fluid therapy and electrolyte replacement guided by point-of-care laboratory testing.[41,42]

Vaccines/Experimental Therapies

Development of vaccines and therapeutics was a high priority once the magnitude of the outbreak became apparent. The WHO convened a meeting in September 2014 to assess efforts under way to evaluate and produce safe and effective vaccines as rapidly as possible (Table 7.2). Two candidate vaccines, ChAd3-ZEBOV and rVSV-ZEBOV, were rapidly assessed in phase I clinical trials in October/November,[57,58] which facilitated the development of phase II and III clinical trials with these vaccines in early 2015. However, rapidly falling incident cases will make it challenging to determine the clinical efficacy of these vaccines.

In November 2014, the WHO convened a meeting of the Scientific and Technical Advisory Committee for Ebola Experimental Interventions (STAC-EE) to accelerate clinical testing of potential therapeutic interventions for EVD. Following much debate about study design of clinical trials, multiple products commenced phase I, II, and III clinical trials in December 2014 and are ongoing.

No FDA-approved diagnostic assays were available prior to the 2014 EVD outbreak; multiple assays, largely PCR-based, have been developed and have attained Emergency Use Authorization.[59] With a large range and number of assays in use, comparison of various assays used in the field is needed, as well as the establishment of control panels and standards.

TABLE 7.2 Vaccine Candidates and Locations

Product/Company	Clinical Trial Phase	Clinical Trial Location
Vaccine Candidates		
ChAd3-ZEBOV (GlaxoSmithKline and PHAC)	Phase I	VRC at NIH, USA; Oxford University, UK; CVD, Mali; University of Lausanne, Lausanne, Switzerland
rVSV-ZEBOV NewLink Genetics and Merck Vaccines USA	Phase I	WRAIR, USA; NIAID, USA; CTC North GmbH, Hamburg, Germany; Albert Schweitzer Hospital, Lambarene, Gabon; University of Geneva, Geneva, Switzerland; IWK Health Centre, Halifax, Canada; KEMRI Wellcome Trust Kilifi, Kenya
Ad26-EBOV and MVA-EBOV Johnson & Johnson and Bavarian Nordic	Phase I	Jenssen Institute, UK; Ghana; Kenya; Uganda; United Republic of Tanzania
Recombinant protein Ebola vaccine candidate Novavax	Phase I	Australia
ChAd3-ZEBOV GlaxoSmithKline and PHAC	Phase II	Cameroon; Ghana; Mali; Nigeria; Senegal
rVSV-ZEBOV NewLink Genetics and Merck Vaccines USA	Phase III	WHO and MOH Guinea, Conakry, Guinea
ChAd3-ZEBOV GlaxoSmithKline and PHAC	Phase III	US NIH and MOH Liberia, Monrovia, Liberia
rVSV-ZEBOV NewLink Genetics and Merck Vaccines USA	Phase III	US CDC and MOH Sierra Leone, Freetown, Sierra Leone
Convalescent Blood and Plasma		
Convalescent plasma	Phase II/III	MSF ETU, Donka Hospital, Conakry, Guinea; ITM Antwerp and 15 partners; funded by European Commission and Wellcome Trust
Convalescent plasma	Phase II/III	Liberia; ClinRM and Duke University; funded by Bill and Melinda Gates Foundation (BMGF)
Convalescent plasma	Phase II/III	Sierra Leone; London School of Hygiene and Tropical Medicine in collaboration with 15 other partners; funded by Wellcome Trust and BMGF
Drugs and Medicines		
Favipiravir Fujifilm/Toyama, Japan	Phase II	INSERM in Guinea: Conakry, Gueckedou, Macenta, Nzerekore

TABLE 7.2 Continued

Product/Company	Clinical Trial Phase	Clinical Trial Location
Drugs and Medicines		
TKM-100802 (siRNA) Tekmira, Canada	Phase II	Oxford University in Kerry Town, Sierra Leone
ZMapp MappBio USA	Phase II	NIAID in Monrovia, Liberia
BCX-4430 Biocryst, USA	Phase I	Quotient Clinic, UK
Interferons		Guinea MOH in Coyah, Guinea
Amiodarone		Lakka & Goderich ETU in Sierra Leone
Atorvostatin + Irbesartan +/− Clomiphene		Sierra Leone
FX06		
Zmab		
Brincidofovir Chimerix, USA	Phase II	Oxford University; ELWA 3, Monrovia, Liberia Trial halted and abandoned

Source: http://www.who.int/medicines/emp_ebola_q_as/en/

Development of point-of care diagnostics, vaccines, and potential therapeutics for Ebola has occurred at a rapid pace and has required the coordination of a range of diverse international partners including governments and nongovernmental organizations, public health and regulatory agencies, pharmaceutical companies, and academic researchers. Multiple challenges have been faced in creating and delivering both diagnostics and therapeutics in the setting of the current outbreak, including from scientific and ethical challenges about study design, community acceptance of research, availability of investigational therapeutic products, compassionate use of therapies, lack of uniformity of laboratory platforms and sharing of knowledge in a rapid but scientifically accurate manner. For several months, investigational products have been assessed in field-based studies across multiple sites. As incident cases decrease, it becomes more difficult to complete this research and reach efficacy endpoints. The ability of regulatory authorities to license vaccines and approve drugs in the absence of definitive efficacy data will be a major challenge and may need to occur via use of the US FDA's accelerated pathway, or "animal rule,"[60] leveraging animal models and our understanding of virus species, dose, routes of administration, supportive interventions, correlates of protection, and pharmacokinetics of therapeutic interventions.

Conclusion

Lessons should be learned from this outbreak, regarding not only the early detection of cases but also the need for rapid mobilization of health care workers and

logistics personnel to manage patients, work with communities, and inform and trace contacts. There is need for improved national and international coordination in order to build a capacity for rapid detection, response, and research into EBV and other emergent infectious diseases. Multiple questions remain unanswered, including natural history of the virus, immunopathogenesis, immune correlates of protection, the impact of supportive treatment on survival, and transmission, including persistence of the virus in various body fluids. Consideration should be given to identifying diseases of concern, especially those with pandemic potential, in order to facilitate prioritization in terms of response and future research and development of vaccines and therapeutics (Figure 7.3).

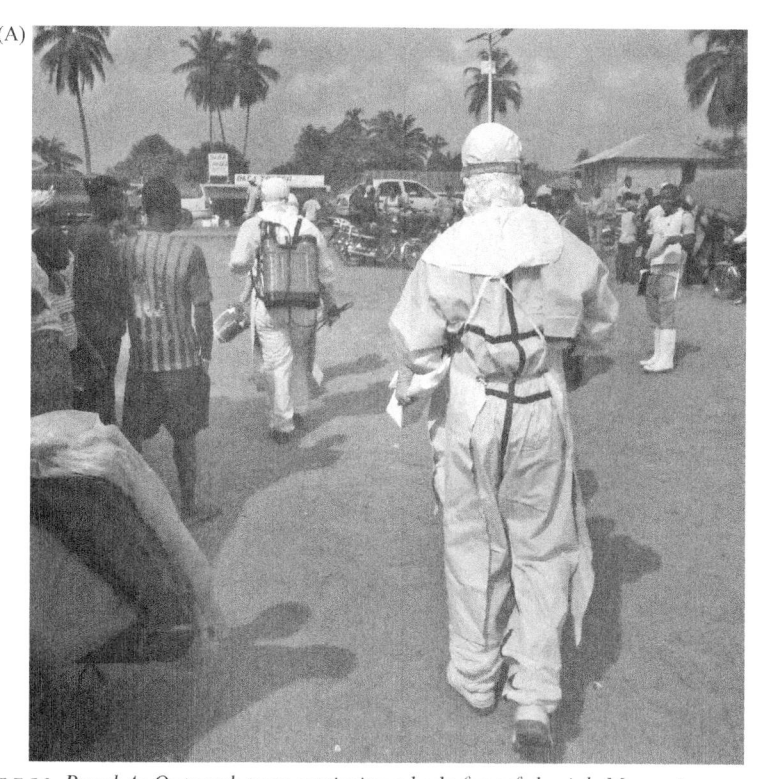

FIGURE 7.3 *Panel A: Outreach team retrieving a body for safe burial. Monrovia, Liberia. Elvis Garcia/MSF Panel B: Medical staff dressing in personal protective equipment before entering the high-risk zone. Monrovia, Liberia. Caitlin Ryan/MSF. Panel C: Two medical staff carrying an unwell contact to the ebola treatment unit (ETU) for assessment. Kailahun, Sierra Leone. Sylvain Cherkaoui/Cosmos for MSF. Panel D: Patients with Ebola and non-Ebola medical conditions arriving at ETU triage for assessment. Clinical staff stand behind a barrier 2 meters away from the patient. Monrovia, Liberia. Mads Geisler/MSF. Panel E: Cannulating a patient for intravenous hydration in the ETU. Sylvain Cherkaoui/Cosmos for MSF. Panel F: A patient drinking to rehydrate himself while being watched by a nurse. Sylvain Cherkaoui/Cosmos for MSF.*

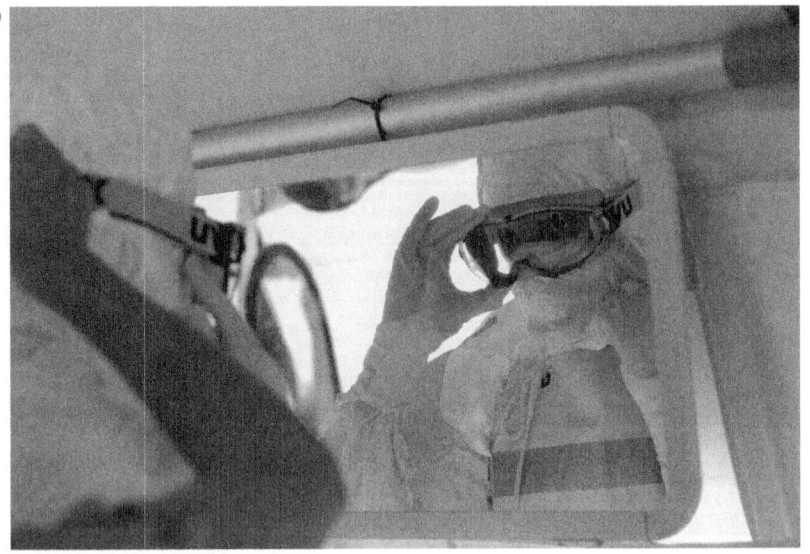

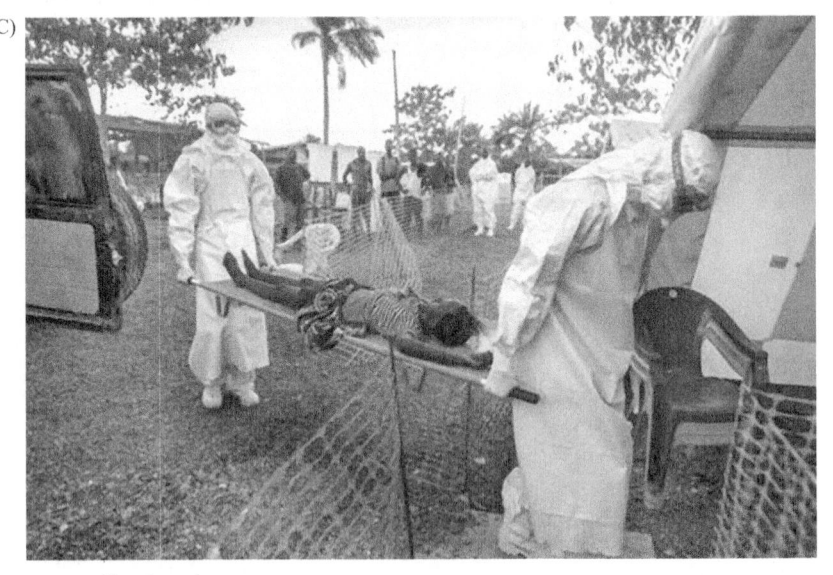

FIGURE 7.3 *Continued*

(D)

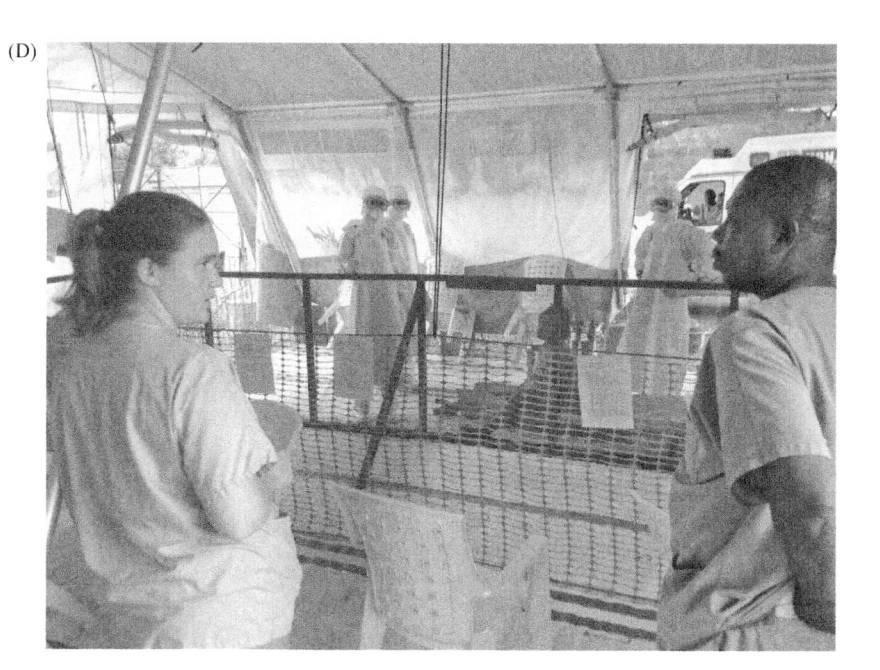

(E)

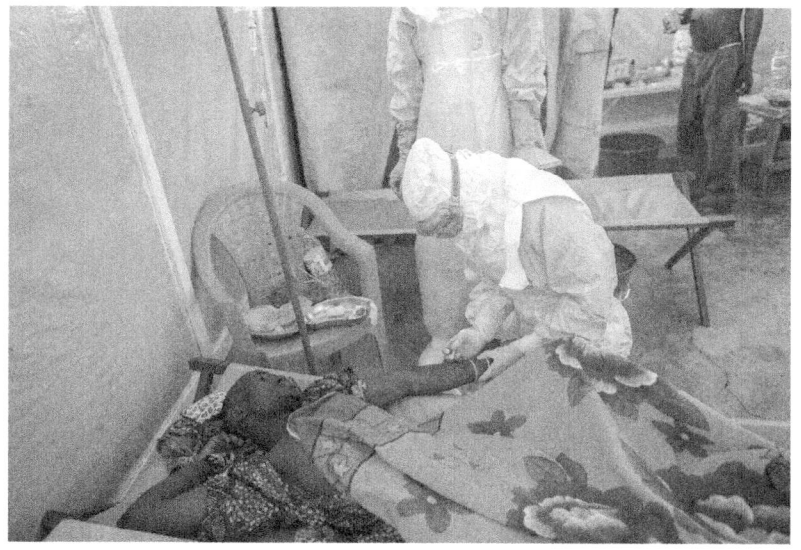

FIGURE 7.3 *Continued*

(F)

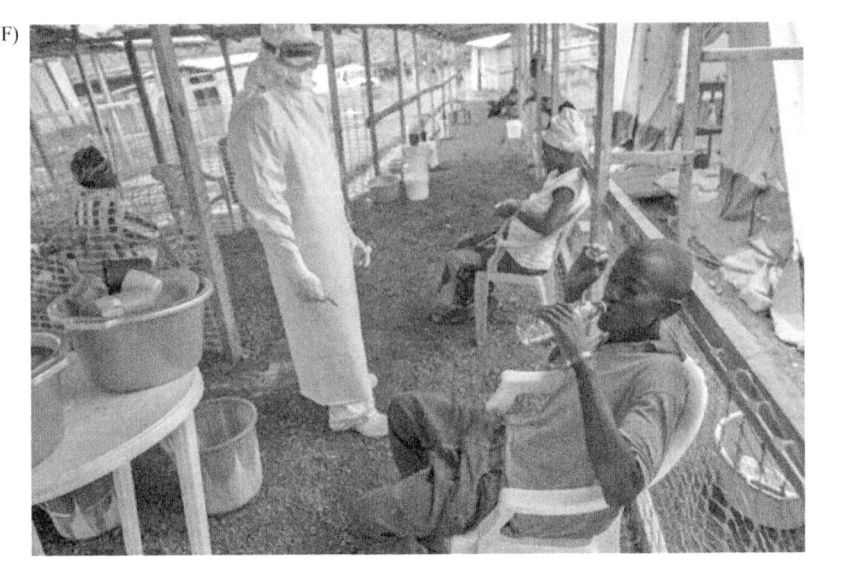

FIGURE 7.3 *Continued*

References

1. World Health Organization. Ebola haemorrhagic fever in Zaire, 1976. Report of an International Convention. Bulletin of the World Health Organization. 1978;56(2):271–293.
2. World Health Organization. Ebola haemorrhagic fever in Sudan, 1976. Report of a WHO/International Study Team. Bulletin of the World Health Organization. 1978;56(2):247–270.
3. Feldmann H, Geisbert TW. Ebola haemorrhagic fever. *Lancet* 2011;377:849–862.
4. Centers for Disease Control and Prevention. Outbreaks Chronology: Ebola Virus Disease. http://www.cdc.gov/vhf/ebola/resources/outbreak-table.html#two
5. Schoepp RJ, Rossi CA, Khan SH, Goba A, Fair JN. Undiagnosed acute viral febrile illnesses, Sierra Leone. *Emerg Infect Dis* 2014;20:1176–1182.
6. Boisen ML, Schieffelin JS, Goba A, et al. Multiple circulating infections can mimic the early stages of viral hemorrhagic fevers and possible human exposure to filoviruses in Sierra Leone prior to the 2014 outbreak. *Vir Immunol* 2015;28:19–31.
7. Baize S, Pannetier D, Oestereich L, et al. Emergence of Zaire Ebola virus disease in Guinea. *N Engl J Med* 2014;371:1418–1425.
8. World Health Organization. Factors that contributed to undetected spread of Ebola virus and impeded rapid containment. http://www.who.int/csr/disease/ebola/one-year-report/factors/en/.
9. Medecins Sans Frontieres. Pushed to the Limit and Beyond: A year into the largest ever Ebola outbreak. http://www.msf.org/article/ebola-pushed-limit-and-beyond.
10. World Health Organization. Successful Ebola responses in Nigeria, Senegal and Mali. http://www.who.int/csr/disease/ebola/one-year-report/nigeria/en/.

11. Maganga GD, Kapetshi J, Berthet N, et al. Ebola virus disease in the Democratic Republic of Congo. *N Engl J Med* 2014;371:2083–2091.

12. Lyon GM, Mehta AK, Varkey JB, et al. Clinical care of two patients with Ebola virus disease in the United States. *N Engl J Med* 2014;371:2402–2409.

13. World Health Organization. WHO statement on the meeting of the International Health Regulations Emergency Committee regarding the 2014 Ebola outbreak in West Africa. http://www.who.int/mediacentre/news/statements/2014/ebola-20140808/en/.

14. Team WHOER. Ebola virus disease in West Africa—the first 9 months of the epidemic and forward projections. *N Engl J Med* 2014;371:1481–1495.

15. United Nations. With Spread of Ebola Outpacing Response, Security Council Adopts Resolution 2177 (2014) Urging Immediate Action, End to Isolation of Affected States. http://www.un.org/press/en/2014/sc11566.doc.htm.

16. Meltzer MI, Atkins CY, Santibanez S, et al. Estimating the future number of cases in the Ebola epidemic—Liberia and Sierra Leone, 2014-2015. *MMWR Surv Summ* 2014;63(Suppl 3):1–14.

17. World Health Organization. Key events in the WHO response to the Ebola outbreak. http://www.who.int/csr/disease/ebola/one-year-report/who-response/en/.

18. Parra JM, Salmeron OJ, Velasco M. The first case of Ebola virus disease acquired outside Africa. *N Engl J Med* 2014;371:2439–2440.

19. Centers for Disease Control and Prevention. Infection Prevention and Control Recommendations for Hospitalized Patients Under Investigation (PUIs) for Ebola Virus Disease (EVD) in U.S. Hospitals. http://www.cdc.gov/vhf/ebola/healthcare-us/hospitals/infection-control.html.

20. Drazen JM, Kanapathipillai R, Campion EW, et al. Ebola and quarantine. *N Engl J Med* 2014;371:2029–2030.

21. World Health Organization. Modernizing the arsenal of control tools: Ebola vaccines. http://www.who.int/csr//disease/ebola/one-year-report/vaccines/en/.

22. Team WHOER, Agua-Agum J, Ariyarajah A, et al. West African Ebola epidemic after one year—slowing but not yet under control. *N Engl J Med* 2015;372:584–587.

23. Doctors of the World. Beyond Ebola: rebuilding health services in Moyamba, Sierra Leone. http://b.3cdn.net/droftheworld/54befeb29ddee73fa1_s4m62058i.pdf.

24. World Health Organization. Ebola Situation Report- 1 July 2015. http://apps.who.int/ebola/current-situation/ebola-situation-report-1-july-2015.

25. Feldmann H, Geisbert TW, Jahrling PB, et al. Virus taxonomy: VIIIth Report of the International Committee on Taxonomy of Viruses. London: Elsevier/Academic Press, 2004;645–653.

26. Muhlberger E, Weik M, Volchkov VE, Klenk HD, Becker S. Comparison of the transcription and replication strategies of marburg virus and Ebola virus by using artificial replication systems. *J Virol* 1999;73:2333–2342.

27. Lee JE, Saphire EO. Ebola virus glycoprotein structure and mechanism of entry. *Future Virol* 2009;4:621–635.

28. Groseth A, Feldmann H, Strong JE. The ecology of Ebola virus. *Trends Microbiol* 2007;15:408–416.

29. Leroy EM, Kumulungui B, Pourrut X, et al. Fruit bats as reservoirs of Ebola virus. *Nature* 2005;438:575–576.

30. Pourrut X, Delicat A, Rollin PE, Ksiazek TG, Gonzalez JP, Leroy EM. Spatial and temporal patterns of Zaire ebolavirus antibody prevalence in the possible reservoir bat species. *J Infect Dis* 2007;196(Suppl 2):S176–S183.

31. Morvan JM, Deubel V, Gounon P, et al. Identification of Ebola virus sequences present as RNA or DNA in organs of terrestrial small mammals of the Central African Republic. *Microbes and Infection/Institut Pasteur* 1999;1:1193–1201.

32. Reiter P, Turell M, Coleman R, et al. Field investigations of an outbreak of Ebola hemorrhagic fever, Kikwit, Democratic Republic of the Congo, 1995: arthropod studies. *J Infect Dis* 1999;179(Suppl 1):S148–S154.

33. Leroy EM, Epelboin A, Mondonge V, et al. Human Ebola outbreak resulting from direct exposure to fruit bats in Luebo, Democratic Republic of Congo, 2007. *Vector borne and Zoonotic Diseases* 2009;9:723–728.

34. Barrette RW, Metwally SA, Rowland JM, et al. Discovery of swine as a host for the Reston ebolavirus. *Science* 2009;325:204–206.

35. Dowell SF, Mukunu R, Ksiazek TG, Khan AS, Rollin PE, Peters CJ. Transmission of Ebola hemorrhagic fever: a study of risk factors in family members, Kikwit, Democratic Republic of the Congo, 1995. Commission de Lutte contre les Epidemies a Kikwit. *J Infect Dis* 1999;179(Suppl 1):S87–S91.

36. Akerlund E, Prescott J, Tampellini L. Shedding of Ebola virus in an asymptomatic pregnant woman. *N Engl J Med* 2015;372:2467–2469.

37. Heffernan RT, Pambo B, Hatchett RJ, Leman PA, Swanepoel R, Ryder RW. Low seroprevalence of IgG antibodies to Ebola virus in an epidemic zone: Ogooue-Ivindo region, Northeastern Gabon, 1997. *J Infect Dis* 2005;191:964–968.

38. Leroy EM, Baize S, Volchkov VE, et al. Human asymptomatic Ebola infection and strong inflammatory response. *Lancet* 2000;355:2210–2215.

39. Ksiazek TG, Rollin PE, Williams AJ, et al. Clinical virology of Ebola hemorrhagic fever (EHF): virus, virus antigen, and IgG and IgM antibody findings among EHF patients in Kikwit, Democratic Republic of the Congo, 1995. *J Infect Dis* 1999;179(Suppl 1):S177–S187.

40. Towner JS, Rollin PE, Bausch DG, et al. Rapid diagnosis of Ebola hemorrhagic fever by reverse transcription-PCR in an outbreak setting and assessment of patient viral load as a predictor of outcome. *J Virol* 2004;78:4330–4341.

41. Chertow DS, Kleine C, Edwards JK, Scaini R, Giuliani R, Sprecher A. Ebola virus disease in West Africa—clinical manifestations and management. *N Engl J Med* 2014;371:2054–2057.

42. Kreuels B, Wichmann D, Emmerich P, et al. A case of severe Ebola virus infection complicated by gram-negative septicemia. *N Engl J Med* 2014;371:2394–2401.

43. Bausch DG, Towner JS, Dowell SF, et al. Assessment of the risk of Ebola virus transmission from bodily fluids and fomites. *J Infect Dis* 2007;196(Suppl 2):S142–S147.

44. Baggi FM, Taybi A, Kurth A, et al. Management of pregnant women infected with Ebola virus in a treatment centre in Guinea, June 2014. *Euro surveillance: bulletin Europeen sur les maladies transmissibles = European communicable disease bulletin* 2014;19.

45. Christie A, Davies-Wayne GJ, Cordier-Lasalle T, et al. Possible sexual transmission of Ebola virus—Liberia, 2015. *MMWR* 2015;64:479–481.

46. Varkey JB, Shantha JG, Crozier I, et al. Persistence of Ebola virus in ocular fluid during convalescence. *N Engl J Med* 2015;372(25):2423–2427.

47. Francesconi P, Yoti Z, Declich S, et al. Ebola hemorrhagic fever transmission and risk factors of contacts, Uganda. *Emerg Infect Dis* 2003;9:1430–1437.

48. Sagripanti JL, Rom AM, Holland LE. Persistence in darkness of virulent alphaviruses, Ebola virus, and Lassa virus deposited on solid surfaces. *Arch Virol* 2010;155:2035–2039.

49. Fischer R, Judson S, Miazgowicz K, Bushmaker T, Prescott J, Munster VJ. Ebola virus stability on surfaces and in fluids in simulated outbreak environments. *Emerg Infect Dis* 2015;21:1243–1246.

50. Bah EI, Lamah MC, Fletcher T, et al. Clinical Presentation of Patients with Ebola Virus Disease in Conakry, Guinea. *N Engl J Med* 2015;372(1):40–47.

51. Schieffelin JS, Shaffer JG, Goba A, et al. Clinical illness and outcomes in patients with Ebola in Sierra Leone. *N Engl J Med* 2014;371:2092–2100.

52. Mahanty S, Bray M. Pathogenesis of filoviral haemorrhagic fevers. *Lancet Infect Dis* 2004;4:487–598.

53. Fitzpatrick G, Vogt F, Gbabai OB, et al. The contribution of Ebola viral load at admission and other patient characteristics to mortality in a Medecins Sans Frontieres (MSF) Ebola Case Management Centre (CMC), Kailahun, Sierra Leone, June-October, 2014. *J Infect Dis* 2015. Epub 22 May 2015.

54. Rollin PE, Bausch DG, Sanchez A. Blood chemistry measurements and D-Dimer levels associated with fatal and nonfatal outcomes in humans infected with Sudan Ebola virus. *J Infect Dis* 2007;196(Suppl 2):S364–S371.

55. Mupapa K, Mukundu W, Bwaka MA, et al. Ebola hemorrhagic fever and pregnancy. *J Infect Dis* 1999;179(Suppl 1):S11–S12.

56. http://www.nytimes.com/interactive/2014/07/31/world/africa/ebola-virus-outbreak-qa.html?_r=0.

57. Regules JA, Beigel JH, Paolino KM, et al. A Recombinant vesicular stomatitis virus Ebola vaccine—preliminary report. *N Engl J Med* 2015. Epub 2015 Apr 1.

58. Ledgerwood JE, DeZure AD, Stanley DA, et al. Chimpanzee adenovirus vector Ebola vaccine—preliminary report. *N Engl J Med* 2014. Epub 2014 Nov 26.

59. U.S. Food and Drug Administration. Ebola Virus EUA Information. http://www.fda.gov/EmergencyPreparedness/Counterterrorism/MedicalCountermeasures/MCMLegalRegulatoryandPolicyFramework/ucm182568.htm#ebola.

60. U.S. Food and Drug Administration. Vaccines and Related Biological Products Advisory Committee Meeting. May 12, 2015. http://www.fda.gov/downloads/AdvisoryCommittees/CommitteesMeetingMaterials/BloodVaccinesandOtherBiologics/VaccinesandRelatedBiologicalProductsAdvisoryCommittee/UCM445819.pdf.

Designing Tomorrow's Vaccines
Gary J. Nabel

Vaccines are among the most effective interventions in modern medicine. Ever since Edward Jenner's first use of a vaccine against smallpox in 1796 (see text box), the use of vaccines has become indispensable to the eradication of disease. In the 20th century alone, smallpox claimed an estimated 375 million lives, but since 1978, after the completion of a successful eradication campaign, not a single person has died from smallpox. Today, more than 70 vaccines have been licensed for use against approximately 30 microbes, sparing countless lives (Fig. 8.1A and 8.1B).[1,2] Diseases including poliomyelitis, measles, mumps, rubella, and others caused an estimated 39 million infections in the 20th century in the United States, but vaccines have since rendered them uncommon (Table 8.1).[3,4] The success of this public health intervention emanates not only from the identification of effective vaccines but also from a robust infrastructure for vaccine manufacturing, regulatory and safety oversight, and organized approaches to delivery. Vaccines represent the least expensive and most facile way to protect against devastating epidemics. Society derives economic benefits by preventing hospitalization, avoiding long-term disability, and reducing absence from work. In brief, vaccines provide the most cost-effective means to save lives, preserve good health, and maintain a high quality of life.

Despite this legacy, infectious diseases still extract an extraordinary toll on humans. Vaccines have yet to realize their full potential for several reasons. First, effective vaccines are often not available in developing countries. The Global Alliance for Vaccines and Immunization (GAVI) estimates that every year more than 1.5 million children (3 per minute) die from vaccine-preventable diseases. Second, effective vaccines have not yet been developed for diseases such as human immunodeficiency virus (HIV) infection, tuberculosis, and malaria, which claim the lives of more than 4 million people worldwide each year.[5–7] For nearly all successful licensed vaccines, natural immunity to infection has been shown, and the vaccine mimics the protective immune response. In contrast, for HIV infection, tuberculosis, and malaria, it has been difficult to show preventive immunity. Protection against these pathogens requires a distinct approach to

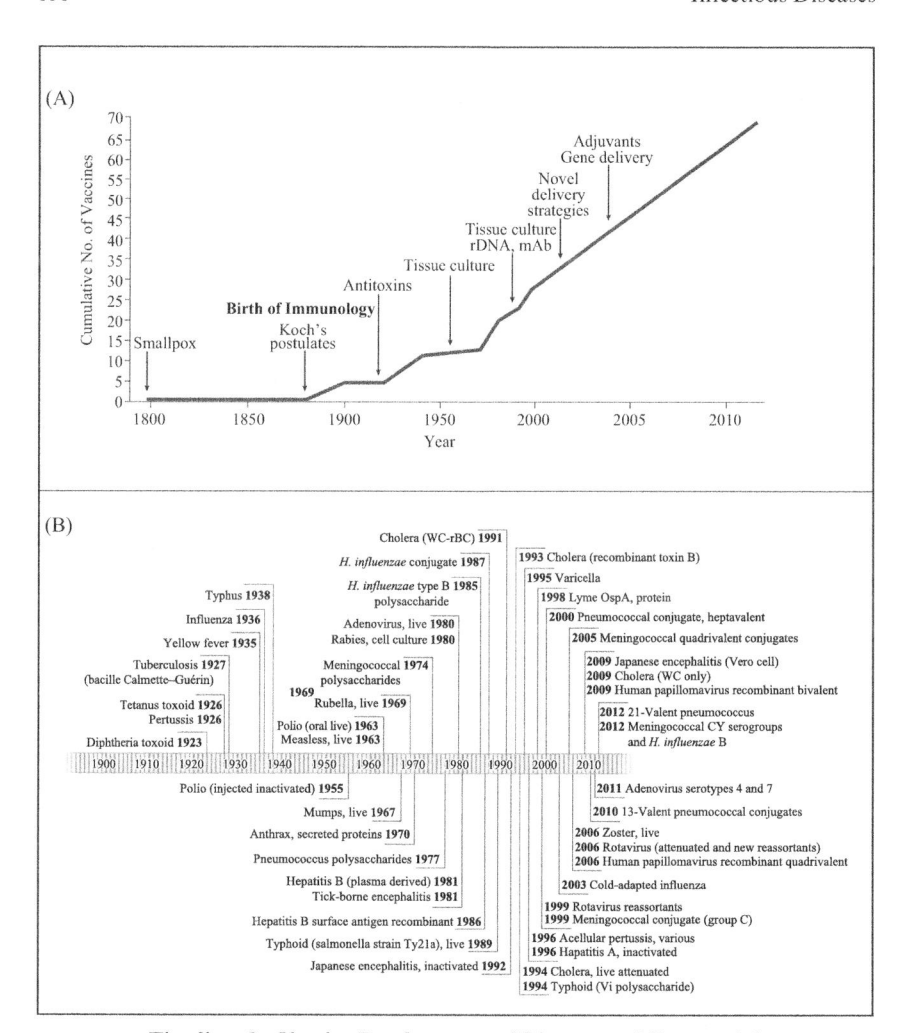

FIGURE 8.1 **Timelines for Vaccine Development and Licensure of Commercial Vaccines** *Panel A shows major milestones and advances in vaccine development and the cumulative number of licensed vaccines since the time of Edward Jenner's first use of a vaccination against smallpox in 1796.[1] Panel B shows the timeline for licensure of commercial vaccines against the indicated pathogens.[2] The abbreviation mAb denotes monoclonal antibody, OspA outer surface protein A, rBS recombinant B subunit of cholera toxin, rDNA recombinant DNA, and WC whole-cell Vibrio cholerae O1.*

vaccine design, based on an understanding of immunopathogenesis and reliance on animal models. In these cases, the challenge is greater, the development path longer, and the outcome less certain.

Finally, many vaccine technologies are old and ill-suited for a rapid response to emerging outbreaks. For example, influenza vaccines rely largely on 50-year-old technology. Current seasonal influenza vaccines are not always well matched and effective against circulating viral strains.[8] Furthermore, when new strains

TABLE 8.1 Estimated Cumulative Number of Cases of Selected Infectious Diseases in the United States in the 20th Century before the Advent of a Vaccine, as Compared with Mortality after Utilization[*]

Disease	Estimated Prevaccine Cases in 20th Century	Deaths in 2002
	number	
Smallpox	4.81 million	0
Poliomyelitis	1.63 million	0
Diphtheria	17.60 million	2
Haemophilus influenzae	2.00 million	22
Measles	5.03 million	36
Mumps	1.52 million	236
Pertussis	1.47 million	6632
Rubella	4.77 million	20
Tetanus	0.13 million	13

[*]Data are from the Centers for Disease Control and Prevention[3] and Roush and Murphy.[4]

emerged unexpectedly from an animal reservoir in the 2009 influenza A (H1N1) pandemic, vaccine developers were unprepared for rapid deployment of a new vaccine strain. Thus, although the triumphs of yesterday's vaccines have been heartening, a variety of challenges remain for the vaccines of tomorrow. Yet there are reasons to be optimistic that these challenges can be addressed.

Scientific Discovery in the Current Vaccine Era

STRUCTURAL BIOLOGY AND PATHOGEN ENTRY

Progress in virology, genetics, synthetic biology, and biotechnology has provided a new set of tools to approach current-day vaccinology. Among currently licensed vaccines, the most consistent biomarker for vaccine efficacy has been the presence of antibodies that neutralize the pathogen. These antibodies are often elicited by natural infection or immunization. Our understanding of the molecular structure of viruses has led to a sophisticated understanding of viral glycoproteins and the specific interactions of antibodies that can inactivate them. The field of structural biology has provided new insights into how such antibodies protect against infection by poliomyelitis, measles, and influenza viruses, as well as human papillomavirus (HPV), among others. This detailed knowledge of the mechanism by which viral glycoproteins mediate entry into host cells can now be applied to pathogens that have not been susceptible to this therapeutic approach (Fig. 8.2).[9-11] Thus, an understanding of the steps related to entry and survival of pathogens that cause illnesses such as HIV type 1 (HIV-1) infection, tuberculosis, and malaria offers molecular targets that serve both to understand natural infection and to identify highly conserved and invariant structures as targets for broadly neutralizing antibodies.

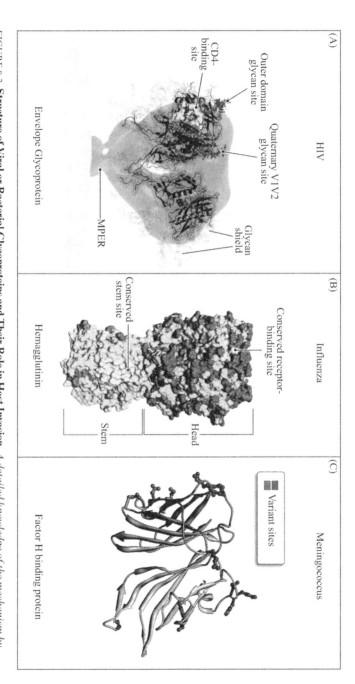

(A) HIV

Envelope Glycoprotein

Outer domain
glycan site

CD4-
binding
site

Quaternary V1V2
glycan site

Glycan
shield

MPER

(B) Influenza

Hemagglutinin

Conserved receptor-
binding site

Conserved
stem site

Stem

Head

(C) Meningococcus

Factor H binding protein

■ Variant sites

FIGURE 8.2 **Structure of Viral or Bacterial Glycoproteins and Their Role in Host Invasion** *A detailed knowledge of the mechanism by which viral glycoproteins mediate entry into host cells can now be applied to pathogens that once were not susceptible to vaccines, including human immunodeficiency virus (HIV) (Panel A, Protein Data Bank code 3J5M), influenza virus (Panel B, Protein Data Bank code 1RU7), and meningococcus (Panel C, adapted with permission from Scarselli et al.; Protein Data Bank code 2Y7S).[9–11] MPER denotes membrane proximal external region, and V1V2 variable regions 1 and 2. The Protein Data Bank is accessible at www.pdb.org*

RATIONAL VACCINE DESIGN

The definition of conserved sites of vulnerability on pathogens provides the basis for structure-based vaccine design. Broadly neutralizing antibodies often recognize highly conserved sites that are susceptible to antibody inactivation. Two pathogens, HIV-1 and influenza virus, have proved to be particularly informative in this regard. For example, analysis of the HIV-1 envelope has revealed at least four discrete sites that represent potential targets for the designs of immunogens (i.e., agents capable of inducing an immune response). These include the CD4-binding site, a glycosylated site in variable regions 1 and 2 (V1V2), glycans on the outer domain, and the membrane proximal external region.

Progress in HIV-vaccine research has been advanced recently by the identification of exceptionally broad and potent neutralizing antibodies to each of these sites. Some monoclonal antibodies neutralize more than 90% of circulating viral strains,[12–17] creating new opportunities for HIV-vaccine development. Similar progress has been made in the identification of broadly neutralizing antibodies directed against diverse influenza viruses. At least two independent sites of vulnerability have been identified, one in the stem region of the viral spike that helps to stabilize the trimer, the three identical viral hemagglutinin glycoproteins that form this structure, and the other in the receptor-binding region that recognizes sialic acid.[18] The existence of such antibodies provides conceptual support and tools that facilitate the development of universal influenza vaccines intended to protect against a wide array of viruses, not only the circulating seasonal strain.

Knowledge of atomic structure also defines viral proteins to elicit these broadly neutralizing antibodies. For HIV infection, alternative forms of envelope glycoproteins include trimers, monomers, subdomains, and specific peptide loops transplanted onto scaffolds.[19] These candidate vaccines are further modified with the use of protein-design algorithms that are based on bioinformatics[10] in efforts to stabilize the immunogen, better expose the conserved sites, and mask or remove undesired epitopes. Similar strategies are under development for influenza viruses, respiratory syncytial virus, and group B meningococcal strains.[9,11,18,20,21]

Although structure-based rational design offers a promising tool for developing vaccines against recalcitrant pathogens, substantial challenges remain. The proper antigenic structure will not necessarily provide all the information needed to produce a potent immunogen that will elicit an antibody response. Furthermore, many broadly neutralizing antibodies are atypical, with an unusually high degree of somatic mutation or long CDRH3 (third complementarity determining regions of heavy-chain variable) regions; such antibodies may not be readily elicited. Finally, a successful vaccine candidate must be designed to bind the germline antibody precursor, select for the appropriate primary recombinational events, and direct its somatic mutations toward the appropriate mature form.[19]

INTERACTIONS BETWEEN HOST AND PATHOGEN

Progress in the field of therapeutic monoclonal antibodies has facilitated the identification of effective targets and led to strategies for their successful use

in humans.[22] Dozens of new antibodies directed against HIV-1,[18,19] influenza virus,[21] respiratory syncytial virus,[20] hepatitis C virus,[18] and other microbes have identified critical viral structures and enabled structure-based vaccine design. Moreover, deep sequencing, the ability to generate millions of independent sequences of a gene product (e.g., immunoglobulin), has identified intermediates that are critical for the evolution of broadly neutralizing antibodies and has guided vaccine development.[23] Millions of gene sequences encoding heavy and light chains (the polypeptide subunits of an antibody) within a single individual can be analyzed with the use of bioinformatics to trace a potential critical path for vaccine design (Fig. 8.3).[23] The overarching goal is to use knowledge of structural biology and antibody evolution to design vaccines that will elicit antibodies of known specificity.[24]

Genomewide sequencing of microbes has also allowed for the rational selection of targets for vaccine development. This approach has identified specific gene products of pathogens as vaccine targets. The expression and evaluation of these immunogens have led to the development of a successful vaccine for group B meningococcal strains through a process known as reverse vaccinology.[25]

IMMUNE BIOMARKERS OF PROTECTION

The human immune response has been analyzed with sensitive high-throughput technologies that allow for systems biologic analysis of gene-expression patterns in lymphocytes and in microbes. Such information not only identifies susceptible microbial targets but also has the potential to define new biomarkers of protective immune responses, termed systems vaccinology.[26] Mechanisms of protection and correlates of immunity can be rigorously explored in relevant animal models, but these properties can be definitively established in humans only through clinical trials and postlicensure surveillance. Such information enables precise immune activation, minimizes unintended side effects, and maximizes clinical efficacy. Successful protection may require neutralizing antibodies,[18] effective T-cell responses,[27] or possibly a combination of the two.

DENDRITIC CELLS AND ADJUVANTS

Critical to the modulation of the immune response is the presentation of specific antigens to the immune system. Dendritic cells play a central role in this process. Three subgroups of such cells, including two forms of myeloid dendritic cells and one plasmacytoid dendritic cell, each with distinct sets of toll receptors, modulate the response to specific antigens and adjuvants. Traditional vaccines have relied on live-attenuated or inactivated organisms, attenuated bacteria or capsules, or inactivated toxins.[28,29] Progress has been made recently in enhancing immunity through a mechanistic understanding of the biology of dendritic cells and their response to adjuvants.[30] Alternative delivery, including viruslike particles or structured arrays with the use of phage or nanoparticles, also stimulate

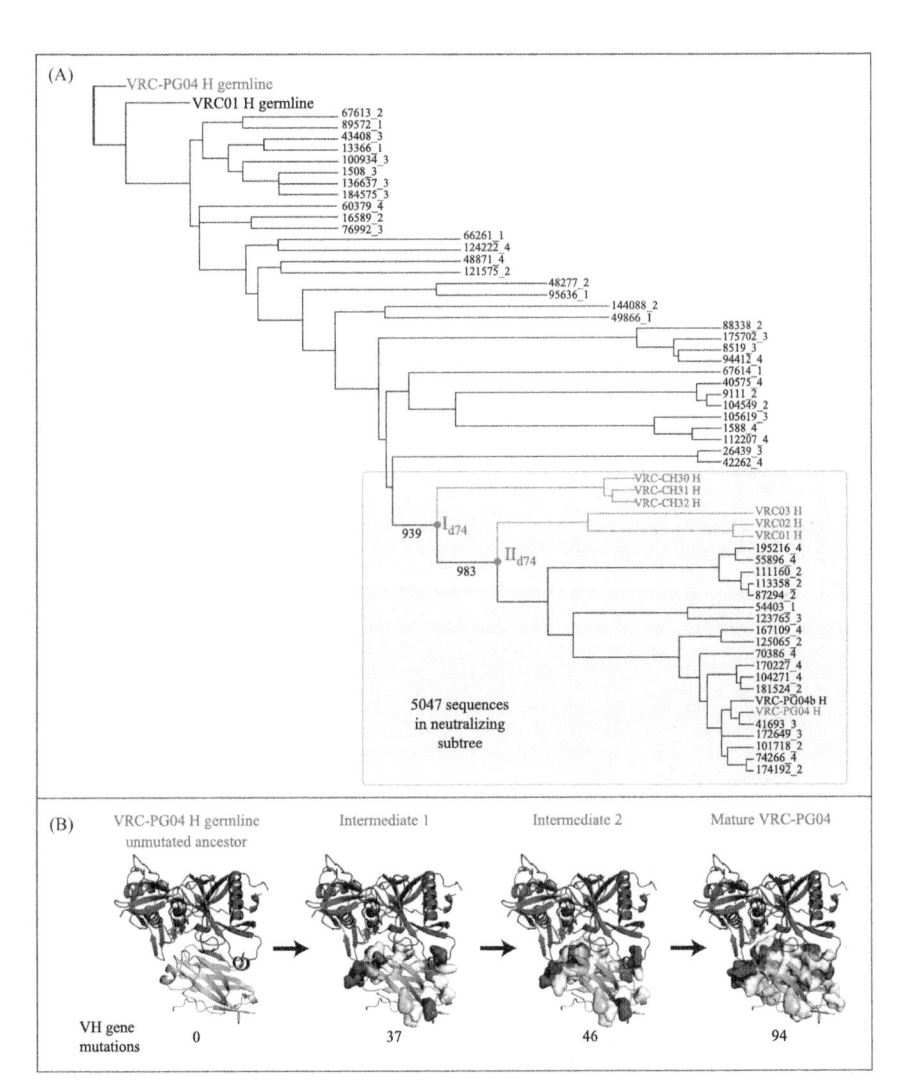

FIGURE 8.3 **Molecular Evolution of a Successful Broadly Neutralizing Antibody** *Deep sequencing (i.e., the ability to generate millions of independent sequences of a gene product) identifies critical intermediates for the evolution of broadly neutralizing antibodies and guides vaccine development. In Panel A, maximum-likelihood trees of heavy-chain sequences were derived from the IGHV1-2 gene that gives rise to a broadly neutralizing antibody, VRC01, in a representative patient, donor 74, as described previously.[23] The donor 74 tree is rooted in the putative reverted unmutated ancestor of the heavy chain of a specific broadly neutralizing CD4-binding site monoclonal antibody, VRC-PG04 (as shown in Panel B, Protein Data Bank code 3SE9). Sequences from other donors are included in the cross-donor phylogenetic analysis. Bars representing 0.1 changes per nucleotide site are shown. Sequences within the shaded box include autologous VRC01-like heavy-chain sequences that neutralize HIV with good potency and breadth and are probably clonal relatives of VRC-PG04. Sequences highlighted represent broadly neutralizing antibodies isolated with structural probes.*

effective immunity and provide powerful tools to confer protection for a specific pathogen (Fig. 8.4).

MODES AND SITES OF VACCINE DELIVERY

An increasing number of vaccine vectors have become available to induce potent humoral or cellular immunity. Gene-based delivery of vaccine antigens effectively elicits immune responses by synthesizing proteins within antigen-presenting cells for endogenous presentation on major histocompatibility complex class I and II molecules. DNA-expression vectors, replication-defective viruses, or prime-boost combinations of the two[31–35] have proved to be effective in eliciting broadly neutralizing antibodies, especially for influenza viruses.[36,37]

Prime-boost vaccine regimens that use DNA and viral vectors[33] have increased both humoral immunity and memory CD8 T-cell responses.[38] For example, a study of a vaccine regimen consisting of a poxvirus vector prime and protein boost (known as the RV144 trial) provided evidence that the vaccine prevented HIV-1 infection among persons in Thailand.[39] Eliciting immune responses at portals of infection (e.g., in the respiratory and intestinal epithelial surfaces for pathogens such as influenza virus and rotavirus, respectively) may generate more efficient mucosal immunity. Similarly, waning vaccine responses require periodic boosting at defined times, requiring more integrated management of vaccines at

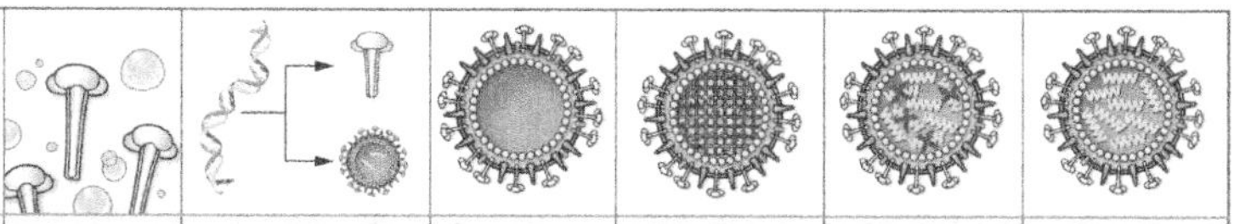

Class:	Proteins or Adjuvants	Gene-based Vectors or Replicons	VLP	Inactivated Viruses	Attenuated Virus	Live Virus
Examples:	Alum MF59 AS01 CpG	VEE Sindbis	HPV HBV	Polio (Salk) Influenza (split)	Polio (Sabin) Adenovirus Vaccinia Yellow fever Flumist	Polio (WT) Smallpox Influenza

Genetic Complexity and Replication Potential →

FIGURE 8.4 **The Spectrum of Costimulation from Adjuvants to Viruses** *A cellular and molecular understanding of dendritic-cell biology has facilitated improvements in vaccine-induced immune responses. Rather than generating responses through infection, immune stimulation can be achieved by increasingly complex modes of antigen presentation that range from introduction of selected proteins, with or without adjuvants, to gene-delivered immunogens, viruslike particles (VLP), structured arrays, or attenuated viruses. These approaches represent a spectrum of complexity and mimicry that elicits protective immunity without inflicting the adverse consequences of natural infection. HBV denotes hepatitis B virus, HPV human papillomavirus, VEE Venezuelan equine encephalitis, and WT wild type.*

all ages. Immunization in the elderly is of substantial concern because immune senescence can lead to a decrease in the responsiveness to vaccination.[40]

Clinical Translation and Implementation

CORRELATES OF PROTECTION AND INNOVATIVE CLINICAL TRIAL DESIGN

The effectiveness of vaccines can be tested only in clinical efficacy trials. In the past, advanced clinical development has been undertaken largely by pharmaceutical companies in an effort to obtain licensure. This process is long, costly, and risky with respect to the likelihood of successful protection. For diseases with a major impact on human health but a limited commercial market, there has been little incentive for drug companies to advance these vaccines. For this reason, government involvement can facilitate success. Funding from the Australian government, for example, catalyzed major advances for cholera and HPV vaccines, along with investments from the U.S. National Institutes of Health. Vaccine trials for HIV infection, tuberculosis, and malaria have been facilitated by clinical and translational infrastructure from the National Institute of Allergy and Infectious Diseases, from the European Union, and by nonprofit organizations including the Bill and Melinda Gates Foundation and the Wellcome Trust. Similarly, the Food and Drug Administration (FDA), the European Medicines Agency, the World Health Organization, and the Centers for Disease Control and Prevention (CDC) provide regulatory, safety, and efficacy oversight. The infrastructure for clinical trials is costly but can be applied to studies of multiple infectious agents and can reduce impediments to vaccine development by facilitating logistically challenging trials in the developing world and supporting the collection of serum samples and lymphocytes for further scientific analysis.

New strategies are sometimes needed to facilitate licensure. For infections that are sporadic or intermittent, such as West Nile, Ebola, and Chikungunya viruses, it is often not possible to perform field trials to demonstrate clinical efficacy. To address this problem, the FDA has proposed the animal rule,[41] according to which efficacy can be shown in relevant animal species, and immune correlates of protection can be defined. Separate phase 2 studies are then performed in humans with the aim of achieving the same level of immunity, and the bridged immune correlate is used as a criterion for licensure. Although uncertainty would remain about vaccine efficacy in a field setting, this approach allows for the development of vaccines that show a high likelihood of protection but that otherwise would not be developed.

Another impediment has been the inability to identify promising vaccine candidates early in development. Definitive efficacy trials take years to perform, and the ability to advance efficacious vaccines represents a key to success for diverse vaccines, a problem evident in the development of vaccines for HIV infection, tuberculosis, and malaria. A potential solution is to use innovative testing, such as adaptive clinical trial designs.[42–44] This approach allows for the evaluation

of multiple vaccine candidates in parallel, looking in real time for early efficacy signals to select candidates for more complete and definitive evaluation.[45]
Innovations in clinical trial design may therefore accelerate early decision making and increase the likelihood of identifying successful vaccines.

The RV144 trial of a candidate HIV vaccine in Thailand showed the value
of efficacy testing for identifying efficacy signals and correlates of immunity in
humans. Despite the modest vaccine efficacy of 31%,[39] investigators found that
antibodies to the V1V2 regions of envelope glycoproteins correlated inversely with
the risk of infection,[46] an unexpected biomarker that may guide product development. Thus, one way to facilitate implementation of successful efficacy trials is to
identify promising candidates in phase 1 trials after defining relevant biomarkers
through efficacy trials and from relevant vaccine studies in animals, at the same
time maintaining stable support and infrastructure for further testing.

FROM LICENSURE TO EFFECTIVE DISTRIBUTION

Many vaccines are intended for use in the developing world, and the development
of clinical infrastructure facilitates the distribution of vaccines in resource-poor
settings. Governmental and international vaccination organizations such as
GAVI and the United Nations Children's Fund (UNICEF) help provide commercial vaccines in these settings. Another impediment is vaccine acceptance by
the public. For example, resistance to vaccination has been encountered during
poliomyelitis eradication campaigns in Nigeria, and unfounded concern related
to autism has proved to be counterproductive for vaccine utilization and in protecting public health in the United States. Increased vigilance and a constructive
response to these concerns are needed to support public confidence in vaccines
and optimize their implementation.[47,48] Public–private partnerships can also
help to address unmet needs, as exemplified in the development of a meningococcal A vaccine in Africa. Modern vaccine development therefore faces challenges beyond biology, and gaps in implementation must be overcome to realize
their full potential.

A Look to the Future

Advances in immunology and microbiology have opened new avenues to improve
vaccine efficacy. New technologies offer alternative products. For example, innovation in manufacturing has allowed a shift from egg-based methods to cell-based
or recombinant methods, including production from insect or plant cells. The following examples illustrate other promising developments.

BEYOND IMMUNOLOGIC MIMICRY

Jenner created the successful smallpox vaccine by building on an observation in
nature: milkmaids who were exposed to cowpox were resistant to smallpox. Most

licensed vaccines similarly use live-attenuated or inactivated natural pathogens (e.g., influenza, measles, mumps, poliomyelitis, or rubella viruses) to elicit protective immune responses. Yet increasingly, microbes that cause diseases such as HIV infection, tuberculosis, and malaria evade human immunity. To counter immune evasion, subdominant immune responses can be generated to highly conserved invariant regions that are vulnerable to the immune system (Fig. 8.1). Vaccines of the future will go beyond mimicking natural immune responses and must generate unnatural immunity.[9] This goal may be achieved by identifying such targets, validating their susceptibility, and using an expanded arsenal of vaccines to target and expand the otherwise subdominant responses to the core vulnerability of these microbes.

LIFE-CYCLE MANAGEMENT OF VACCINES

Whereas vaccines are approved for clinical use in the United States by the FDA, standard practices regarding their efficacy, clinical utility, and public health benefit are made by the Advisory Committee on Immunization Practices (ACIP), through the CDC. The ACIP provides advice intended to reduce the incidence of vaccine-preventable diseases and to increase the safety of vaccines, largely in pediatric populations. Yet there are unmet vaccine needs for persons of varying ages, such as the HPV vaccine recommended for adolescents or the shingles vaccine for the elderly. Immune responses also decline with age and vary according to previous pathogen exposure, suggesting that a systematic view of vaccines be adopted for different stages of life,[40] a life-cycle management concept for vaccines that can maximize protection at all ages.

NEXT-GENERATION VACCINES

While vaccines are under development, the ability of selected antibodies to show protection in humans would validate the antibody target as a protective antigen and provide valuable information about serum levels required for protection. Because techniques with respect to monoclonal antibodies have improved production and bioavailability, such antibodies can be used more broadly for passive prevention. Pilot studies have recently been considered for persons at high risk for HIV infection. If these studies show that such therapy is effective, sustained delivery mechanisms could potentially be achieved with gene-based antibody delivery. Adeno-associated viral vectors have shown efficacy in protecting rodents, nonhuman primates, and humanized mice from lentiviral infection.[49,50] However, widespread implementation of this approach is not without its challenges. Notable among them is the need to regulate or extinguish antibody gene expression in the event of unanticipated adverse events, but should this approach succeed with the incorporation of such safeguards, it could fundamentally change strategies of immune protection and speed the delivery and expand the promise of vaccines.

Conclusions

Traditional vaccines have shown unprecedented success in preventing human infectious diseases and preserving public health by alleviating death and suffering from numerous microbial threats. The success of such therapies has heralded the arrival of a new era for vaccines. Increased understanding of human immunity and microbes has catalyzed unprecedented advances that can be adopted to improve public health. Despite continuing challenges, the collective effort of governments and nonprofit organizations to expand the utilization of effective vaccines throughout the world has grown. Scientific, medical, and biotechnologic advances promise to improve the utilization of existing vaccines and expand the horizons for tomorrow's vaccines.

Since this article was accepted for publication in NEJM, the author moved from the National Institutes of Health to Sanofi.

I thank Drs. Anthony S. Fauci, Harvey Fineberg, Peter Kwong, John Mascola, and Stanley Plotkin for helpful comments and discussions; Dr. Jeffrey Boyington for structural modeling of influenza hemagglutinin; Greg Folkers for advice regarding the composition of the original figures; Ati Tislerics and Mythreyi Shastri for assistance in the preparation of the manuscript; and Brenda Hartman and Jonathan Stuckey for assistance with molecular graphics.

References

1. Landry S, Heilman C. Future directions in vaccines: the payoffs of basic research. Health Aff (Millwood) 2005;24:758–69.
2. Berkley S. Getting the miracle of vaccines to those who most need them. Presented at the John Ring LaMontagne Memorial Lecture, National Institutes of Health, Bethesda, MD, May 22, 2012 (http://videocast.nih.gov/summary.asp?live=11173).
3. Impact of vaccines universally recommended for children—United States, 1900–1998. MMWR Morb Mortal Wkly Rep 1999;48:243–48.
4. Roush SW, Murphy TV. Historical comparisons of morbidity and mortality for vaccine-preventable diseases in the United States. JAMA 2007;298:2155–63.
5. World malaria report 2011: fact sheet. Geneva: World Health Organization (http://www.who.int/malaria/world_malaria_report_2011/WMR2011_factsheet.pdf).
6. 2011/2012 Tuberculosis global facts. Geneva: World Health Organization (http://www.who.int/tb/publications/2011/factsheet_tb_2011.pdf).
7. Joint United Nations Programme on HIV/AIDS. World AIDS Day report 2012 (http://www.slideshare.net/UNAIDS/unaids-world-aids-day-report-2011-core-slides-10250153).
8. Osterholm MT, Kelley NS, Sommer A, Belongia EA. Efficacy and effectiveness of influenza vaccines: a systematic review and meta-analysis. Lancet Infect Dis 2012;12:36–44. [Erratum, Lancet Infect Dis 2012;12:655.]
9. Nabel GJ, Fauci AS. Induction of unnatural immunity: prospects for a broadly protective universal influenza vaccine. Nat Med 2010;16:1389–91.

10. Nabel GJ, Kwong PD, Mascola JR. Progress in the rational design of an AIDS vaccine. Philos Trans R Soc Lond B Biol Sci 2011;366:2759–65.

11. Scarselli M, Arico B, Brunelli B, et al. Rational design of a meningococcal antigen inducing broad protective immunity. Sci Transl Med 2011;3:91ra62.

12. Walker LM, Phogat SK, Chan-Hui PY, et al. Broad and potent neutralizing antibodies from an African donor reveal a new HIV-1 vaccine target. Science 2009;326:285–89.

13. Wu X, Yang ZY, Li Y, et al. Rational design of envelope identifies broadly neutralizing human monoclonal antibodies to HIV-1. Science 2010;329:856–61.

14. Zhou T, Georgiev I, Wu X, et al. Structural basis for broad and potent neutralization of HIV-1 by antibody VRC01. Science 2010;329:811–17.

15. Pejchal R, Doores KJ, Walker LM, et al. A potent and broad neutralizing antibody recognizes and penetrates the HIV glycan shield. Science 2011;334:1097–103.

16. Scheid JF, Mouquet H, Ueberheide B, et al. Sequence and structural convergence of broad and potent HIV antibodies that mimic CD4 binding. Science 2011;333:1633–37.

17. Walker LM, Huber M, Doores KJ, et al. Broad neutralization coverage of HIV by multiple highly potent antibodies. Nature 2011;477:466–70.

18. Burton DR, Poignard P, Stanfield RL, Wilson IA. Broadly neutralizing antibodies present new prospects to counter highly antigenically diverse viruses. Science 2012;337:183–86.

19. Kwong PD, Mascola JR, Nabel GJ. Rational design of vaccines to elicit broadly neutralizing antibodies to HIV-1. Cold Spring Harb Perspect Med 2011;1(1):a007278.

20. McLellan JS, Yang Y, Graham BS, Kwong PD. Structure of respiratory syncytial virus fusion glycoprotein in the postfusion conformation reveals preservation of neutralizing epitopes. J Virol 2011;85:7788–96.

21. Ekiert DC, Wilson IA. Broadly neutralizing antibodies against influenza virus and prospects for universal therapies. Curr Opin Virol 2012;2:134–41.

22. Nelson AL, Dhimolea E, Reichert JM. Development trends for human monoclonal antibody therapeutics. Nat Rev Drug Discov 2010;9:767–74.

23. Wu X, Zhou T, Zhu J, et al. Focused evolution of HIV-1 neutralizing antibodies revealed by structures and deep sequencing. Science 2011;333:1593–602.

24. Burton DR, Desrosiers RC, Doms RW, et al. HIV vaccine design and the neutralizing antibody problem. Nat Immunol 2004;5:233–36.

25. Kelly DF, Rappuoli R. Reverse vaccinology and vaccines for serogroup B Neisseria meningitidis. Adv Exp Med Biol 2005;568:217–23.

26. Rappuoli R, Aderem A. A 2020 vision for vaccines against HIV, tuberculosis and malaria. Nature 2011;473:463–69.

27. Sullivan NJ, Hensley L, Asiedu C, et al. CD8+ cellular immunity mediates rAd5 vaccine protection against Ebola virus infection of nonhuman primates. Nat Med 2011;17:1128–31.

28. Lauring AS, Jones JO, Andino R. Rationalizing the development of live attenuated virus vaccines. Nat Biotechnol 2010;28:573–79.

29. Delrue I, Verzele D, Madder A, Nauwynck HJ. Inactivated virus vaccines from chemistry to prophylaxis: merits, risks and challenges. Expert Rev Vaccines 2012;11:695–719.

30. Levitz SM, Golenbock DT. Beyond empiricism: informing vaccine development through innate immunity research. Cell 2012;148:1284–92.

31. Benmira S, Bhattacharya V, Schmid ML. An effective HIV vaccine: a combination of humoral and cellular immunity? Curr HIV Res 2010;8:441–49.

32. Hu SL, Abrams K, Barber GN, et al. Protection of macaques against SIV infection by subunit vaccines of SIV envelope glycoprotein gp160. Science 1992;255:456–59.

33. Mascola JR, Sambor A, Beaudry K, et al. Neutralizing antibodies elicited by immunization of monkeys with DNA plasmids and recombinant adenoviral vectors expressing human immunodeficiency virus type 1 proteins. J Virol 2005;79:771–79.

34. Wang S, Kennedy JS, West K, et al. Cross-subtype antibody and cellular immune responses induced by a polyvalent DNA prime-protein boost HIV-1 vaccine in healthy human volunteers. Vaccine 2008;26:3947–57.

35. Tomaras GD, Haynes BF. Strategies for eliciting HIV-1 inhibitory antibodies. Curr Opin HIV AIDS 2010;5:421–27.

36. Wei CJ, Boyington JC, McTamney PM, et al. Induction of broadly neutralizing H1N1 influenza antibodies by vaccination. Science 2010;329:1060–64.

37. Ledgerwood JE, Wei CJ, Hu Z, et al. DNA priming and influenza vaccine immunogenicity: two phase 1 open label randomised clinical trials. Lancet Infect Dis 2011;11:916–24.

38. Butler NS, Nolz JC, Harty JT. Immunologic considerations for generating memory CD8 T cells through vaccination. Cell Microbiol 2011;13:925–33.

39. Rerks-Ngarm S, Pitisuttithum P, Nitayaphan S, et al. Vaccination with ALVAC and AIDSVAX to prevent HIV-1 infection in Thailand. N Engl J Med 2009;361:2209–20.

40. Rappuoli R, Mandl CW, Black S, De Gregorio E. Vaccines for the twenty-first century society. Nat Rev Immunol 2011;11:865–72. [Erratum, Nat Rev Immunol 2012;12:225.]

41. Burns DL. Licensure of vaccines using the Animal Rule. Curr Opin Virol 2012;2:353–56.

42. Emerson SS. Issues in the use of adaptive clinical trial designs. Stat Med 2006;25:3270–96.

43. Chow S-C, Chang M. Adaptive design methods in clinical trials. Boca Raton, FL: Chapman and Hall/CRC, 2007.

44. Coffey CS, Kairalla JA. Adaptive clinical trials: progress and challenges. Drugs R D 2008;9:229–42.

45. Corey L, Nabel GJ, Dieffenbach C, et al. HIV-1 vaccines and adaptive trial designs. Sci Transl Med 2011;3(79):79ps13.

46. Haynes BF, Gilbert PB, McElrath MJ, et al. Immune-correlates analysis of an HIV-1 vaccine efficacy trial. N Engl J Med 2012;366:1275–86.

47. Black S, Rappuoli R. A crisis of public confidence in vaccines. Sci Transl Med 2010;2(61):61mr1.

48. Larson HJ, Cooper LZ, Eskola J, Katz SL, Ratzan S. Addressing the vaccine confidence gap. Lancet 2011;378:526–35.

49. Johnson PR, Schnepp BC, Zhang J, et al. Vector-mediated gene transfer engenders long-lived neutralizing activity and protection against SIV infection in monkeys. Nat Med 2009;15:901–906.

50. Balazs AB, Chen J, Hong CM, Rao DS, Yang L, Baltimore D. Antibody-based protection against HIV infection by vectored immunoprophylaxis. Nature 2012;481:81–84.

"I have received a copy of the evidence at large respecting the discovery of the vaccine inoculation which you have been pleased to send me, and for which I return you my thanks. ... I avail myself of this occasion of rendering you a portion of the tribute of gratitude due to you from the whole human family. Medicine has never before produced any single improvement of such utility. Harvey's discovery of the circulation of the blood was a beautiful addition to our knowledge of the animal economy, but on a review of the practice of medicine before and since that epoch, I do not see any great amelioration which has been derived from that discovery. You have erased from the calendar of human afflictions one of its greatest. Yours is the comfortable reflection that mankind can never forget that you have lived. Future nations will know by history only that the loathsome small-pox has existed and by you has been extirpated."

Letter to Dr. Edward Jenner from Thomas Jefferson, Monticello (May 14, 1805)

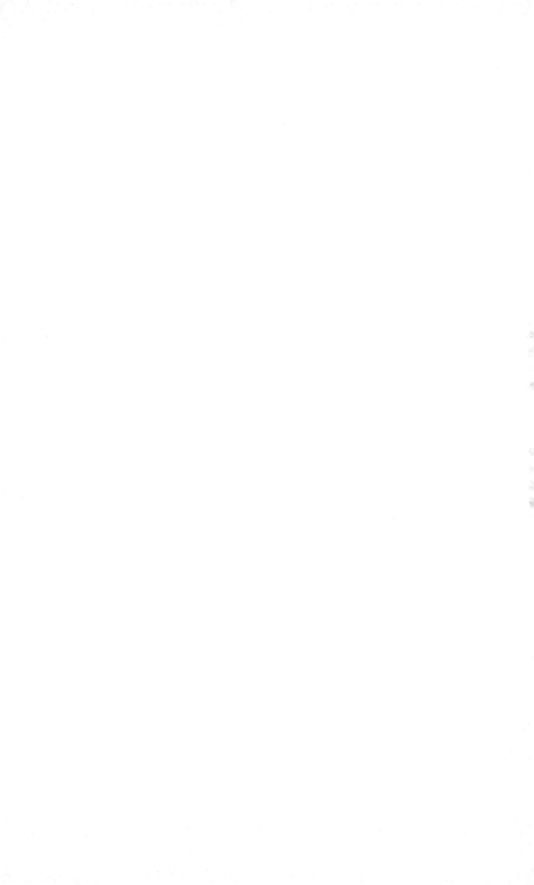

{ 9 }

Disease Eradication
Donald R. Hopkins

Since the last case of naturally occurring smallpox, in 1977, there have been three major international conferences devoted to the concept of disease eradication.[1-3] Several other diseases have been considered as potential candidates for eradication,[4] but the World Health Organization (WHO) has targeted only two other diseases for global eradication after smallpox. In 1986, WHO's policymaking body, the World Health Assembly, adopted the elimination of dracunculiasis (guinea worm disease) as a global goal,[5] and it declared the eradication of poliomyelitis a global goal in 1988.[6] Although both diseases now appear to be close to eradication, the fact that neither goal has been achieved after more than two decades, and several years beyond the initial target dates for their eradication, underscores the daunting challenge of such efforts, as does the failure of previous attempts to eradicate malaria, hookworm, yaws, and other diseases.[1]

The word "eradicate" is defined as "to pull or tear up by the roots" and "to remove entirely, extirpate, get rid of."[7] Definitions of eradication and elimination have also been suggested by various international bodies (and are used herein), and the International Task Force for Disease Eradication uses certain scientific and social criteria when evaluating candidate diseases (see box 9.1).[1,2,4] Eradication of a disease means worldwide interruption of transmission, whereas elimination means interruption of transmission in a limited geographic area. The term "elimination" is often used imprecisely.[8] For example, the World Health Assembly resolutions in 1986 and 1989 referred to the "elimination" of dracunculiasis but changed the term to "eradication" for the same global goal in a 1991 resolution.

A brief review of five diseases selected for eradication or elimination will illustrate the potential benefits of such efforts and some of the challenges they pose (see the interactive graphic available at NEJM.org). Although dracunculiasis and poliomyelitis are now the only officially sanctioned targets of eradication campaigns, the WHO has designated the campaign against lymphatic filariasis as the Global Program to Eliminate Lymphatic Filariasis. These three programs represent different levels of international commitment to disease eradication. The

BOX 9.1   Definitions and Eradicability

Definitions

Eradication

Zero disease globally as a result of deliberate efforts

Control measures no longer needed

Elimination

Zero disease in a defined geographic area as a result of deliberate efforts

Control measures needed to prevent reestablishment of transmission

Criteria for Assessing the Eradicability of a Disease

Scientific feasibility

Epidemiologic susceptibility (e.g., no nonhuman reservoir, ease of spread, naturally induced immunity, ease of diagnosis)

Effective, practical intervention available (e.g., vaccine, curative treatment)

Demonstrated feasibility of elimination (e.g., documented elimination from -island or other geographic unit)

Political will and popular support

Perceived burden of the disease (e.g., extent, deaths, other effects; relevance to rich and poor countries)

Expected cost of eradication

Synergy of eradication efforts with other interventions (e.g., potential for added benefits or savings)

Need for eradication rather than control

---

program to eliminate onchocerciasis (river blindness) from the Americas is an example of a highly successful regional initiative, whereas the effort to eliminate malaria and lymphatic filariasis from Hispaniola is an example of a compelling, binational initiative that might suggest the feasibility of a global eradication effort.

Several key principles are inherent in an eradication or elimination campaign: the need to intervene everywhere the disease occurs, no matter how remotely located or difficult to access occurrences of disease are or how minor the perceived problem is in an individual country or area; the importance of monitoring the target disease and the extent of interventions closely; the need for flexibility and urgency in response to ongoing monitoring and operational research; and the need for an intense focus on the goal of stopping transmission of the targeted disease, even when the costs per case rise sharply as the number of cases declines. Common difficulties faced by such campaigns include sporadic or widespread political insecurity in areas where the disease is endemic, inadequate or delayed funding, and the challenges of motivating officials, health workers, and affected populations.

Dracunculiasis

The global campaign to eradicate dracunculiasis began in 1980 at the Centers for Disease Control and Prevention (CDC)[9] and since 1986 has been led by the Carter

Center in close cooperation with the WHO, the CDC, and the United Nations Children's Fund (UNICEF).[10] The life cycle of the parasite *Dracunculus medinensis* is shown in Figure 9.1A. When exposed to water, the adult worms discharge thousands of larvae, which are ingested by tiny crustaceans (cyclops). About a year after a person has drunk water from ponds or open wells contaminated with these crustaceans, adult worms measuring about 1 m in length slowly begin to emerge through the infected person's skin.

(A)

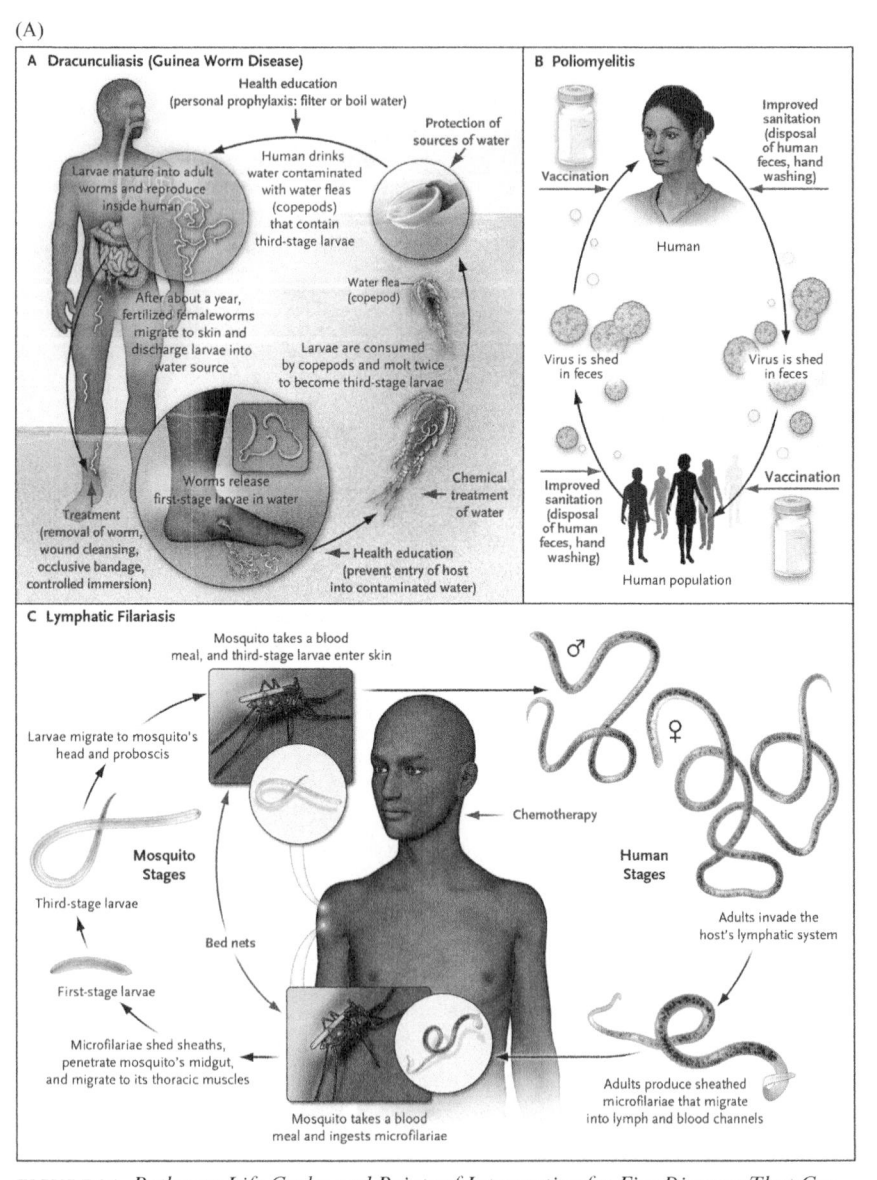

FIGURE 9.1 *Pathogen Life Cycles and Points of Intervention for Five Diseases That Can Be Eradicated or Eliminated*

(B)

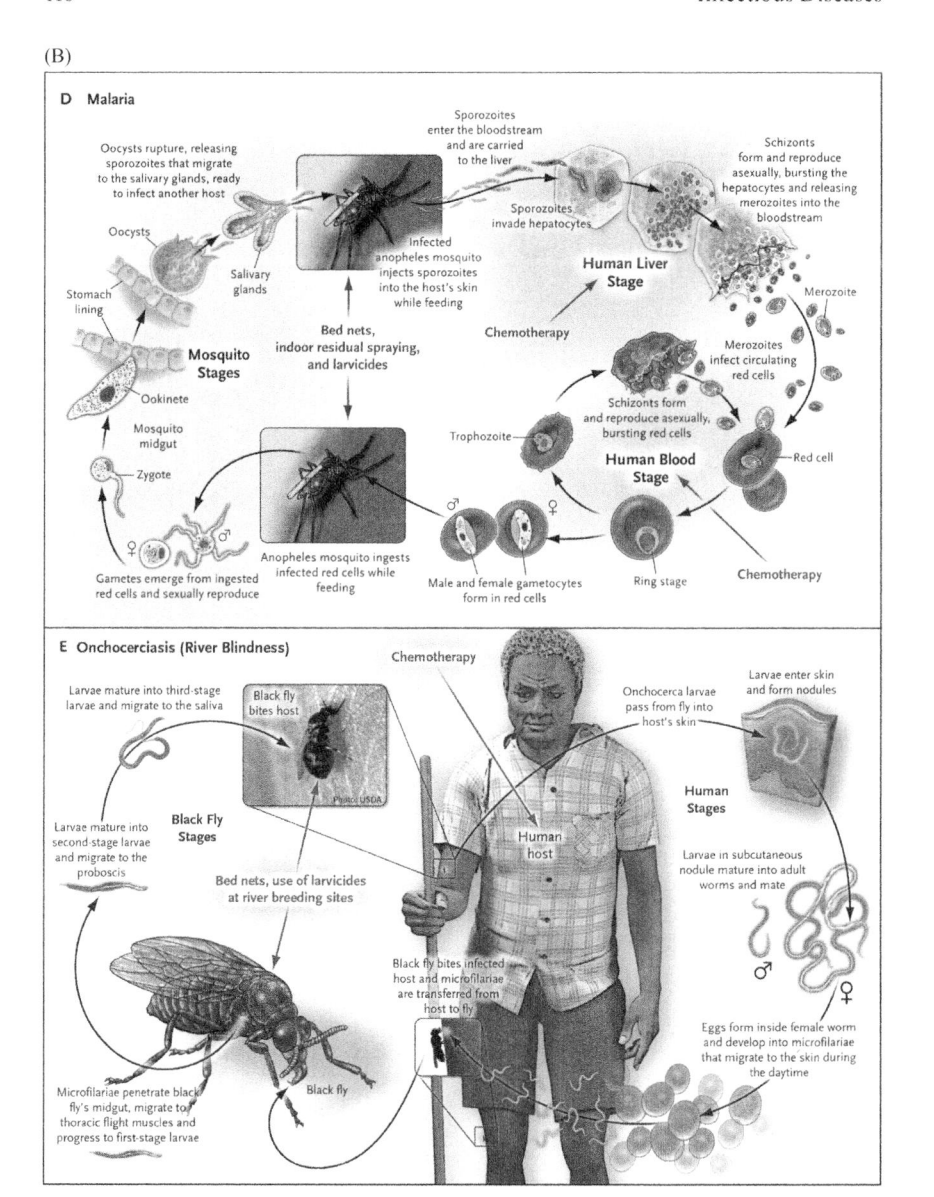

FIGURE 9.1 *Continued*

Dracunculiasis met the scientific criteria for eradication (see box), although the campaign was handicapped by the 1-year incubation period of the parasite and the lack of a vaccine or curative treatment. The true extent and burden of the disease among neglected populations were unknown because cases of dracunculiasis were greatly underreported. The adverse effects of this disease on health, agriculture, and school attendance were easy to imagine, however, since the pain and secondary infections associated with the emergence of the worms incapacitated many affected persons for several weeks during the agricultural

season. The main interventions included health education focused on teaching villagers how to filter their drinking water and avoid contaminating the water, application of a mild larvicide to water sources, voluntary isolation of patients (case containment), and provision of safe water sources when possible.[11] Synergistic benefits of this campaign have included the development of village-based active case surveillance and health education and improved supplies of drinking water.

Down from an estimated 3.5 million cases in 20 African and Asian countries in 1986,[12] the number of cases reported in 2014 was only 126, most of which were in the new Republic of South Sudan, with a few in Mali (40 cases) and Ethiopia (3 cases), as well as Chad (13 cases), in which a new outbreak was discovered in 2010 (Fig. 9.2).[13,14] The eradication strategy evolved from an emphasis on the provision of safe water supplies to a focus on health education and the use of cloth filters and, later, to case containment. The active leadership of former U.S. President Jimmy Carter, the focus on village-based reporting and interventions, and major funding provided by the Bill and Melinda Gates Foundation all facilitated this program's achievements. Political instability in some affected areas of South Sudan and Mali are the main challenges to eradicating dracunculiasis. The estimated cost for this program (1986–2015) and for certification of eradication, not including provision of a water supply, is approximately $350 million.

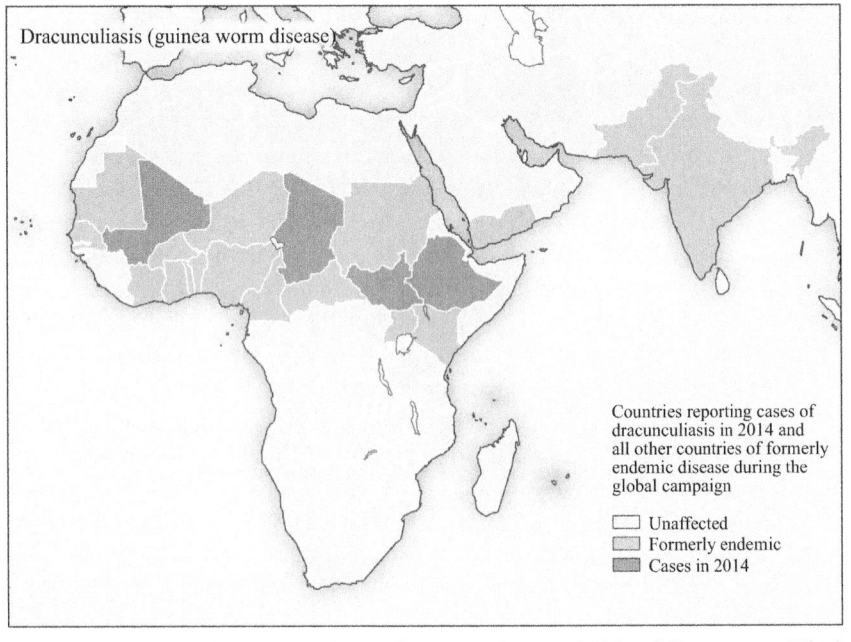

FIGURE 9.2 *Countries Reporting Cases of Dracunculiasis in 2014 and Countries in Which the Disease Was Endemic in 1980*

Poliomyelitis

The Global Polio Eradication Initiative, which began in 1988,[15] was inspired by the successful elimination of this disease in the Americas. An enteroviral infection characterized by influenza-like symptoms, poliomyelitis causes muscle paralysis in one or more limbs or the chest, or both, in less than 1% of infected persons. People are infected by ingesting virus shed in feces or by inhaling viral particles exhaled by those already infected (Fig 1B). Patients may exhale virus for a week and shed virus in feces for a month, beginning just before symptoms develop, 7 to 14 days after they are infected. Persons who recover are then immune to the viral type that infected them (poliovirus 1, 2, or 3). Vaccination to prevent infection requires three or more doses of live attenuated virus administered orally or of killed virus administered by injection. Before polio vaccination was introduced, in the 1950s, the disease killed or paralyzed an estimated 600,000 persons each year worldwide.[16]

The Global Polio Eradication Initiative engendered massive global immunization and surveillance efforts with the support of the WHO, UNICEF, the CDC, Rotary International, the Bill and Melinda Gates Foundation, and others. These efforts have helped strengthen routine immunization in some instances (e.g., measles immunization in the Americas) and the delivery of vitamin A supplements in others. Surveillance for polioviruses, which is performed in health facilities and laboratories, involves the use of sophisticated methods for characterizing polioviruses detected in specimens from sewage or from patients with suspected infection.[17] Type 2 wild poliovirus was eradicated worldwide by 1999.[18] By 2006, transmission of indigenous wild virus had been halted in all but four countries. In India, suboptimal seroconversion due to poor sanitation and high population density required immunization with many more doses than expected; parts of Afghanistan and Pakistan became inaccessible after 2002, owing to political conflict; and rumors of side effects from vaccination compromised the acceptance of immunization in Nigeria. Additional problems included the discoveries that immunosuppressed persons could excrete virus indefinitely and that the virus in the live-virus vaccine could, in rare cases, regain virulence and spread to others, just as the virus in the attenuated vaccine did, although spread of the attenuated virus was beneficial, augmenting herd immunity.[18]

By 2011, after setbacks that resulted in cases being exported to other countries, 650 confirmed cases of poliomyelitis were reported provisionally from 16 polio-affected countries: 4 countries where the disease was endemic and 12 countries with reestablished transmission (lasting ≥12 months) or outbreaks (lasting <12 months) after importations (Fig. 9.3).[15,17,19] Global coverage of infants with three doses of oral trivalent vaccine was about 85% in 2010 but is uneven at the national and subnational levels.[15] In January 2012, India celebrated a full year with no cases of poliomyelitis, leaving Nigeria, Afghanistan, and Pakistan as countries with endemic disease where eradication was problematic because of political instability or fear of immunization.[20-22] Among countries with reestablished transmission, Chad and the Democratic Republic of Congo reported

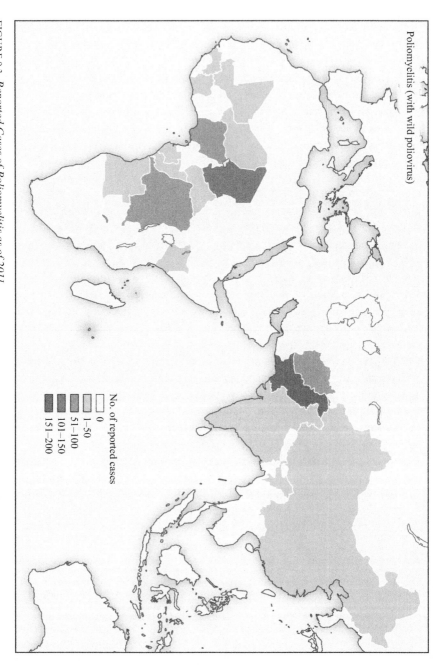

Poliomyelitis (with wild poliovirus)

No. of reported cases
0
1–50
51–100
101–150
151–200

FIGURE 9.3 *Reported Cases of Poliomyelitis as of 2011*
Adapted from the World Health Organization.[1]

the most cases (132 and 93, respectively) in 2011.[19] The goal is to interrupt transmission of poliovirus types 1 and 3 by December 2012. The main challenges to poliomyelitis eradication are donor fatigue; political instability in parts of Afghanistan, Pakistan, and some other affected countries; public fatigue with repeated immunizations against poliomyelitis alone; and weak routine immunization systems. This program is estimated to cost $9.5 billion for the period from 1988 through 2013.[23]

Lymphatic Filariasis

In 1997, after the International Task Force for Disease Eradication had first suggested the potential eradicability of lymphatic filariasis, the World Health Assembly formally targeted the disease for global elimination.[24] Characterized by painful adenolymphangitis, damage to kidneys and other organs, and grotesque swelling of limbs and genital organs, lymphatic filariasis is caused by the filarial parasites *Wuchereria bancrofti, Brugia malayi*, and *B. timori* and is transmitted to humans by repeated bites of mosquitoes that previously ingested microfilariae from the blood of an infected person (Fig. 9.1C). In Africa, lymphatic filariasis is transmitted by the same anopheles species of mosquitoes that transmit malaria (Fig. 9.1D). Annual oral mass drug administration with ivermectin and albendazole or with diethylcarbamazine and albendazole suppresses microfilaremia and interrupts transmission. About 6 years of treatment are required before the adult worms die. Mass drug administration with ivermectin is contraindicated in African areas where the parasite *Loa loa* occurs (because treatment of persons with heavy *L. loa* infections may have fatal side effects), but bed nets to thwart nocturnal, indoor-biting mosquitoes such as anopheles also prevent the transmission of lymphatic filariasis.[25] In 2010, about 120 million people were infected and almost 1.4 billion were at risk for lymphatic filariasis in 72 countries of Asia, Africa, and Latin America (Fig. 9.4).[26]

In 2000, generous donations of drugs helped launch the Global Program to Eliminate Lymphatic Filariasis, which aims to eliminate lymphatic filariasis "as a public health problem" by 2020. In 2010, a total of 466 million (34%) of the persons at risk for lymphatic filariasis received treatment, and mapping was complete in 59 countries.[26] India, Indonesia, and Nigeria have the most cases. Scaling up mass drug administration for lymphatic filariasis has been slowest in Africa, where the expanding use of long-lasting impregnated nets provides synergy between efforts to eliminate lymphatic filariasis and efforts to control malaria. Mass drug administration for lymphatic filariasis also treats onchocerciasis and several soil-transmitted helminths.[27] There is evidence that mass drug administration has interrupted the transmission of lymphatic filariasis in some parts of Nigeria where the disease is heavily endemic,[28] in Egypt[29] and in Togo[30] and has reduced microfilariae levels to less than 1% in 12 Asian and Pacific Island countries.[26] There is also evidence from Nigeria that widespread use of long-lasting impregnated nets can halt transmission of the disease (Richards

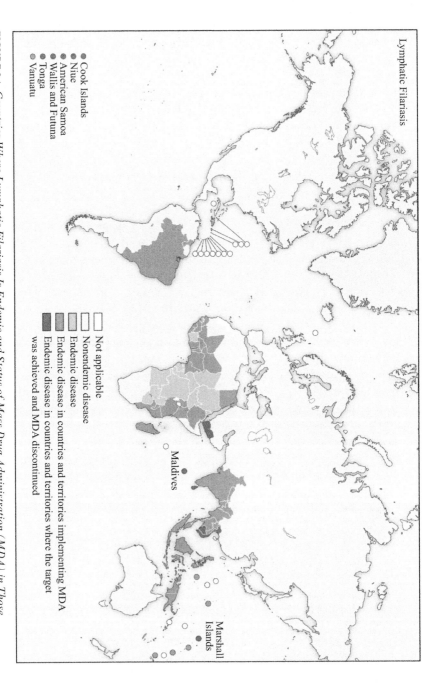

Lymphatic Filariasis

● Cook Islands
● Niue
● American Samoa
● Wallis and Futuna
● Tonga
● Vanuatu

Not applicable
Nonendemic disease
Endemic disease
Endemic disease in countries and territories implementing MDA
Endemic disease in countries and territories where the target
was achieved and MDA discontinued

Maldives

Marshall
Islands

FIGURE 9.4 *Countries Where Lymphatic Filariasis Is Endemic and Status of Mass Drug Administration (MDA) in Those Countries, 2010*

Adapted from the World Health Organization.[26]

F: personal communication). The main challenges to a full-scale campaign for lymphatic filariasis eradication are inadequate political and financial support for scaling up mass drug administration, constraints on such treatment because of the presence of *L. loa* in certain areas (although the use of impregnated nets may eliminate this constraint), and political insecurity in certain countries. The overall costs of this program have not been estimated, although limited studies have suggested that interventions against lymphatic filariasis are very beneficial in relation to their cost.[31,32]

Onchocerciasis in the Americas

The Americas was the first WHO region to eliminate smallpox, poliomyelitis, and measles. Since 1992, the region has pursued a program to eliminate onchocerciasis from 13 foci in six countries of Central and South America with the use of mass administration of ivermectin twice a year.[33,34] The parasite *Onchocerca volvulus* is spread to humans by the bites of tiny black flies, after which the adult worms cluster in nodules and release millions of microfilariae that migrate to the skin, causing intense itching, and to the eyes, where they may impair sight and, after many years, cause blindness (Fig. 9.1E). By the end of 2011, onchocerciasis transmission had been halted or suppressed in all but 2 of the 13 foci and in four of the six affected countries (Table 9.1).[35,36] Accessing indigenous populations in remote adjacent areas of Venezuela and Brazil is still a challenge. Progress in the effort to eliminate onchocerciasis in the Americas has inspired a reappraisal of ongoing programs to control the disease in Africa, where most cases occur.[37,38] Over the past two decades, the Onchocerciasis Elimination Program for the Americas has cost approximately $124 million, with $46 million of that amount paid for by the countries themselves, $51 million paid by Merck in the form of donated drugs, and most of the remainder raised by the Carter Center.

Malaria and Lymphatic Filariasis in Hispaniola

A special opportunity also exists in the Americas to apply the principles of disease elimination in Hispaniola, comprising the Dominican Republic and Haiti. These two countries are the only remaining foci of endemic malaria among the Caribbean islands and account for more than 90% of all cases of lymphatic filariasis in the Western Hemisphere. The International Task Force for Disease Eradication highlighted this compelling opportunity in 2006, concluding that eliminating both diseases from Hispaniola "is technically feasible, [is] medically desirable and [would be] economically beneficial."[39] The Dominican Republic has almost eliminated lymphatic filariasis already. Despite the earthquake in 2010, Haiti extended mass drug administration for lymphatic filariasis to all affected districts for the first time in 2011 and

TABLE 9.1 Ocular Morbidity and Transmission Status of Onchocerciasis in the Americas

Focus	Population at Risk no(%)	Blindness Eliminated	Ocular Morbidity Disappeared	Transmission Status*
Santa Rosa, Guatemala	12,208 (2)	Yes	Yes	Eliminated
Lopez de Micay, Colombia	1,366 (0.2)	Yes	Yes	Eliminated
Escuintla, Guatemala	62,590 (11)	Yes	Yes	Eliminated
North Chiapas, Mexico	7,125 (1)	Yes	Yes	Eliminated
Huehuetenango, Guatemala	30,239 (5.5)	Yes	Yes	Interrupted in 2008
Oaxaca, Mexico	44,919 (8)	Yes	Yes	Interrupted in 2008
Esmeraldas, Ecuador	25,863 (4.7)	Yes	Yes	Interrupted in 2009
North-central Venezuela	14,385 (2.6)	Yes	Yes	Interrupted in 2010
South Chiapas, Mexico	114,024 (21)	Yes	Yes	Interrupted in 2011
Central Guatemala	124,498 (22)	Yes	Yes	Interrupted in 2011
Northeastern Venezuela	93,239 (17)	Yes	No	Suppressed
Amazonas, Brazil	12,521 (2)	Yes	No	Ongoing
Southern Venezuela	9,168 (1.7)	Yes	No	Ongoing

*Eliminated means that there has been no recrudescence of infection during a period of 3 or more years since mass drug administration was halted, with ongoing post-treatment surveillance. Interrupted means that there has been no transmission during a period of fewer than 3 years since mass drug administration was halted, with ongoing post-treatment surveillance. Suppressed means that transmission indexes are negative; mass drug administration has not yet been halted. Data are adapted from the WHO.[35,36]

estimates that $49 million will be needed to eliminate the disease by 2020. In 2009, the two countries also announced a binational plan to eliminate malaria by 2020 by combining active case detection and treatment with vector control at an estimated cost of $194 million over the decade.[40] An outbreak of malaria in 2004 cost the Dominican Republic an estimated $200 million in lost revenue from tourism alone.[39]

Some Lessons and Conclusions

Past and current experience confirms that disease eradication is difficult and risky and will probably require more effort, time, and money than initially expected, even when it is successful. It is advisable to start early in the most heavily affected areas, since they will present the most difficult challenges and require the longest effort and because the specific challenges cannot be anticipated on the basis of work in areas that are less heavily affected. The inherent risks of

failure to achieve eradication are offset by the benefits that accrue indefinitely from a successful eradication campaign. The unique power of eradication campaigns derives from their supreme clarity of purpose, their unparalleled ability to inspire dedication and sacrifice among health workers, and their attractiveness to donors, all of which are needed to overcome the barriers to successful eradication. Evidence that disease incidence and intervention coverage are being monitored closely and that progress is being made toward eradication can help secure the resources needed for these demanding campaigns.

Political instability and insecurity, which are usually outside the realm of public health professionals and can be avoided in a program designed to control disease, are inescapable challenges in an eradication program. Smallpox eradication succeeded despite civil wars in Nigeria, Pakistan, and Sudan, and the programs to eradicate dracunculiasis and poliomyelitis face similar challenges. Unlike the dracunculiasis eradication program, the programs to eradicate smallpox and poliomyelitis must address the risk of waning immunity levels, should the virus be reintroduced by bioterrorists after eradication, when routine immunizations have ceased.

In the medical realm, each eradication or elimination program is different and will require its own strategies and tactics. No program will have all the answers from the outset, so ongoing innovation and research are important. The smallpox eradication program switched from mass vaccination to the successful surveillance-containment strategy after it was under way, and the guinea worm and poliomyelitis eradication programs also developed new strategies after they had begun.[41] All eradication programs, however, require an intensive focus. Opportunities for integrating interventions of eradication programs with those of control programs will be scarce, but such opportunities should be seized when it makes sense to do so. Measles immunization was combined with smallpox eradication efforts in West Africa, despite the additional logistic and financial burdens imposed by the need to refrigerate the measles vaccine (but not the smallpox vaccine), because the African governments requested it.[42] Meeting this request added public health value and political virtue to the campaign. Similar opportunities for mutually beneficial, combined interventions against lymphatic filariasis, onchocerciasis, malaria, and soil-transmitted helminths in Africa are also evident.[27]

The successful eradication of dracunculiasis with interventions other than a vaccine will soon validate and expand the concept of disease eradication as we have known it, such as in the use of vaccination to eradicate smallpox (and in the impending eradication of poliomyelitis). That imminent success, generous drug donations for combating lymphatic filariasis, and ongoing elimination efforts in the Americas and elsewhere against other diseases augur well for the future, although the eradication of lymphatic filariasis is not yet an official goal of the WHO. However, the fact that neither dracunculiasis nor poliomyelitis was eradicated by December 2012, as planned, underscores the inherent difficulties of disease eradication. I believe this powerful public health tool will be used to eradicate other carefully selected diseases in the future, provided that inflated promises and failure to deliver on them do not tarnish the concept. In the meantime,

lessons from eradication programs could be adapted to improve control of many other diseases.

References

1. Dowdle WR, Hopkins DR, eds. The eradication of infectious diseases. New York: John Wiley, 1998.
2. Dowdle WR. The principles of disease elimination and eradication. Bull World Health Organ 1998;76:Suppl 2:22–25.
3. Cochi SL, Dowdle WR, eds. Disease eradication in the 21st century: implications for global health. Strungmann forum report. Vol. 7. Cambridge, MA: MIT Press, 2011.
4. Recommendations of the International Task Force for Disease Eradication. MMWR Recomm Rep 1993;42(RR-16):1–38.
5. World Health Assembly. Resolution WHA39.21: elimination of dracunculiasis. Geneva: World Health Organization, 1986.
6. *Idem.* Resolution WHA41.28: global eradication of poliomyelitis by year 2000. Geneva: World Health Organization, 1988.
7. The compact edition of the Oxford English dictionary. Oxford, United Kingdom: Oxford University Press, 1971.
8. Hopkins DR. The allure of eradication. Global Health 2009;3:14–17.
9. Hopkins DR, Foege WH. Guinea worm disease. Science 1981;212:495.
10. Hopkins DR, Ruiz-Tiben E. Strategies for eradication of dracunculiasis. Bull World Health Organ 1991;69:533–40.
11. Ruiz-Tiben E, Hopkins DR. Helminthic diseases: dracunculiasis. In: Heggenhougen K, Quah S, eds. International encyclopedia of public health. San Diego, CA: Academic Press, 2008:294–311.
12. Watts SJ. Dracunculiasis in Africa: its geographic extent, incidence, and at-risk population. Am J Trop Med Hyg 1987;37:119–25.
13. Progress toward global eradication of dracunculiasis, January 2010–June 2011. MMWR Morb Mortal Wkly Rep 2011;60:1450–53.
14. Renewed transmission of dracunculiasis—Chad, 2010. MMWR Morb Mortal Wkly Rep 2011;60:744–48.
15. Progress towards interrupting wild poliovirus transmission worldwide: January 2010–March 2011. Wkly Epidemiol Rec 2011;86:199–204.
16. Pigman HA. Conquering polio. Evanston, IL: Rotary International, 2005.
17. Tracking progress toward global polio eradication—worldwide, 2009–2010. MMWR Morb Mortal Wkly Rep 2011;60:441–45.
18. Heymann DL. Disease eradication and control. In: Guerrant RL, Walker DH, Weller PF, eds. Tropical infectious diseases. Edinburgh: Saunders Elsevier, 2011:40–44.
19. Progress towards global interruption of wild poliovirus transmission, January 2011–March 2012. Wkly Epidemiol Rec 2012;87:195–200.
20. Progress toward poliomyelitis eradication—India, January 2010–September 2011. MMWR Morb Mortal Wkly Rep 2011;60:1482–86.
21. Progress toward poliomyelitis elimination—Nigeria, January 2010–June 2011. MMWR Morb Mortal Wkly Rep 2011;60:1053–57.

22. Progress toward poliomyelitis eradication—Afghanistan and Pakistan, January 2010–September 2011. MMWR Morb Mortal Wkly Rep 2011;60:1523–27.

23. Global Polio Eradication Initiative. Financial resource requirements 2012–2013 (http://www.polioeradication.org/financing.aspx).

24. World Health Assembly. WHA50.29: elimination of lymphatic filariasis as a public health problem. Geneva: World Health Organization, 1997.

25. Nutman TB, Kazura JW. Lymphatic filariasis. In: Guerrant RL, Walker DH, Weller PF, eds. Tropical infectious diseases. Edinburgh: Saunders Elsevier, 2011:729–34.

26. Global Programme to Eliminate Lymphatic Filariasis: progress report on mass drug administration, 2010. Wkly Epidemiol Rec 2011;86:377–87.

27. Meeting of the International Task Force for Disease Eradication, April 2011. Wkly Epidemiol Rec 2011;86:341–51.

28. Richards FO, Eigege A, Miri ES, et al. Epidemiological and entomological evaluations after six years or more of mass drug administration for lymphatic filariasis elimination in Nigeria. PLoS Negl Trop Dis 2011;5(10):e1346.

29. Molyneux DH. Elimination of transmission of lymphatic filariasis in Egypt. Lancet 2006;367:966–68.

30. Progress toward elimination of lymphatic filariasis—Togo, 2000–2009. MMWR Morb Mortal Wkly Rep 2011;60:989–91.

31. Goldman AS, Guisinger VH, Aikins M, et al. National mass drug administration costs for lymphatic filariasis elimination. PLoS Negl Trop Dis 2007;1(1):e67.

32. Ottesen EA, Hooper PJ, Bradley M, Biswas G. The Global Programme to Eliminate Lymphatic Filariasis: health impact after 8 years. PLoS Negl Trop Dis 2008;2(10):e317.

33. Working to overcome the global impact of neglected tropical diseases. Geneva: World Health Organization, 2010.

34. InterAmerican Conference on Onchocerciasis, 2010: progress towards eliminating river blindness in the WHO Region of the Americas. Wkly Epidemiol Rec 2011;86:417–23.

35. Progress towards eliminating onchocerciasis in the WHO Region of the Americas in 2011: interruption of transmission in Guatemala and Mexico. Wkly Epidemiol Rec 2012;87:309–14.

36. Report from the 2009 Inter-American Conference on Onchocerciasis: progress towards eliminating river blindness in the Region of the Americas. Wkly Epidemiol Rec 2010;85:321–26.

37. Hopkins DR, Richards FO, Katabarwa M. Whither onchocerciasis control in Africa? Am J Trop Med Hyg 2005;72:1–2.

38. Mackenzie CD, Homeida MM, Hopkins AD, et al. Elimination of onchocerciasis from Africa: possible? Trends Parasitol 2012;28:16–22.

39. Meeting of the International Task Force for Disease Eradication—12 May 2006. Wkly Epidemiol Rec 2007;82:25–30.

40. Roberts L. Elimination meets reality in Hispaniola. Science 2010;328:850–51.

41. Stepan NL. Eradication: ridding the world of diseases forever? Ithaca, NY: Cornell University Press, 2011.

42. Ogden HG. CDC and the smallpox crusade. Washington, DC: Government Printing Office, 1987. (HHS publication no. (CDC) 87-8400.)

{ PART III }

Noncommunicable Diseases

INTRODUCTION

The term *noncommunicable diseases* (NCDs) is a misnomer. It has come to stand for a "cluster" of disparate diseases including cardiovascular disease and stroke, cancers, diabetes and chronic respiratory diseases. However, several types of cancer are caused by communicable viral infections (e.g., human papillomavirus infection and cervical cancer, hepatitis B and C viruses and liver cancer), bacterial infections (e.g., *Helicobacter pylori* and stomach cancer), and parasites (e.g., schistosomiasis and bladder cancer). Similarly, the leading cause of cardiomyopathy in some Central and Latin American countries is infection with *Trypanosoma cruzi*, the parasite that causes Chagas disease. Furthermore, rheumatic fever due to streptococcal infection causes pericarditis and heart valve damage and is estimated to be responsible for more deaths globally than prostate cancer.[1]

A second problem is that the list of diseases conventionally considered NCDs omits many conditions of consequence that are not due to communicable causes, such as cirrhosis of the liver; digestive diseases; neurological diseases; mental and behavioral disorders; urogenital, blood, and endocrine diseases; and musculoskeletal and miscellaneous disorders. If these multiple diseases were included, then NCDs would account for approximately 2 of every 3 of deaths throughout the world.[1] If only cardiovascular disease and stroke, cancers, diabetes and chronic respiratory diseases were included, these would account for 54% of all deaths. When measured in terms of morbidity, the failure to include mental and behavioral disorders has an even greater impact. Although this category accounts for 0.4% of deaths, it accounts for 7.4% of disability-adjusted life years (DALYs) lost.[2]

A common misconception is that NCDs, by conventional or inclusive definition, are "diseases of affluence." To the contrary, about 80% of NCDs

occur in low- and middle-income countries, and many of them are more prevalent among the lower-socioeconomic-status groups within countries. The greatest driver of the increases in the number of people with NCDs is the increasing proportion of the populations that are living into later life. Age-specific rates of many of these diseases are falling,[2] presumably owing to declining risk-factor prevalence and/or improved access to treatments. At the same time, the absolute number of cases is increasing owing to longer life expectancies and the "bulge" of older people as population pyramids invert. Years of life lived with disability are increasing as non-fatal causes of disability-adjusted life-years (DALYs) lost become more common, and fatal causes decline.[2] Behind these global generalizations are very large differences in regional disease and disability rates, reflecting great heterogeneity of epidemiological, demographic, and sociocultural circumstances.

In this section, we have adopted a broadly inclusive definition of NCDs. We begin with a piece by Riboli and Ezzati that, in accordance with the classic, narrower construct of NCDs, examines the geographic distribution and temporal changes in risk factors that substantially determine the prevalence and incidence of cancers, cardiovascular disease, strokes and diabetes. The impact of these NCDs along with strategies for prevention and control is reviewed by Hunter and Reddy. Jha and Peto consider approaches to the single greatest environmental cause of morbidity and mortality from cancers, cardiovascular disease, and stroke—cigarette smoking—with a focus on policy interventions to reduce cigarette consumption. For those who live in North America, Australia, and the United Kingdom, it is easy to assume that the corner has been turned on tobacco consumption, but the number of cigarettes produced worldwide annually is still increasing. If the 20th century was the "tobacco century" in the United States,[3] then the 21st century will see a global reprise of that phenomenon. Approximately 100 million deaths were caused by tobacco in the 20th century. On the basis of current trends, 1 billion tobacco-related deaths will occur in the present century.

Also often underestimated is the mortality and morbidity due to injuries, responsible for about 10% of deaths and 11% of DALYs lost in 2010,[1,2] as discussed by Norton and Kobusingye. Over 20 years, from 1990 to 2010, road injury deaths are estimated to have increased by 46%, most notably in low- and middle-income countries with rapidly increasing numbers of motor vehicles but poor roads and little emergency response infrastructure. Road traffic injuries are the leading cause of death among men in the 15- to 24-year age group, and the highest mortality rate is in Sub-Saharan Africa.

The rise in absolute numbers of people with NCDs, however defined, has substantial implications for the design and management of health systems, the subject of the next section of this book.

References

1. Lozano R, Naghavi M, Foreman K, et al. (2012). Global and regional mortality from 235 causes of death for 20 age groups in 1990 and 2010: a systematic analysis for the Global Burden of Disease Study 2010. *Lancet* 380(9859):2095–2128.
2. Murray CJ, Vos T, Lozano R, et al. (2012). Disability-adjusted life years (DALYs) for 291 diseases and injuries in 21 regions, 1990-2010: a systematic analysis for the Global Burden of Disease Study 2010. *Lancet* 380(9859):2197–2223.
3. Brandt AM (2007). *The cigarette century: the rise, fall, and deadly persistence of the product that defined America*. New York, NY: Basic Books.

Behavioral and Dietary Risk Factors for Noncommunicable Diseases

Majid Ezzati and Elio Riboli

Except in eastern Europe and parts of Africa, mortality among adults has declined in most countries for decades.[1] Lower rates of death from infectious diseases were the early driver of this improvement, but there have been subsequent declines in mortality from cardiovascular disease and some cancers.[2,3] There have also been important trends in various cancers[2]—for example, the rise and subsequent decline in lung-cancer incidence and mortality among men in many high-income countries, a decline in stomach-cancer incidence and mortality as economies develop, and the worldwide increase in breast-cancer incidence.

The hazardous effects of behavioral and dietary risk factors on noncommunicable diseases, and the metabolic and physiological conditions that mediate their effects, have been established in prospective cohort studies and randomized trials. This knowledge, together with data from risk-factor surveillance, has helped to establish the mortality and disease burden attributable to risk factors, globally and by region and country.[4-7] There is less information on risk-factor trends, which makes it difficult to assess how they have affected population health in the past or how they may do so in the future.

In this article, we summarize the available data on trends in selected behavioral and dietary risk factors for noncommunicable diseases and examine the effects they have had, or may have in the future, on the health of populations around the world. Risk factors such as smoking, alcohol consumption, excess weight, and dietary factors are responsible for a large share of the global disease burden, directly or through conditions such as high blood pressure and elevated blood glucose and cholesterol levels (Fig. 10.1).[4,5]

Smoking

The hazardous effects of smoking on mortality from cancers and cardiovascular and respiratory diseases have been known for decades. Effects on other globally

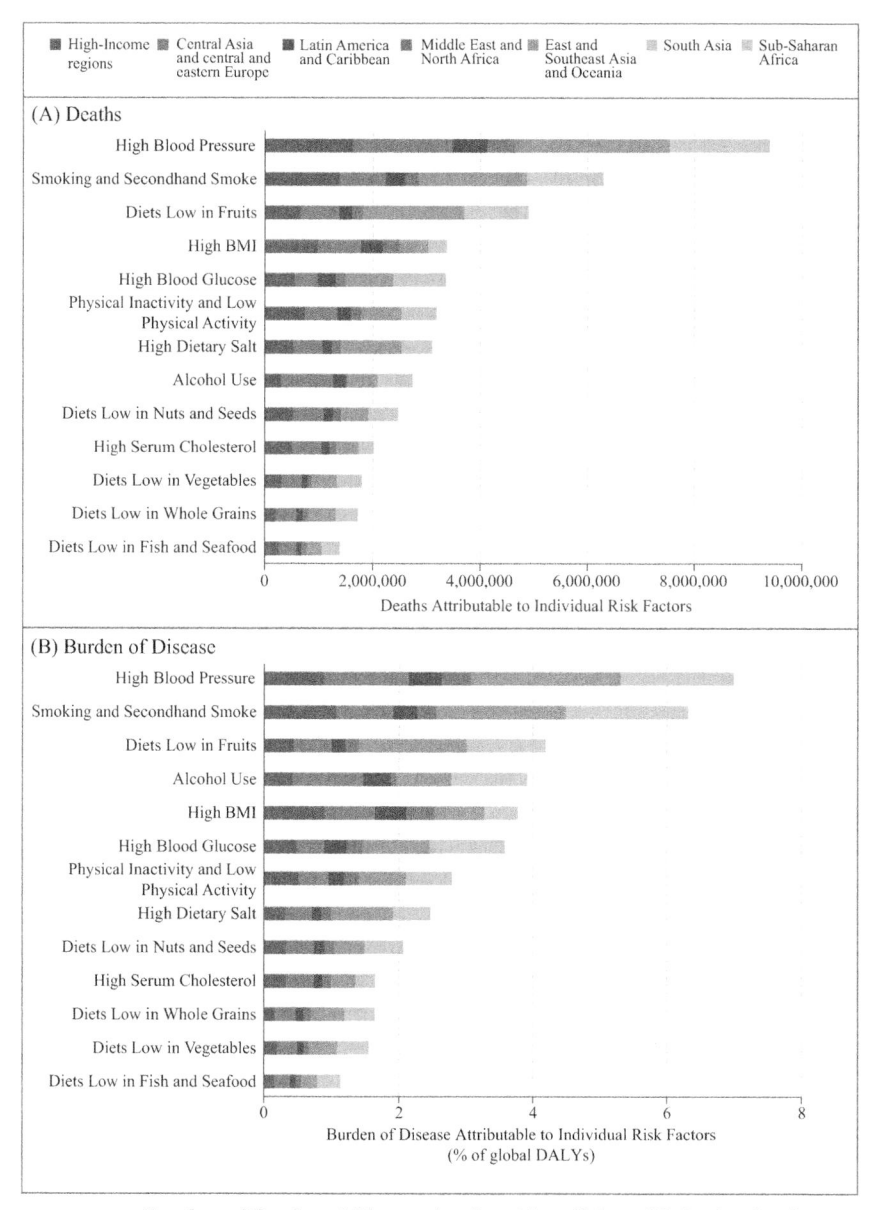

FIGURE 10.1 **Deaths and Burden of Disease Attributable to Selected Behavioral and Dietary Risk Factors in 2010 and the Metabolic and Physiological Mediators of Their Hazardous Effects** *High-income regions are Australasia, the Asia–Pacific region, North America, and western Europe. The figure shows deaths (Panel A) and disease burden (Panel B) attributable to the total effects of each individual risk factor. There is overlap among the effects of risk factors because of multicausality and because the effects of some risk factors (e.g., physical inactivity) are partly mediated through other risk factors (e.g., high body-mass index [BMI]). Therefore, the deaths and disease burden attributable to individual risk factors cannot simply be added together. DALYs denotes disability-adjusted life-years. Data are from Lim et al.[5]*

important diseases such as diabetes[8] and tuberculosis[9] have also been shown. In parallel, evidence of the hazards of smoking in Asian countries has established that it is a global problem.[10–12] Moreover, exposure of pregnant women, children, and nonpregnant adults to secondhand smoke at home and in public places is associated with adverse birth outcomes, childhood respiratory diseases, and many of the same diseases that are associated with active smoking.[13]

In most Western high-income countries, the prevalence of smoking increased among men in the first half of the 20th century and peaked in the post–World War II decades, with 80% of men having smoked at some point in their adult lives. Smoking among men subsequently declined in English-speaking countries and in northern Europe, followed by more than two decades of decline in age-standardized mortality from lung cancer (Fig. 10.2A) and in deaths from other diseases attributable to smoking.[15] The prevalence of smoking among women rose throughout the second half of the 20th century, first in English-speaking countries and northern European countries, then in Japan and countries in Latin America and central and southern Europe. The more recent declines in the United Kingdom, North America, and Australia are beginning to translate into a plateau or decline in lung-cancer mortality (Fig. 10.2B) and in smoking-attributable deaths from other diseases among women.[15] However, lung-cancer mortality continues to rise among continental European women (Fig. 10.2B).

The majority of the more than 1 billion smokers worldwide now live in low- and middle-income countries. The prevalence of smoking has fallen below 20% in Australia and Canada but has plateaued at high levels among men and women in central and eastern Europe, among women in some western and southern European countries, and among men in East Asia (Fig. 10.2C).[14] An estimated 60% of men in some countries in eastern Europe and East Asia smoke. The prevalence of smoking among women is still highest in Western societies, with a prevalence of about 40% in some European countries.[14] The prevalence of smoking remains relatively low in sub-Saharan Africa (Fig. 10.2C), and smokers there tend to smoke fewer cigarettes than do their Western and Asian counterparts.

In addition to shifting patterns of smoking prevalence, there have been changes in the type of cigarettes available, including the introduction of "low-tar" and "light" cigarettes. A recent review concluded that "five decades of evolving cigarette design had not reduced overall disease risk among smokers."[16] Prevention and cessation remain the only effective public health measures to reduce the harmful effects of smoking.

Tobacco smoking and exposure to secondhand smoke together are responsible for about 6.3 million annual deaths worldwide and 6.3% of the global burden of disease, mostly in low- and middle-income countries (Fig. 10.1).[5] The death toll from smoking is especially large in eastern Europe, where the prevalence of smoking and the prevalence of other cardiovascular risk factors are concurrently high; this death toll is increasing in the large populations of Asia and slowly declining in Western countries. In addition to smoking, oral tobacco use and betel-nut chewing are highly prevalent in South Asia and are responsible for a large number of cases of oral cancer and deaths from this disease.[17]

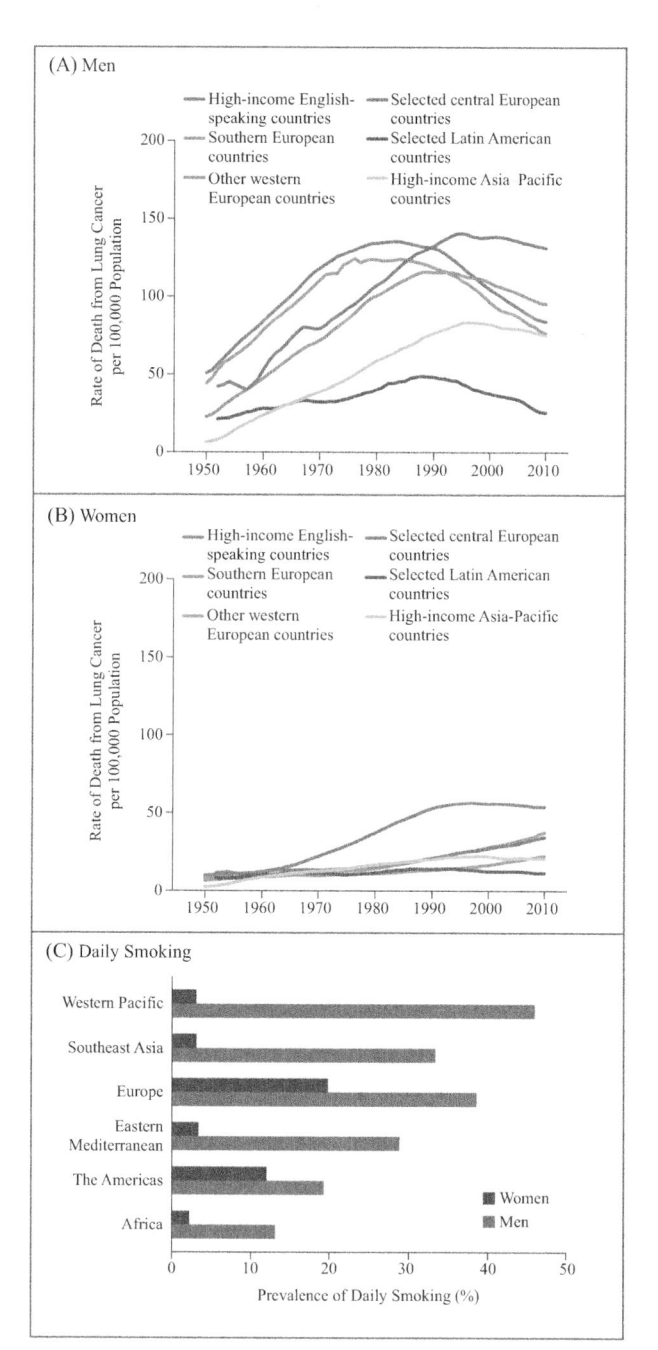

FIGURE 10.2 **Trends in Lung-Cancer Mortality and Prevalence of Daily Tobacco Smoking in 2008** *Panels A and B show trends in age-standardized mortality from lung cancer among men and women, respectively, 30 years of age or older. Death rates are age-standardized to the World Health Organization (WHO) standard population. Data are from the WHO database of vital statistics, with adjustment for completeness of death registration and for validity and comparability of cause-of-death assignment. Panel C shows the age-standardized prevalence of daily tobacco smoking among adults in 2008, according to WHO region. Data are from the WHO.[14]*

Alcohol Consumption

Alcohol consumption is associated with numerous diseases and injuries. Moderate alcohol consumption has been inversely associated with the risk of cardiovascular diseases and diabetes, although the benefits may be greater for persons with existing cardiovascular risk factors than for those without such risk factors.[18] Epidemiologic studies that have measured both the amount and patterns of alcohol consumption have shown that heavy episodic (or binge) drinking not only substantially raises the risk of injuries but can also increase the risk of or exacerbate cardiovascular disease and liver disease.[19–21]

Although cultural factors are important determinants of alcohol consumption, including harmful drinking, social change and policy interventions have modified alcohol-drinking behaviors in some countries.[22,23] For example, per capita alcohol consumption has decreased by about one half in traditional wine-producing and wine-drinking countries such as Italy and France during the past few decades[22,23]; during the same period, it has doubled in the United Kingdom and Denmark, and levels of consumption in the two groups of countries have converged (Fig. 10.3). Alcohol consumption has increased steadily in Japan, China, and many other countries in Asia, where it was previously low.

Alcohol consumption is responsible for about 2.7 million annual deaths and 3.9% of the global burden of disease (Fig. 10.1).[5] The major contributors to the alcohol-attributable disease burden are cancers, chronic liver disease, unintentional injuries, alcohol-related violence, neuropsychiatric conditions, and, in some regions (especially eastern Europe) that have a high prevalence of binge and harmful drinking, a large death toll from cardiovascular diseases.[4,5,24,25] The role of alcohol consumption in injuries and violence among young adults and in nonfatal neuropsychiatric conditions makes its contribution to the disease burden larger than its contribution to mortality, relative to other risk factors for noncommunicable diseases (Fig. 10.1).

Alcohol consumption is the leading single cause of the disease burden in eastern Europe and is one of the top three risk factors, along with high blood pressure and overweight or obesity, in much of Latin America, where it ranks ahead of smoking.[4,5,7] The effects of alcohol on population health are greatest in Russia and some other former Soviet republics. Though recorded per capita alcohol consumption in Russia is the same as or only slightly higher than consumption in western European countries, the health effects are substantially larger. In traditional wine-producing countries, most alcohol is consumed as wine during meals, in relatively modest daily amounts, by a large proportion of the population. In contrast, in Russia and neighboring countries, men (especially those of low socio-economic status) consume very large amounts of spirits, either as a regular daily habit or by binge drinking. A substantial proportion of consumed alcohol is from unrecorded and nonbeverage sources such as medicinal and industrial ethanol. Alcohol consumption may be responsible for one third to one half of deaths among young and middle-aged men in Russia.[24,26] In contrast to the current, enormous death toll, mortality declined temporarily in the 1980s,

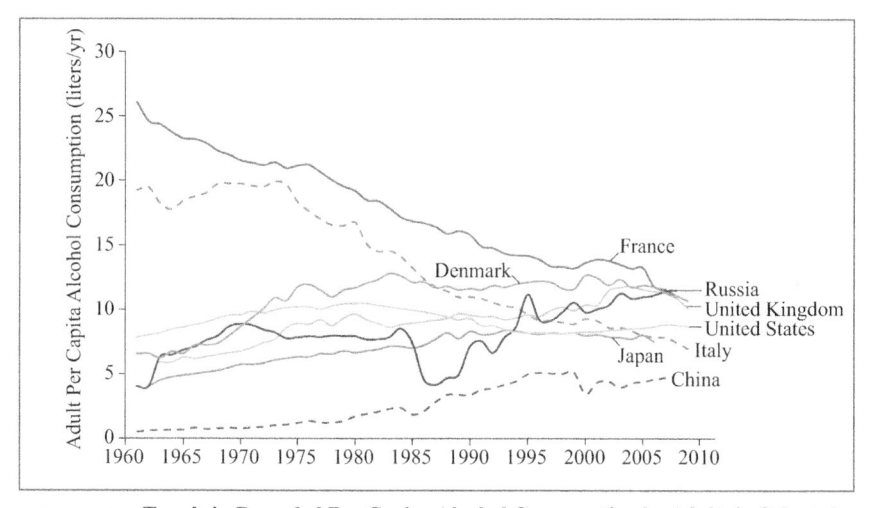

FIGURE 10.3 **Trends in Recorded Per Capita Alcohol Consumption by Adults in Selected Countries** *In addition to recorded consumption, there is unrecorded consumption in some countries. For example, in 2005, adult per capita unrecorded consumption was estimated to be less than 0.5 liters per year in Japan and France; 1 to 2 liters per year in China, the United Kingdom, and the United States; and close to 5 liters per year in Russia. Data are from the WHO Global Information System on Alcohol and Health (http://apps.who.int/gho/data/node.main.GISAH).*

when policies introduced under Mikhail Gorbachev reduced alcohol consumption by about one half (Fig. 10.3).[25]

Excess Weight and Obesity

Numerous observational studies in Western and Asian populations have associated different measures of adiposity and excess body weight with increased total mortality and increased risks of disease or death from diabetes, ischemic heart disease and ischemic stroke, cancers, chronic kidney disease, and osteoarthritis.[27-32] The risks of diabetes and ischemic heart disease increase monotonically with an increase in the body-mass index (BMI, the weight in kilograms divided by the square of the height in meters), starting at a BMI in the low 20s. In contrast, the association with hemorrhagic stroke, which is more common in Asian populations than in other populations, has been observed only at a BMI of 25 or higher.[27,31] Currently, excess weight is responsible for about 3.4 million annual deaths and 3.8% of the global burden of disease, with diseases that have low mortality and long periods of disability, such as diabetes and musculoskeletal diseases, accounting for a proportion of this burden (Fig. 10.1).[5]

In recent decades, men and women in all but a few countries have gained weight, with the age-standardized mean BMI increasing by more than 2 units per decade in some Pacific islands (Fig. S1 in the Supplementary Appendix, available

at NEJM.org). In high-income regions, the BMI is higher in English-speaking countries than in continental Europe and the Asia–Pacific region, especially for women. The global prevalence of obesity (defined as a BMI ≥30) doubled between 1980 and 2008, to 9.8% among men and 13.8% among women—equivalent to more than half a billion obese people worldwide (205 million men and 297 million women) (Fig. 10.4).[33,34] An additional 950 million adults have a BMI of 25 to less than 30. The United States has had the largest absolute increase in the number of obese people since 1980, followed by China, Brazil, and Mexico.[33] Currently, the age-standardized mean BMI ranges from less than 22 in parts of sub-Saharan Africa and Asia to 30 to 35 in some Pacific islands and countries in the Middle East and North Africa.[34] The prevalence of obesity ranges from less than 2% in Bangladesh to more than 60% in some Pacific islands.[33]

Diet and Nutrition

Centuries after the effects of specific dietary intakes on conditions such as scurvy were discovered, nutritional epidemiology has established the associations of specific foods and nutrients or overall dietary patterns with cancers, cardiovascular diseases, and diabetes[35,36] and with intermediate outcomes such as weight gain, increased blood pressure, and insulin resistance and hyperglycemia.[37–39] The large body of observational studies is increasingly complemented

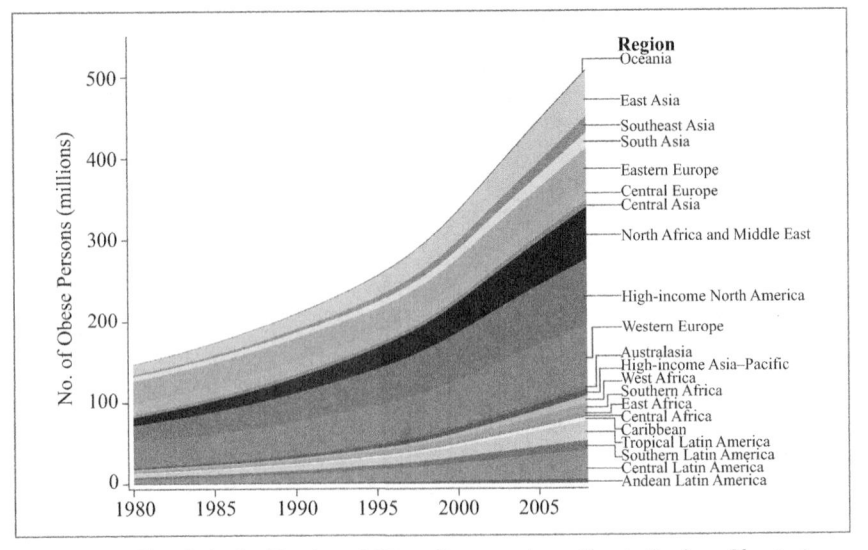

FIGURE 10.4 **Trends in the Number of Obese Persons, According to Region** *Obesity is defined as a BMI of 30 or higher. High-income North America includes Canada and the United States; high-income Asia–Pacific includes Brunei, Japan, Singapore, and South Korea. See Figure S1 in the Supplementary Appendix, available at NEJM.org, for the rise in BMI by country. Data are from Stevens et al.[33]*

by well-designed randomized trials that have, for example, shown the benefits of lower salt intake, the replacement of saturated fats with polyunsaturated fats, and healthy dietary patterns.[37,38,40,41] Low dietary intakes of fruits, vegetables, whole grains, or nuts and seeds or a high dietary intake of salt are individually responsible for 1.5% to more than 4% of the global disease burden (Fig. 10.1).[5]

There have so far been few population-based analyses of trends in specific dietary risk factors. Administrative data, such as the United Nations Food and Agriculture Organization (FAO) food balance sheets, provide a broad picture of dietary patterns and trends based on the availability of different food types for human consumption. FAO data show that consumption of animal fats and high-calorie foods is increasing in Mediterranean countries, such as Greece, but declining slightly in Nordic countries and New Zealand,[42] with consumption in these countries converging at similar levels (Fig. 10.5A). These changes may also partly explain trends in serum cholesterol levels, which have declined more rapidly in Nordic countries and New Zealand than in southern Europe, with cholesterol levels now lower in Sweden and Finland than in Italy.[45] Dietary change has been even more drastic in parts of Asia, with China rapidly adopting a Western, animal-based diet (Fig. 10.5A) and having one of the largest worldwide increases in serum cholesterol levels.[45]

Parallel to this westernization trend, fruits, vegetables, nuts, and cereals have become more available in Nordic and English-speaking Western countries and in Asia, partly because technological and economic developments have increased year-around availability through expanded production, imports, and storage capacity (Fig. 10.5B). Similarly, there has been a modest increase in the availability of fish and other marine products in some Western and Asian countries (Fig. 10.5C).

The FAO data, which are based on agricultural production and trade statistics, do not capture food waste or subsistence production, nor do they account for food processing. For example, these data do not include specific information about consumption of refined flour versus whole grains, sugar-sweetened beverages, and partially hydrogenated vegetables oils (and hence trans-fat consumption), all of which are important dietary risk factors. The FAO databases also do not record consumption of salt, which is common in the diets of countries at all stages of economic development.[46] A high intake of salt is a risk factor for stomach cancer and also for elevated blood pressure, which in turn increases the risk of stroke, other cardiovascular diseases, chronic kidney disease, and kidney cancer. A decrease in dietary salt in Japan and Finland, countries in which salt intake was previously more than 20 g per day in some areas, has been associated with a decline in rates of stomach cancer and hemorrhagic stroke.[47,48]

Physical Activity

Studies of the beneficial health effects of physical activity date back to the 1950s[49] and have been replicated in large cohorts.[50] Physical activity at work, walking, and, in some populations, bicycling used to be major contributors to total energy

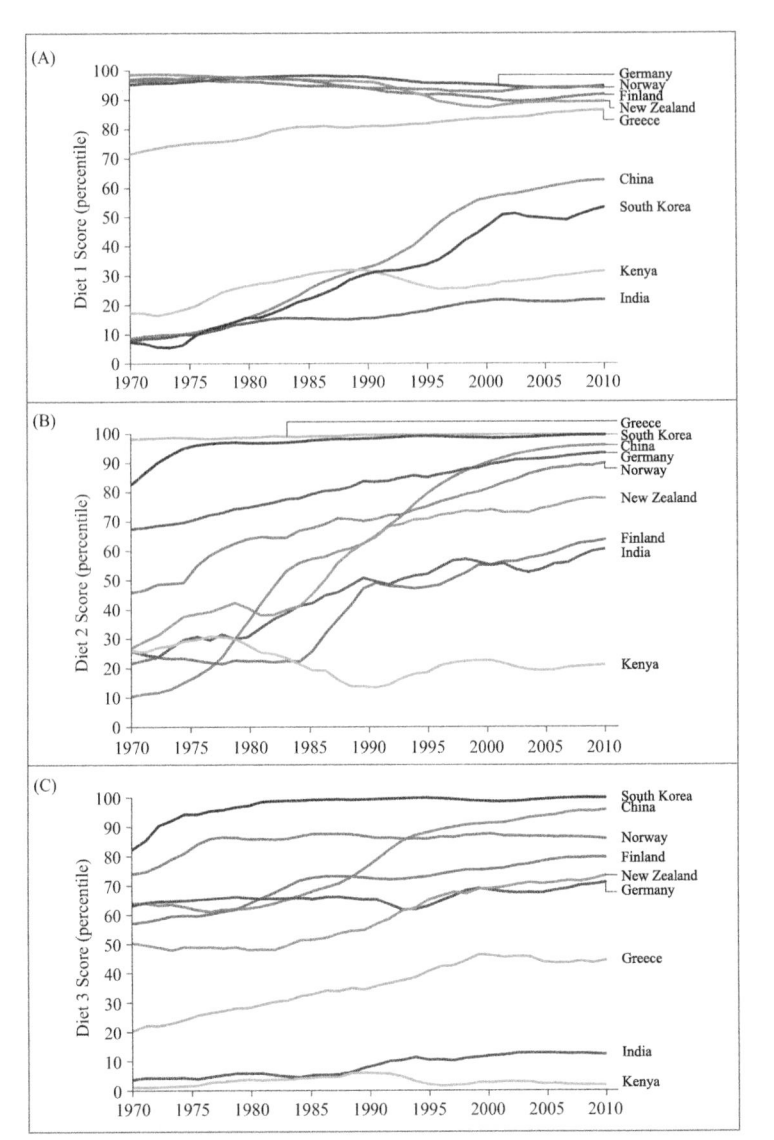

FIGURE 10.5 **Trends in Composite Dietary Scores in Selected Countries** *Each dietary score is a composite indicator that captures the availability of 21 food types in the United Nations Food and Agriculture Organization food balance sheets. A high Diet 1 score (Panel A) indicates a high availability of sugars; meat, animal products, animal fats, milk, and eggs; and total calories, as well as a low availability of pulses (legumes) and cereals. A high Diet 2 score (Panel B) indicates a high availability of nuts; fruits, vegetables, and vegetable oils; cereals; and total calories. A high Diet 3 score (Panel C) indicates a high availability of fish, aquatic products, and oil crops (e.g., soybeans, coconuts, and olives) and a relatively low availability of milk and pulses. Scores were calculated with the use of principal-component analysis, an approach that aggregates food types on the basis of the degree of correlation to each other within the data set.[43,44] Because principal components do not have a directly interpretable scale, we used percentiles of values (smoothed using a 5-year moving average) for presentation. The re-scaled values therefore range from 0% (lowest value observed in any country in the world between 1970 and 2009) to 100% (highest value observed in any country in the world between 1970 and 2009).*

expenditure but have declined dramatically in industrial and urban societies. Paralleling this shift, more recent epidemiologic studies in high-income countries have focused on leisure-time activity, with less emphasis on work and methods of local transportation, which are important in developing countries.[51] Only recently has attention been given to population-based measurement of physical activity in countries at all stages of urbanization and economic development. The limited available global data nonetheless show low levels of activity and long periods in sedentary conditions in high-income and urbanized countries and higher activity levels in rural populations that engage in agricultural activity and walk or bicycle long distances for daily activities.

The Global Risk-Factor Transition

Thus far, the epidemiologic transition has been viewed as a process through which the share of noncommunicable diseases as causes of death increases with declining mortality and rising longevity. As population-based data on medical causes of death and, more recently, on risk factors have become available, a more complete picture of the epidemiologic transition is emerging—one in which the interplay among risk factors and medical care leads to distinct disease patterns in different populations, with variations even among noncommunicable diseases.[2] Despite this diversity, an increasingly salient feature of risk-factor transitions is that many behavioral and dietary risks, and their metabolic and physiological mediators, that have been prominent in high-income countries are now at the same or higher levels in low- and middle-income countries.[44] This pattern parallels the higher prevalence of most risk factors and higher mortality from noncommunicable diseases in lower socioeconomic groups than in higher socioeconomic groups within high-income countries.[52]

Knowledge of risk-factor trends provides a more complete picture of the epidemiologic transition as well as lessons for how the risk factors can be reduced and managed in countries at all levels of economic development, with the use of various preventive strategies.[2] From a public health perspective, smoking is currently the most policy-responsive behavioral risk factor, with major successes in tobacco control in a number of high- and middle-income countries but with a shifting burden to low- and middle-income nations. Harmful alcohol consumption has been curbed in some Western countries but remains a major public health burden or is even worsening in others, especially in eastern Europe and Latin America.[25] Curbing its current harms and preventing its rise in Asia and other developing regions with the use of interventions known to be effective[2] should be a priority.

Although dietary patterns are shaped by cultural, environmental, technological, and economic factors, they can also be modified through mechanisms that range from broad food and agricultural policies to targeted pricing and regulatory interventions related to specific harmful or beneficial dietary components. Such mechanisms are reviewed elsewhere.[2,53]

The availability of population-based and personal interventions for tobacco smoking, excessive alcohol consumption, and elevated blood pressure or lipid levels has made overweight, obesity, and high blood glucose levels the wild cards of noncommunicable-disease risks globally. Some have argued that the obesity epidemic may reverse life-expectancy gains in high-income nations.[54] At the same time, blood pressure and cholesterol levels, which partially mediate the hazardous effects of excess weight on cardiovascular diseases, have declined in most high-income countries and in parts of Latin America.[43,45] This has probably helped dampen or delay the effects of weight gain on cardiovascular diseases, which have declined impressively in industrialized countries.[55] However, there are currently few effective measures against the harms of overweight and obesity with respect to hyperglycemia, diabetes, and cancers, making the concurrent epidemic of diabetes a global health challenge.[56] Randomized trials of dietary changes (in some cases combined with exercise) have shown moderate weight-loss benefits for up to 2 years,[57] but the long-term and large-scale community effectiveness of such interventions has not been established.[58] Similarly, studies have modeled or qualitatively assessed the potential benefits of physical-activity interventions,[59] but the empirical evidence of their effectiveness at the population level remains limited. As a result, policy options and recommendations for weight control[60] and increased physical activity remain broad and untested but are needed to avoid a slowdown or even reversal of the progress in mortality reduction.[2]

Although the behaviors of individuals are important factors in the patterns of risk factors for noncommunicable diseases, successful efforts to reduce smoking, alcohol consumption, and, more recently, trans-fat and salt consumption show that there is great scope for collective action through policy formulation and implementation.[2] Successful policies, such as tobacco and alcohol taxes and restrictions, should be replicated in all populations. There is also a need for bold and creative policies that address harmful alcohol consumption, improve diet, and increase physical activity.

We thank Alexandra Fleischmann, Colin Mathers, Vladimir Poznyak, Jürgen Rehm, Robin Room, Gitanjali Singh, and Gretchen Stevens for data sources and advice on references; and Mariachiara Di Cesare, Jessica Ho, Yuan Lu, and Anne-Claire Vergnaud for assistance with figures.

References

1. Wang H, Dwyer-Lindgren L, Lofgren KT, et al. Age-specific and sex-specific mortality in 187 countries, 1970-2010: a systematic analysis for the Global Burden of Disease Study 2010. Lancet 2012;380:2071–94.

2. Ezzati M, Riboli E. Can noncommunicable diseases be prevented? Lessons from studies of populations and individuals. Science 2012;337:1482–87.

3. Lozano R, Naghavi M, Foreman K, et al. Global and regional mortality from 235 causes of death for 20 age groups in 1990 and 2010: a systematic analysis for the Global Burden of Disease Study 2010. Lancet 2012;380:2095–128.

4. Ezzati M, Lopez AD, Rodgers A, Vander Hoorn S, Murray CJ. Selected major risk factors and global and regional burden of disease. Lancet 2002;360:1347–60.

5. Lim SS, Vos T, Flaxman AD, et al. A comparative risk assessment of burden of disease and injury attributable to 67 risk factors and risk factor clusters in 21 regions, 1990-2010: a systematic analysis for the Global Burden of Disease Study 2010. Lancet 2012;380:2224–60. [Erratum, Lancet 2013;381:1276.]

6. Danaei G, Ding EL, Mozaffarian D, et al. The preventable causes of death in the United States: comparative risk assessment of dietary, lifestyle, and metabolic risk factors. PLoS Med 2009;6(4):e1000058.

7. Stevens G, Dias RH, Thomas KJ, et al. Characterizing the epidemiological transition in Mexico: national and subnational burden of diseases, injuries, and risk factors. PLoS Med 2008;5(6):e125.

8. Willi C, Bodenmann P, Ghali WA, Faris PD, Cornuz J. Active smoking and the risk of type 2 diabetes: a systematic review and meta-analysis. JAMA 2007;298:2654–64.

9. Lin HH, Ezzati M, Murray M. Tobacco smoke, indoor air pollution and tuberculosis: a systematic review and meta-analysis. PLoS Med 2007;4(1):e20.

10. Gu D, Kelly TN, Wu X, et al. Mortality attributable to smoking in China. N Engl J Med 2009;360:150–59. [Erratum, N Engl J Med 2010;363:2272.]

11. Nakamura K, Huxley R, Ansary-Moghaddam A, Woodward M. The hazards and benefits associated with smoking and smoking cessation in Asia: a meta-analysis of prospective studies. Tob Control 2009;18:345–53.

12. Jha P, Jacob B, Gajalakshmi V, et al. A nationally representative case–control study of smoking and death in India. N Engl J Med 2008;358:1137–47.

13. Department of Health and Human Services. The health consequences of involuntary exposure to tobacco smoke: a report of the Surgeon General. Atlanta: National Center for Chronic Disease Prevention and Health Promotion, Office on Smoking and Health, 2006. (DHHS publication no. [CDC] 89-8411.)

14. Global status report on noncommunicable diseases 2010. Geneva: World Health Organization, 2011.

15. Thun M, Peto R, Boreham J, Lopez AD. Stages of the cigarette epidemic on entering its second century. Tob Control 2012;21:96–101.

16. Department of Health and Human Services. A report of the Surgeon General: how tobacco smoke causes disease: the biology and behavioral basis for smoking-attributable disease. Atlanta: National Center for Chronic Disease Prevention and Health Promotion, Office on Smoking and Health, 2010. (DHHS publication no. [CDC] 89-8411.)

17. Secretan B, Straif K, Baan R, et al. A review of human carcinogens—Part E: tobacco, areca nut, alcohol, coal smoke, and salted fish. Lancet Oncol 2009;10:1033–34.

18. Roerecke M, Rehm J. The cardioprotective association of average alcohol consumption and ischaemic heart disease: a systematic review and meta-analysis. Addiction 2012;107:1246–60.

19. Mathurin P, Deltenre P. Effect of binge drinking on the liver: an alarming public health issue? Gut 2009;58:613–17.

20. Rehm J, Baliunas D, Borges GL, et al. The relation between different dimensions of alcohol consumption and burden of disease: an overview. Addiction 2010;105:817–43.

21. Roerecke M, Rehm J. Irregular heavy drinking occasions and risk of ischemic heart disease: a systematic review and meta-analysis. Am J Epidemiol 2010;171:633–44.

22. Allamani A, Prina F. Why the decrease in consumption of alcoholic beverages in Italy between the 1970s and the 2000s? Shedding light on an Italian mystery. Contemp Drug Probl 2007;34:187–97.

23. Cipriani F, Prina F. The research outcome: summary and conclusions on the reduction in wine consumption in Italy. Contemp Drug Probl 2007;34:361–78.

24. Zaridze D, Brennan P, Boreham J, et al. Alcohol and cause-specific mortality in Russia: a retrospective case-control study of 48,557 adult deaths. Lancet 2009;373:2201–14.

25. Leon DA, Chenet L, Shkolnikov VM, et al. Huge variation in Russian mortality rates 1984-94: artefact, alcohol, or what? Lancet 1997;350:383–88.

26. Leon DA, Shkolnikov VM, McKee M. Alcohol and Russian mortality: a continuing crisis. Addiction 2009;104:1630–36.

27. Whitlock G, Lewington S, Sherliker P, et al. Body-mass index and cause-specific mortality in 900 000 adults: collaborative analyses of 57 prospective studies. Lancet 2009;373:1083–96.

28. Wormser D, Kaptoge S, Di Angelantonio E, et al. Separate and combined associations of body-mass index and abdominal adiposity with cardiovascular disease: collaborative analysis of 58 prospective studies. Lancet 2011;377:1085–95.

29. Renehan AG, Tyson M, Egger M, Heller RF, Zwahlen M. Body-mass index and incidence of cancer: a systematic review and meta-analysis of prospective observational studies. Lancet 2008;371:569–78.

30. Ni Mhurchu C, Parag V, Nakamura M, Patel A, Rodgers A, Lam TH. Body mass index and risk of diabetes mellitus in the Asia-Pacific region. Asia Pac J Clin Nutr 2006;15:127–33.

31. Ni Mhurchu C, Rodgers A, Pan WH, Gu DF, Woodward M. Body mass index and cardiovascular disease in the Asia-Pacific Region: an overview of 33 cohorts involving 310 000 participants. Int J Epidemiol 2004;33:751–58.

32. Pischon T, Boeing H, Hoffmann K, et al. General and abdominal adiposity and risk of death in Europe. N Engl J Med 2008;359:2105–20. [Erratum, N Engl J Med 2010;362:2433.]

33. Stevens GA, Singh GM, Lu Y, et al. National, regional, and global trends in adult overweight and obesity prevalences. Popul Health Metr 2012;10:22.

34. Finucane MM, Stevens GA, Cowan MJ, et al. National, regional, and global trends in body-mass index since 1980: systematic analysis of health examination surveys and epidemiological studies with 960 country-years and 9.1 million participants. Lancet 2011;377:557–67.

35. Food, nutrition, physical activity, and the prevention of cancer: a global perspective. Washington, DC: American Institute for Cancer Research, 2007.

36. Mozaffarian D, Appel LJ, Van Horn L. Components of a cardioprotective diet: new insights. Circulation 2011;123:2870–91.

37. He FJ, Li J, Macgregor GA. Effect of longer term modest salt reduction on blood pressure: Cochrane systematic review and meta-analysis of randomised -trials. BMJ 2013;346:f1325.

38. Sacks FM, Bray GA, Carey VJ, et al. Comparison of weight-loss diets with different compositions of fat, protein, and carbohydrates. N Engl J Med 2009;360:859–73.

39. Mozaffarian D, Hao T, Rimm EB, Willett WC, Hu FB. Changes in diet and lifestyle and long-term weight gain in women and men. N Engl J Med 2011;364:2392–404.

40. Mozaffarian D, Micha R, Wallace S. Effects on coronary heart disease of increasing polyunsaturated fat in place of saturated fat: a systematic review and meta-analysis of randomized controlled trials. PLoS Med 2010;(3)7:e1000252.

41. Estruch R, Ros E, Salas-Salvadó J, et al. Primary prevention of cardiovascular disease with a Mediterranean diet. N Engl J Med 2013;368:1279–90.

42. Puska P, Stahl T. Health in All Policies—the Finnish initiative: background, principles, and current issues. Annu Rev Public Health 2010;31:315–28.

43. Danaei G, Finucane MM, Lin JK, et al. National, regional, and global trends in systolic blood pressure since 1980: systematic analysis of health examination surveys and epidemiological studies with 786 country-years and 5.4 million participants. Lancet 2011;377:568–77.

44. Danaei G, Singh GM, Paciorek CJ, et al. The global cardiovascular risk transition: associations of four metabolic risk factors with national income, urbanization, and Western diet in 1980 and 2008. Circulation 2013;127:1493–502.

45. Farzadfar F, Finucane MM, Danaei G, et al. National, regional, and global trends in serum total cholesterol since 1980: systematic analysis of health examination surveys and epidemiological studies with 321 country-years and 3.0 million participants. Lancet 2011;377:578–86.

46. Asaria P, Chisholm D, Mathers C, Ezzati M, Beaglehole R. Chronic disease prevention: health effects and financial costs of strategies to reduce salt intake and -control tobacco use. Lancet 2007;370:2044–53. [Erratum, Lancet 2007;370:2004.]

47. Hirayama T. Epidemiology of stomach cancer in Japan: with special reference to the strategy for the primary prevention. Jpn J Clin Oncol 1984;14:159–68.

48. Tuomilehto J, Geboers J, Joossens JV, Salonen JT, Tanskanen A. Trends in stomach cancer and stroke in Finland: comparison to northwest Europe and USA. Stroke 1984;15:823–28.

49. Morris JN, Heady JA, Raffle PA, Roberts CG, Parks JW. Coronary heart-disease and physical activity of work. Lancet 1953;265:1053–57.

50. Sattelmair J, Pertman J, Ding EL, Kohl HW III, Haskell W, Lee IM. Dose response between physical activity and risk of coronary heart disease: a meta-analysis. Circulation 2011;124:789–95.

51. Levine JA, Weisell R, Chevassus S, Martinez CD, Burlingame B, Coward WA. The work burden of women. Science 2001;294:812.

52. Di Cesare M, Khang YH, Asaria P, et al. Inequalities in non-communicable diseases and effective responses. Lancet 2013;381:585–97.

53. Mozaffarian D, Afshin A, Benowitz NL, et al. Population approaches to improve diet, physical activity, and smoking habits: a scientific statement from the American Heart Association. Circulation 2012;126:1514–63.

54. Olshansky SJ, Passaro DJ, Hershow RC, et al. A potential decline in life expectancy in the United States in the 21st century. N Engl J Med 2005;352:1138–45.

55. Di Cesare M, Bennett JE, Best N, Stevens GA, Danaei G, Ezzati M. The contributions of risk factor trends to cardiometabolic mortality decline in 26 indus-trialized countries. Int J Epidemiol 2013;42:838–48.

56. Danaei G, Finucane MM, Lu Y, et al. National, regional, and global trends in fasting plasma glucose and diabetes prevalence since 1980: systematic analysis of

health examination surveys and epidemiological studies with 370 country-years and 2.7 million participants. Lancet 2011;378:31–40.

57. Nordmann AJ, Nordmann A, Briel M, et al. Effects of low-carbohydrate vs low-fat diets on weight loss and cardiovascular risk factors: a meta-analysis of randomized controlled trials. Arch Intern Med 2006;166:285–93. [Erratum, Arch Intern Med 2006;166:932.]

58. Douketis JD, Macie C, Thabane L, Williamson DF. Systematic review of long-term weight loss studies in obese adults: clinical significance and applicability to clinical practice. Int J Obes (Lond) 2005;29:1153–67.

59. Cobiac LJ, Vos T, Barendregt JJ. Cost-effectiveness of interventions to promote physical activity: a modelling study. PLoS Med 2009;6(7):e1000110.

60. Gortmaker SL, Swinburn BA, Levy D, et al. Changing the future of obesity: science, policy, and action. Lancet 2011;378:838–47.

Global Effects of Smoking, of Quitting, and of Taxing Tobacco

Prabhat Jha and Richard Peto

On the basis of current smoking patterns, with a global average of about 50% of young men and 10% of young women becoming smokers and relatively few stopping, annual tobacco-attributable deaths will rise from about 5 million in 2010 to more than 10 million a few decades hence,[1-3] as the young smokers of today reach middle and old age. This increase is due partly to population growth and partly to the fact that, in some large populations, generations in which few people smoked substantial numbers of cigarettes throughout adult life are being succeeded by generations in which many people did so. There were about 100 million deaths from tobacco in the 20th century, most in developed countries.[2,3] If current smoking patterns persist, tobacco will kill about 1 billion people this century, mostly in low- and middle-income countries. About half of these deaths will occur before 70 years of age.[1-4]

The 2013 World Health Assembly called on governments to reduce the prevalence of smoking by about a third by 2025,[5] which would avoid more than 200 million deaths from tobacco during the remainder of the century.[2,3] Price is the key determinant of smoking uptake and cessation.[6-9] Worldwide, a reduction of about a third could be achieved by doubling the inflation-adjusted price of cigarettes, which in many low- and middle-income countries could be achieved by tripling the specific excise tax on tobacco. Other interventions recommended by the World Health Organization (WHO) Framework Convention on Tobacco Control (FCTC) and the WHO six-point MPOWER initiative[4] could also help reduce consumption[7,8] and could help make substantial increases in specific excise taxes on tobacco politically acceptable. Without large price increases, a reduction in smoking by a third would be difficult to achieve.

The WHO has also called for countries to achieve a 25% reduction between 2008 and 2025 in the probability of dying from noncommunicable disease between 30 and 70 years of age.[10] Widespread cessation of smoking is the most important way to help achieve this goal, because smoking throughout adulthood

substantially increases mortality from several major noncommunicable diseases (and from tuberculosis).[1–3,11–19]

To help achieve a large reduction in smoking in the 2010s or 2020s, governments, health professionals, journalists, and other opinion leaders should appreciate the full eventual hazards of smoking cigarettes from early adulthood, the substantial benefits of stopping at various ages, the eventual magnitude of the epidemic of tobacco-attributable deaths if current smoking patterns persist, and the effectiveness of tax increases and other interventions to reduce cigarette consumption.

Three Key Messages for Smokers in the 21st Century

First, the risk is big. Large studies in the United Kingdom, the United States, Japan, and India have examined the eventual effects on mortality in populations of men and of women in which many began to smoke in early adult life and did not quit.[11–16] All these studies showed that in middle age (about 30 to 69 years of age), mortality among cigarette smokers was two to three times the mortality among otherwise similar persons who had never smoked, leading to a reduction in life span by an average of about 10 years (Fig. 11.1). This average reduction combines zero loss for those not killed by tobacco with an average loss of well over a decade for those who are killed by it.

Second, many of those killed are still in middle age, losing many years of life. Some of those killed in middle age might have died soon anyway, but others might have lived on for decades. On average, those killed in middle age by smoking lose about 20 years of life expectancy as compared with persons who have never smoked.[1]

Third, stopping smoking works. Those who have smoked cigarettes since early adulthood but stop at 30, 40, or 50 years of age gain about 10, 9, and 6 years of life expectancy, respectively, as compared with those who continue smoking.

Eventual Hazards of Smoking

Tobacco is the biggest external cause of noncommunicable disease and is responsible for even more deaths than adiposity both in high-income countries such as the United States[20] and globally.[21] The risks in middle age are much greater for smokers who started in early adulthood than for those who started later. This means that the ratio of mortality among smokers to that among persons who have never smoked is much more extreme now (Fig. 11.1, and the 50-year trends shown in the Supplementary Appendix, available at NEJM.org) than it was half a century earlier, when the epidemic of smoking-attributable deaths was at an earlier stage.[11–15]

Cigarette smoking was uncommon throughout the world in 1900, but smoking rates increased substantially in many high-income countries during the first half of the 20th century, first among men and then, in some countries, among

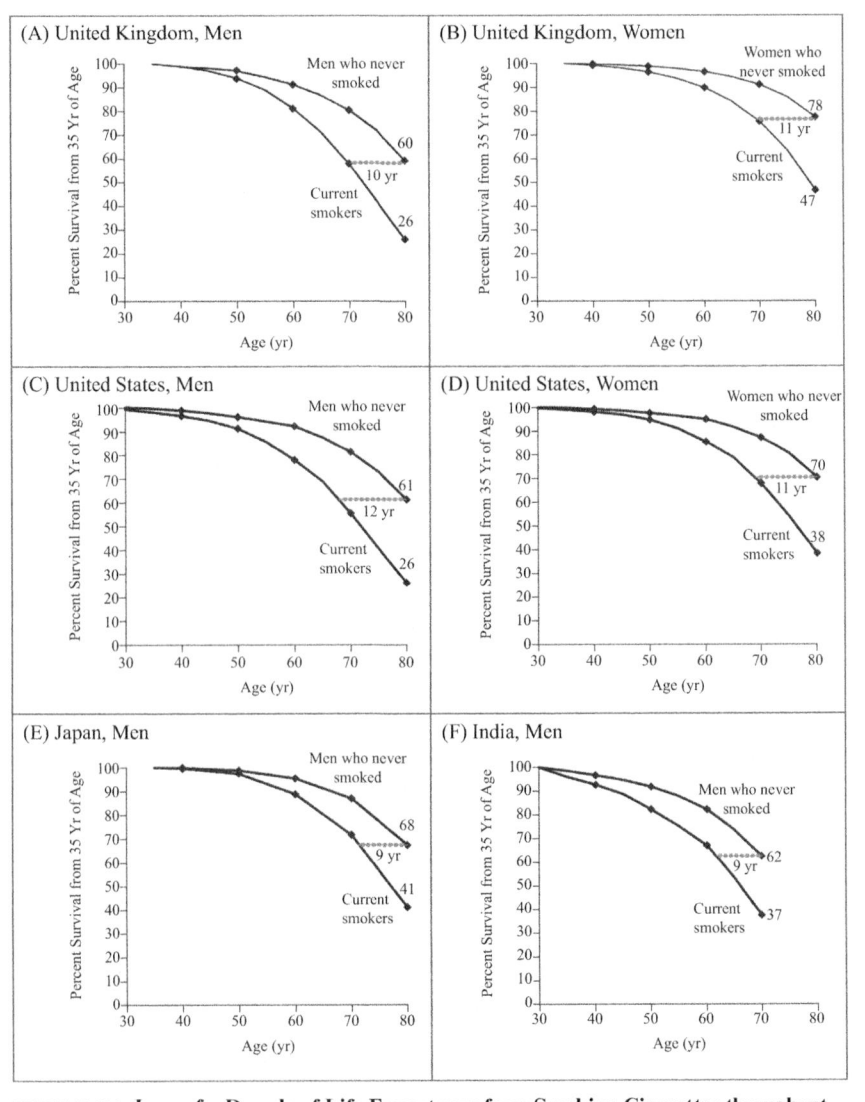

FIGURE 11.1 **Loss of a Decade of Life Expectancy from Smoking Cigarettes throughout Adulthood** *Shown are probabilities of survival from 30 or 35 years of age (current smokers vs. persons who never smoked, linked by dots representing 1 year each) among U.K. men[11] and women,[12] U.S. men and women,[13] Japanese men,[15] and Indian men.[16]*

women.[22] By 1950 in the United States and the United Kingdom, substantial numbers not only of men but also of women smoked, and rates of lung cancer were increasing steeply, particularly among men.[1] In 1950, major studies in both countries[23,24] showed that smoking was a cause of most deaths from lung cancer, and subsequent reports showed that smoking caused even more deaths from other diseases than from lung cancer.[25,26]

After 1950, cigarette consumption continued to rise for some decades in high-income countries, and it has risen among men (though generally not among women) in many low- and middle-income countries. Although there has been widespread cessation in many high-income countries (in some, consumption per adult has been halved since the 1970s),[22] about 1.3 billion people worldwide now smoke, most in low- and middle-income countries where cessation is uncommon.[4] Two thirds of all smokers live (in descending order of numbers of smokers) in China, India, the European Union (in which central tobacco legislation can influence 28 countries), Indonesia, the United States, Russia, Japan, Brazil, Bangladesh, and Pakistan (Table 11.1).[27,28] In India, manufactured cigarettes are now displacing bidis (locally manufactured small cigarettes).[29] Cigarette consumption in China continues to rise steeply and now accounts for more than 2 trillion of a worldwide total of about 6 trillion cigarettes smoked per year.[30] A useful approximation suggested by studies in high-income countries is that 1 ton of tobacco yields about 1 million cigarettes and causes about 1 death, so just 1 trillion cigarettes consumed a year will eventually cause about 1 million deaths a year.

One reason why the mid-century evidence of hazard was not at first taken seriously, even in countries where it was generated, is the delay of about half a century between widespread adoption of smoking by young adults and the main effect on mortality in later life.[1–3] Among all U.S. adults, for example, cigarette consumption averaged 1, 4, and 10 per day in 1910, 1930, and 1950, respectively, after which it stabilized. The long-delayed result of this increase in consumption during the first half of the century was seen only in the second half of the

TABLE 11.1 Current and Former Smokers in Selected Areas, 2008–2012[*]

Region or Country	≥15 Yr of Age		45–64 Yr of Age		
	Current Smokers no. in millions	Former Smokers no. in millions	Current Smokers %	Former Smokers	Stopped Smoking[†]
European Union	115	83	37	36	49
United States	50	54	18	22	55
Japan	28	14	9	5	36
Low- and middle-income countries[‡]					
China	317	42	115	21	15
India	122	15	46	7	13
Indonesia	115	6	17	2	11
Russia	47	10	15	4	21
Brazil	26	21	9	10	53
Bangladesh	25	5	7	2	22

[*]Data are from Giovino et al.[27] and Zatoński and Mańczuk,[28] combined with United Nations population estimates for 2012.

[†]The percentage of persons who have stopped smoking is calculated as former smokers divided by the sum of current smokers and former smokers.

[‡]There are approximately 25 million current smokers in Pakistan[4] but no standardized surveys.[27]

century; tobacco caused about 12% of all U.S. deaths in middle age in 1950 but about 33% of such deaths in 1990.[1] A similar pattern was seen about 40 years later among Chinese men, who consumed about 1, 4, and 10 cigarettes per day in 1952, 1972, and 1992, respectively. In 1990, tobacco caused about 12% of all deaths among middle-aged Chinese men, and it could well cause about 33% in 2030.[31,32] (Tobacco causes few deaths in Chinese women, because less than 1% of Chinese women born in each decade since 1950 smoke.[27,31])

Because men started smoking before women, the effects in middle-aged men are now apparent in most high-income countries. The full eventual effects of persistent smoking in women, however, can be assessed directly in only a few countries (e.g., the United States and the United Kingdom) and only in the present (21st) century. The ratio of mortality from lung cancer among U.S. women who currently smoke to the (constant) mortality among women who have never smoked has increased greatly during the past half-century: it was only 3 in the 1960s, but it was 13 in the 1980s and 26 (similar to that among men) in the 2000s.[14] The reason for the jump from a ratio of 3 to a ratio of 26 is that in the 2000s many U.S. women in their 60s who were smokers had smoked ever since early adulthood, whereas in the 1960s few women in their 60s who were smokers had done so.

Even though mortality from lung cancer among U.S. women was still low in the 1960s, women who were then in their 20s and who continued to smoke without quitting faced substantial hazards 40 years later.[13,14] Similarly, among men in low- and middle-income countries where many smoke but the death rates in middle age from smoking are not yet substantial, a full decade of life expectancy will eventually be lost by young adults who continue to smoke. Tobacco already accounts for about 12 to 25% of deaths among men in low- and middle-income countries such as China,[31,32] India,[16–18] Bangladesh,[33] and South Africa[34]; given current smoking patterns, these proportions are likely to increase. Worldwide, about half a billion of the children and adults younger than 35 years of age already smoke or will do so if current uptake rates persist, and given current cessation patterns, relatively few will quit.[27] In all countries, young adults who smoke face about a decade of life lost if they continue and hence have much to gain by stopping.

Rapid Benefits of Stopping

Whereas tobacco-attributable mortality increases slowly after the uptake of smoking, the effects of cessation emerge more rapidly.[11–15] Persons who began smoking in early adulthood but stopped before 40 years of age avoid more than 90% of the excess risk during their next few decades of life, as compared with those who continue to smoke, and even those who stop at 50 years of age avoid more than half the excess risk, although substantial hazards persist (Fig. 11.2).[11–15]

The ratio of former smokers to current smokers in middle age is a useful measure of the success of tobacco control. Among persons 45 to 64 years of age in

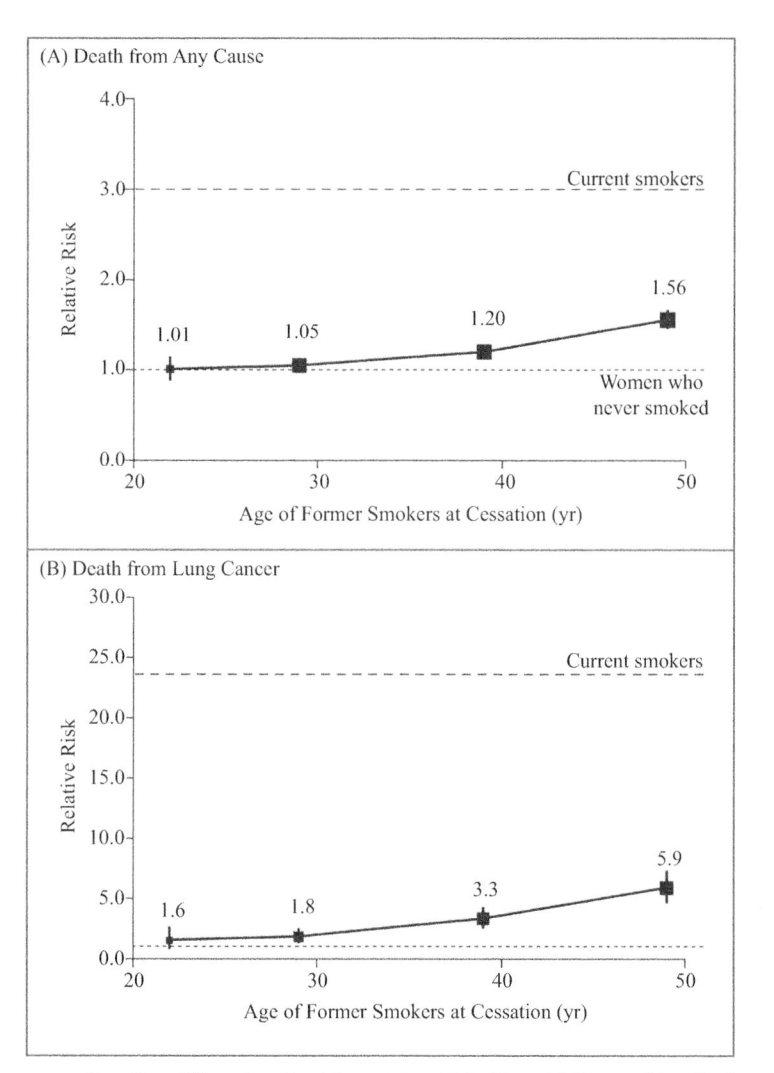

FIGURE 11.2 **Benefits of Stopping Smoking at about 30, 40, or 50 Years of Age in the United Kingdom Million Women Study** *Shown are multivariate-adjusted relative risks of death among former smokers according to age at which they stopped and among current smokers. (Persons who never smoked had a relative risk of 1.0.) Both former smokers and current smokers had on average begun to smoke at 19 years of age, and the number of cigarettes smoked per day was similar in the two groups. Vertical bars represent 95% confidence intervals. Data are from Pirie et al.[12]*

the European Union and the United States, there are now about as many former smokers as current smokers[28,35]; by contrast, in most low- and middle-income countries (with the notable exception of Brazil), there are far fewer former smokers than current smokers (Table 11.1). Cessation is the only practicable way to avoid a substantial proportion of tobacco-attributable deaths before 2050,

because a substantial reduction by 2025 in uptake by adolescents will have its main effect on mortality only after 2050.[2,3]

Effects of Increasing Cigarette Prices

Comprehensive tobacco-control programs using several price and nonprice interventions can substantially raise smoking-cessation rates and decrease initiation of smoking.[4] Uruguay implemented most of the FCTC provisions and reduced consumption more rapidly than otherwise similar Argentina, which implemented only a few of the provisions.[36] Large increases in specific excise taxes on tobacco are particularly important, because they can have a substantial and rapid effect on consumption.[6-9] Reviews of comprehensive control programs in various U.S. states[37,38] and other high-income areas[39] concur that higher prices account for much, but not all, of the decline in smoking.

Similarly, an International Agency for Research on Cancer review of more than 100 econometric studies confirmed that tobacco taxes and consumption are strongly inversely related.[9] It concluded that a 50% increase in inflation-adjusted tobacco prices reduces consumption by about 20% in both high-income countries and low- and middle-income countries,[6-9] corresponding to a price elasticity (percent consumption change per 1% price change) of about −0.4. Hence, doubling inflation-adjusted prices should reduce consumption by about one third (in which case revenues would increase, because the effect of reduced demand would be outweighed by the extra revenue per pack). Some of the effect among adults is due to quitting (or not starting), and some is due to reduced consumption per smoker.[9] Higher taxes are particularly effective in poorer or less educated groups[6-9,39] and help prevent young people who are experimenting with smoking from becoming regular smokers.[40]

The two major types of tobacco tax are specific excise taxes (which, being based on quantity or weight, are difficult for the industry to manipulate) and ad valorem taxes (which are based on manufacturer-defined price and can be manipulated more easily). In many high-income countries, about 50 to 60% of the retail price of the most-sold brand is a specific excise tax on tobacco or some variation of it (as in the European Union), but in low- and middle-income countries, this proportion is typically only about 35 to 40% (Fig. 11.3).[4,6] A low specific excise tax on tobacco is the main reason that cigarettes are about 70% cheaper (even after adjustment for purchasing power) in many low-income countries than in high-income countries. Moreover, rapid income growth in many low- and middle-income countries is making the lower-priced tobacco products more affordable[41] and helping cigarettes to displace bidis in India.[29]

A low reliance on specific excise taxes on tobacco by China,[42] India,[29] Indonesia,[43] and most low- and middle-income countries[4,6] means that the prices of commonly sold cigarette brands vary greatly within each country (by a factor of more than 10 in China, as compared with a factor of only about 2 in

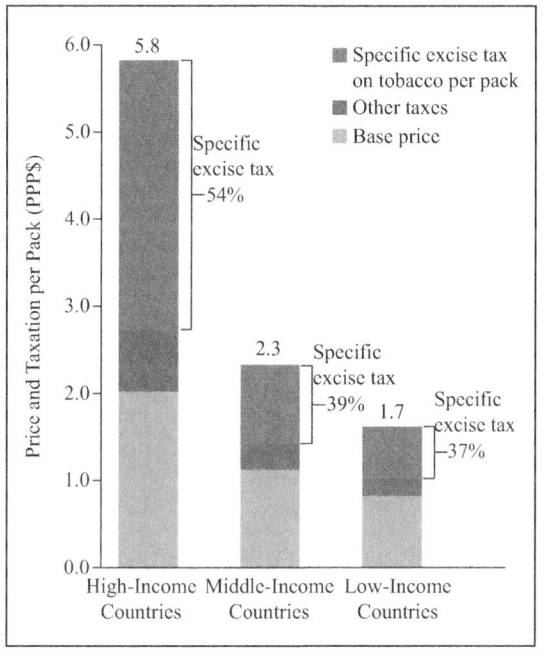

FIGURE 11.3 **Contributions of Specific Excise Taxes on Tobacco and Other Taxes to the Total Cost per Pack of the Most-Sold Brand of Cigarettes in High-, Middle-, and Low-Income Countries** *Prices are expressed in dollars adjusted for purchasing-power parity (PPP). In low- and middle-income countries, tripling specific excise taxes on tobacco would approximately double street prices, because nonexcise taxes (e.g., sales tax) and retailer markup would also rise. In the European Union, more complex variations on specific excise taxes on tobacco are used. Data, which are from the World Health Organization, are for 48 high-income countries, 95 middle-income countries, and 30 low-income countries.*[4]

the United Kingdom and the United States), and this continued availability of low-cost brands discourages smoking cessation. In contrast, high specific excise taxes on tobacco of all brands encourage cessation rather than switching (by narrowing the price gap between the most and least expensive cigarettes), are easier to administer than ad valorem taxes, and produce a steadier revenue stream.[9] In many low- and middle-income countries, although specific excise taxes on tobacco account for less than half the total retail price of cigarettes, tripling them approximately doubles the retail price, partly by triggering smaller increases in other taxes (e.g., sales tax) and markup. In most high-income countries, specific excise taxes on tobacco already account for more than half the retail price, so even just doubling them would approximately double prices.

The United States and the United Kingdom took more than 30 years to halve cigarette consumption per adult.[22] With the use of large tax increases, however, France and South Africa halved consumption in less than 15 years (Fig. 11.4).[3,44,45] From 1990 to 2005, France tripled inflation-adjusted cigarette prices by raising taxes 5% or more every year in excess of inflation, halved cigarette consumption,

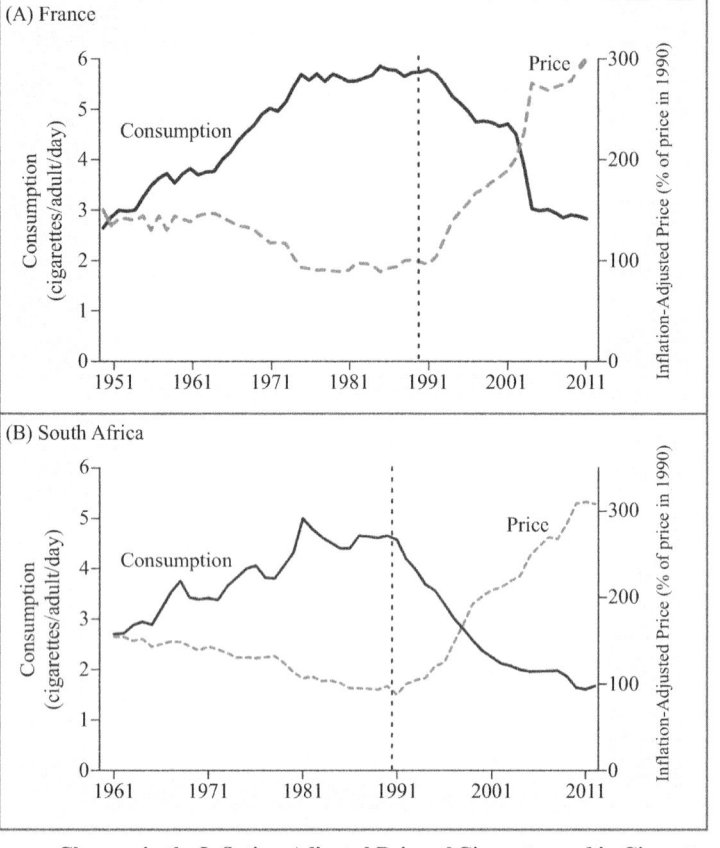

FIGURE 11.4 **Changes in the Inflation-Adjusted Price of Cigarettes and in Cigarette Consumption in France and South Africa** *Prices in both countries are scaled to be 100 in the baseline year of 1990.[44,45] Consumption is expressed as the number of cigarettes per adult per day and takes into account growth in the population.*

and doubled inflation-adjusted tobacco revenues. Today, the ratio of former smokers to current smokers in France comfortably exceeds the European average.[28,35] Over a similar period, South Africa also tripled the inflation-adjusted price of cigarettes, halved cigarette consumption, and doubled tobacco revenues.[45] Additional revenue can be used to fund tobacco-control programs or broader health efforts; much of the revenue from the 2009 U.S. taxation increase of 53 cents per pack of 20 cigarettes is allocated to expand children's health insurance.[46]

Other Effective Interventions

Though tobacco advertising is banned throughout the European Union, China, and some other countries, cigarettes are still among the most heavily advertised and promoted products in the world, with spending on tobacco marketing reaching $8.6 billion annually in the United States alone.[47] In 2011 Australia, which

had already banned advertising, introduced plain packaging for tobacco products, removing all brand imagery. The brand is printed only in small standard lettering below a pictorial warning. Recent evidence suggests that plain packaging increases cessation attempts.[48,49] New Zealand will introduce plain packaging in 2014, and the United Kingdom is considering it. Plain packaging goes beyond the prominent, rotating pictorial warning labels on tobacco products that have helped increase cessation attempts in Canada, Thailand, and elsewhere.[50] Pictorial warnings can reach even illiterate persons, and half the deaths from tobacco in India occur among the illiterate.[29]

In the United States and the United Kingdom, bans on tobacco advertising on television coincided with the start of the long-term downturn in sales,[51] although these partial bans on advertising allowed the industry to shift to other forms of advertising or promotion. More comprehensive bans on all direct and indirect advertising or promotion of any tobacco goods or trademarks further help to reduce consumption[52,53] and have the advantage of severing any dependence of the media on the tobacco industry. Bans on smoking in public places reduce nonsmokers' exposure to tobacco smoke and can also help decrease overall consumption,[54,55] as can mass-media campaigns.[51,56] In populations with many long-term smokers, low-cost epidemiologic studies of various types that monitor the changing extent to which tobacco is causing premature death help to raise political awareness of tobacco hazards and to provide information for the individual smoker.[1,16,33,34]

Throughout the world, most former smokers managed to quit unaided, but physician support or telephone-based or Internet-based counseling and support can increase the likelihood of success.[57] In motivated persons, pharmacologic treatments or electronic cigarettes, or e-cigarettes, can also increase quit rates.[57,58] The eventual role of e-cigarettes remains uncertain, however, particularly if the tobacco industry controls the marketing of both traditional and e-cigarettes.

Death and Taxes

The WHO reports[4] that although many countries now use nonprice interventions, only a few (including Mauritius, Mexico, the Philippines, Poland, and Turkey) have been using large increases in specific excise taxes on tobacco to reduce smoking.[6] A large increase in inflation-adjusted price is, however, a key component of any realistic strategy to reduce smoking substantially during the 2010s or 2020s. The Bill and Melinda Gates Foundation, Bloomberg Philanthropies, the World Bank, and the Asian Development Bank are therefore providing technical advice for some ministries of finance to counter misleading tax advice from the tobacco industry.[29,42,43,59] Manufacturers' worldwide profits of about $50 billion in 2012[60] (approximately $10,000 per tobacco-attributable death) yield enormous political influence that is used, among other things, to try to prevent large tax increases.

Smuggling is a concern when tobacco taxes rise; about 10% of all cigarettes manufactured worldwide are already untaxed.[61] Use of specific excise taxes on tobacco (rather than ad valorem taxes), stronger tax administration, and practicable controls on organized smuggling can, however, limit the problem.[62] Even with some smuggling, large tax increases can substantially reduce consumption and increase revenue (Fig. 11.4), especially if supported by better tax enforcement.[61]

Tripling inflation-adjusted specific excise taxes on tobacco would, in many low- and middle-income countries, approximately double the average price of cigarettes (and more than double prices of cheaper brands), which would reduce consumption by about a third and actually increase tobacco revenues by about a third. In countries in which the government owns most of the industry, as in China, the distinction between taxes and profit is fairly arbitrary, but doubling the average prices would still substantially reduce consumption and increase revenue. Worldwide, raising specific excise taxes on tobacco to double prices would raise about another $100 billion (in U.S. dollars) per year in tobacco revenues, in addition to the approximately $300 billion that the WHO estimates governments already collect on tobacco.[4] Conversely, if a decrease in smoking by about a third were somehow achieved without increasing the inflation-adjusted price, tobacco tax revenues would decrease by about $100 billion.[6]

The main argument for reducing smoking is, however, the hundreds of millions of tobacco-related deaths if current smoking patterns persist. Indeed, in reviewing options to achieve a grand convergence by 2035 among the risks of premature death in low-, middle-, and high-income countries, the *Lancet* Commission on Investing in Health[63] recently identified a substantial increase in specific excise taxes on tobacco as the single most important intervention against noncommunicable diseases, as did the 2013 World Health Assembly.[5] Losses or gains in tobacco revenue are of secondary importance; indeed, tobacco taxes are a small percentage of overall revenue in most countries (except China), and money not spent on tobacco is spent on other taxable goods or services.[7] Attainment of the WHO target of a decrease of about a third in the prevalence of smoking by 2025, involving major decreases not only in high-income countries but also in populous low- and middle-income countries, would prevent several tens of millions of tobacco—attributable deaths during the next few decades[2,3,63] and about 200 million tobacco-attributable deaths during the century as a whole, mostly among people who are already alive, both by helping smokers to quit and by helping adolescents not to start.

We thank Jillian Boreham and Hong-Chao Pan for the Supplementary Appendix on 50-year smoking-attributed mortality trends in the United Kingdom, United States, and Poland (available at NEJM.org); Judith MacKay for comments and Cathy Harwood, Leslie Newcombe, and Joy Pader for editorial assistance on an earlier draft of the manuscript; Catherine Hill and Corne van Walbeek for French and South African data; and Ayda Yurekli for WHO tax-revenue estimates.

References

1. Peto R, Lopez AD, Boreham J, Thun M. Mortality from smoking in developed countries, 1950–2010. Oxford, United Kingdom: Clinical Trial Service Unit and Epidemiological Studies Unit, March 2012 (http://www.ctsu.ox.ac.uk/~tobacco).

2. Peto R, Lopez AD. The future worldwide health effects of current smoking patterns. In: Koop E, Pearson CE, Schwarz MR, eds. Critical issues in global health. San Francisco: Jossey-Bass, 2001:154–61.

3. Jha P. Avoidable global cancer deaths and total deaths from smoking. Nat Rev Cancer 2009;9:655–64.

4. WHO report on the global tobacco epidemic, 2013: enforcing bans on tobacco advertising, promotion and sponsorship. Geneva: World Health Organization, 2013.

5. Draft action plan for the prevention and control of non-communicable diseases 2013–2020. Geneva: World Health Assembly, World Health Organization, 2013.

6. WHO technical manual on tobacco tax administration. Geneva: World Health Organization, 2010.

7. Jha P, Chaloupka FJ. Curbing the epidemic: governments and the economics of tobacco control. Washington DC: World Bank, 1999.

8. Jha P, Chaloupka FJ, Moore J, et al. Tobacco addiction: In: Jamison DT, Breman JG, Measham AR, et al., eds. Disease control priorities in developing countries. 2nd ed. Washington, DC: World Bank and Oxford University Press, 2006:869–86.

9. International Agency for Research on Cancer. Effectiveness of tax and price policies for tobacco control: IARC handbook of cancer prevention, vol. 14. Lyon, France: IARC, 2011.

10. Draft: comprehensive global monitoring framework and targets for the prevention and control of non-communicable diseases. Geneva: World Health Organization, 2013.

11. Doll R, Peto R, Boreham J, Sutherland I. Mortality in relation to smoking: 50 years' observations on male British doctors. BMJ 2004;328:1519–33.

12. Pirie K, Peto R, Reeves GK, Green J, Beral V. The 21st century hazards of smoking and benefits of stopping: a prospective study of one million women in the UK. Lancet 2013;381:133–41.

13. Jha P, Ramasundarahettige C, Landsman V, Rostron B, Thun P, Peto R. 21st-Century hazards of smoking and benefits of cessation in the United States. N Engl J Med 2013;368:341–50.

14. Thun MJ, Carter BD, Feskanich D, et al. 50-Year trends in smoking-related mortality in the United States. N Engl J Med 2013;368:351–64.

15. Sakata R, McGale P, Grant EJ, Ozasa K, Peto R, Darby SC. Impact of smoking on mortality and life expectancy in Japanese smokers: a prospective cohort study. BMJ 2012;345:e7093.

16. Jha P, Jacob B, Gajalakshmi V, et al. A nationally representative case–control study of smoking and death in India. N Engl J Med 2008;358:1137–47.

17. Gupta PC, Pednekar MS, Parkin DM, Sankaranarayanan R. Tobacco associated mortality in Mumbai (Bombay) India: results of the Bombay Cohort Study. Int J Epidemiol 2005;34:1395–402.

18. Gajalakshmi V, Peto R, Kanaka TS, Jha P. Smoking and mortality from tuberculosis and other diseases in India: retrospective study of 43 000 adult male deaths and 35 000 controls. Lancet 2003; 362:507–15.

19. Jha P, Mony P, Moore JA, Zatonski W. Avoidance of worldwide vascular deaths and total deaths from smoking. In: Yusuf S, Cairns JA, Camm AJ, Gallen EL, Gersh BJ, eds. Evidence-based cardiology. Oxford, United Kingdom: Oxford University Press, 2010:111–24.

20. Peto R, Whitlock G, Jha P. Effects of obesity and smoking on U.S. life expectancy. N Engl J Med 2010;362:855–56.

21. Finucane MM, Stevens GA, Cowan MJ, et al. National, regional, and global trends in body-mass index since 1980: systematic analysis of health examination surveys and epidemiological studies with 960 country-years and 9.1 million participants. Lancet 2011;377:557–67.

22. Forey B, Hamling J, Hamling J, Thornton A, Lee PN. International smoking statistics: Web edition. Sutton, United Kingdom: PN Lee Statistics & Computing, 2013 (http://www.pnlee.co.uk/ISS3.htm).

23. Wynder EL, Graham EA. Tobacco smoking as a possible etiologic factor in bronchogenic carcinoma: a study of 684 proved cases. JAMA 1950;143:329–36.

24. Doll R, Hill AB. Smoking and carcinoma of the lung; preliminary report. Br Med J 1950;2:739–48.

25. Smoking and health: summary and report of the Royal College of Physicians of London on smoking in relation to cancer of the lung and other diseases. London: Pitman Publishing, 1962.

26. Smoking and health: report of the Advisory Committee to the Surgeon-General of the Public Health Service. Washington, DC: Department of Health, Education, and Welfare, 1964.

27. Giovino GA, Mirza SA, Samet JM, et al. Tobacco use in 3 billion individuals from 16 countries: an analysis of nationally representative cross-sectional household surveys. Lancet 2012;380:668–79. [Errata, Lancet 2012;380:1908, 2013;382:128.]

28. Zatoński WA, Mańczuk M. Tobacco smoking and tobacco-related harm in the European Union, with special attention to the new EU member states. In: Boyle P, Gray N, Henningfield J, Seffrin J, Zatoński WA, eds. Tobacco: science, policy, and public health. Oxford, United Kingdom: Oxford University Press, 2010:134–55.

29. Jha P, Guindon E, Joseph RA, et al. A rational taxation system of bidis and cigarettes to reduce smoking deaths in India. Econ Polit Wkly 2011;42:44–51.

30. Market research for the tobacco industry: cigarettes. London: Euromonitor International, 2012 (http://www.euromonitor.com/tobacco).

31. Liu BQ, Peto R, Chen ZM, et al. Emerging tobacco hazards in China: 1. Retrospective proportional mortality study of one million deaths. BMJ 1998;317:1411–22.

32. Gu D, Kelly TN, Wu X, et al. Mortality attributable to smoking in China. N Engl J Med 2009;360:150–59. [Erratum, N Engl J Med 2010;363:2272.]

33. Alam DS, Jha P, Ramasundarahettige C, et al. Smoking-attributable mortality in Bangladesh: proportional mortality study. Bull World Health Organ 2013;91:757–64.

34. Sitas F, Egger S, Bradshaw D, et al. Differences among the coloured, white, black, and other South African populations in smoking-attributed mortality at ages 35-74 years: a case-control study of 481,640 deaths. Lancet 2013;382:685–93.

35. Jha P. The 21st century benefits of smoking cessation in Europe. Eur J Epidemiol 2013;28:617–19.

36. Abascal W, Esteves E, Goja B, et al. Tobacco control campaign in Uruguay: a population-based trend analysis. Lancet 2012;380:1575–82.

37. Decline in cigarette consumption following implementation of a comprehensive tobacco prevention and education program—Oregon, 1996–1998. MMWR Morb Mortal Wkly Rep 1999;48:140–43.

38. Levy DT, Hyland A, Higbee C, Remer L, Compton C. The role of public policies in reducing smoking prevalence in California: results from the California tobacco policy simulation model. Health Policy 2007;82:167–85.

39. Chaloupka FJ, Hu T-W, Warner KE, Jacobs R, Yurekli A. The taxation of tobacco products. In: Jha P, Chaloupka FJ, eds. Tobacco control in developing countries. Oxford, United Kingdom: Oxford University Press, 2000:237–72.

40. Kostova D, Ross H, Blecher E, Marko-witz S. Is youth smoking responsive to cigarette prices? Evidence from low- and middle-income countries. Tob Control 2011;20:419–24. [Erratum, Tob Control 2012;21:64.]

41. Blecher E. Targeting the affordability of cigarettes: a new benchmark for taxation policy in low-income and middle-income countries. Tob Control 2010;19:325–30.

42. Hu TW, Mao Z, Shi J, Chen W. Tobacco taxation and its potential impact in China. Paris: International Union Against Tuberculosis and Lung Disease, 2008.

43. Barber S, Adioetomo SM, Ahsan A, Setyonaluri D. Tobacco economics in Indonesia. Paris: International Union Against Tuberculosis and Lung Disease, 2008.

44. Hill C. Impact de l'augmentation des prix sur la consummation de tabac. Paris: Institut Gustave Roussy, 2013 (http://www.igr.fr/doc/cancer/pdf/prevention/prixtab2013.pdf).

45. Van Walbeek CP. Industry responses to the tobacco excise tax increases in South Africa. S Afr J Econ 2006;74:110–22.

46. Baumgardner JR, Bilheimer LT, Booth MB, Carrington WJ, Duchovny NJ, Werble EC. Cigarette taxes and the federal budget—report from the CBO. N Engl J Med 2012;367:2068–70.

47. Federal Trade Commission. Cigarette report for 2011. Washington, DC: FTC, 2013 (http://www.ftc.gov/os/2013/05/130521cigarettereport.pdf).

48. Wakefield MA, Hayes L, Durkin S, Borland R. Introduction effects of the Australian plain packaging policy on adult smokers: a cross-sectional study. BMJ Open 2013;3:e003175.

49. Cancer Research UK. The answer is plain—campaign for plain cigarette packaging (http://www.youtube.com/watch?feature=player_embedded&v=c_z-4S8iicc).

50. Hammond D. "Plain packaging" regulations for tobacco products: the impact of standardizing the color and design of cigarette packs. Salud Publica Mex 2010;52:Suppl 2:S226–32.

51. Kenkel D, Chen L. Consumer information and tobacco use. In: Jha P, Chaloupka FJ, eds. Tobacco control in developing countries. Oxford, United Kingdom: Oxford University Press, 2000:177–214.

52. Saffer H. Tobacco advertising and promotion. In: Jha P, Chaloupka FJ, eds. Tobacco control in developing countries. Oxford, United Kingdom: Oxford University Press, 2000:215–36.

53. Blecher E. The impact of tobacco advertising bans on consumption in developing countries. J Health Econ 2008;27:930–42.

54. Callinan JE, Clarke A, Doherty K, Kelleher C. Legislative smoking bans for reducing secondhand smoke exposure, smoking prevalence and tobacco consumption. Cochrane Database Syst Rev 2010;4:CD005992.

55. Fichtenberg CM, Glantz SA. Effect of smoke-free workplaces on smoking behaviour: systematic review. BMJ 2002;325:188–99.

56. Bala MM, Strzeszynski L, Topor-Madry R, Cahill K. Mass media interventions for smoking cessation in adults. Cochrane Data-base Syst Rev 2013;6:CD004704.

57. Hartmann-Boyce J, Stead LF, Cahill K, Lancaster T. Efficacy of interventions to combat tobacco addiction: Cochrane update of 2012 reviews. Addiction 2013;108:1711–21.

58. Bullen C, Howe C, Laugesen M, et al. Electronic cigarettes for smoking cessation: a randomised controlled trial. Lancet 2013;382:1629–37.

59. Jha P, Joseph RC, Moser P, et al. Tobacco taxes: a win–win measure for fiscal space and health. Manila, Philippines: Asian Development Bank, 2012 (http://www.adb.org/publications/tobacco-taxes-win-win-measure-fiscal-space-and-health).

60. Eriksen M, Mackay J, Ross H. The tobacco atlas. American Cancer Society and World Lung Foundation, 2012 (http://www.TobaccoAtlas.org).

61. Yürekli A, Sayginosoy Ö. Worldwide organized cigarette smuggling: an empirical analysis. Appl Econ 2010;42:545–61.

62. Joossens L, Merriman D, Ross H, Raw M. How eliminating the global illicit cigarette trade would increase tax revenue and save lives. Paris: International Union Against Tuberculosis and Lung Disease, 2009.

63. Jamison DT, Summers LH, Alleyne G, et al. Global health 2035: a world converging within a generation. Lancet 2013;382:1898–955.

Noncommunicable Diseases

David J. Hunter
and K. Srinath Reddy

The United Nations has held only two meetings of heads of state on a health-related issue. The first, in 2001, was on human immunodeficiency virus infection and the acquired immunodeficiency syndrome. The second, in September 2011, was on noncommunicable diseases. Although noncommunicable diseases were ignored during the framing of the Millennium Development Goals in 2000, their leading and growing contribution to preventable deaths and disability across the globe has compelled policymakers to pay attention and initiate action. The United Nations and the World Health Organization (WHO) have called for a 25% reduction by 2025 in mortality from noncommunicable diseases among persons between 30 and 70 years of age, in comparison with mortality in 2010, adopting the slogan "25 by 25."[1,2] We review the burden of noncommunicable diseases and issues in prevention, detection, and treatment that must be addressed in order to meet this goal.

Disease and Economic Burdens

DISEASE BURDEN

Noncommunicable diseases have been a difficult group to define. Even the term "noncommunicable diseases" is a misnomer, because it includes some diseases—notably, cancers of the liver, stomach, and cervix—that are at least partly caused by infectious organisms, and it usually excludes mental illnesses, despite their large contribution to long-term disability. However, four common behavioral risk factors (tobacco use, excessive alcohol consumption, poor diet, and lack of physical activity) are associated with four disease clusters (cardiovascular diseases, cancers, chronic pulmonary diseases, and diabetes) that account for about 80% of deaths from noncommunicable diseases.[3] According to WHO estimates, noncommunicable diseases contributed to 36 million deaths globally in 2008, accounting for 63% of 57 million total deaths (Fig. 12.1).[4] The Global

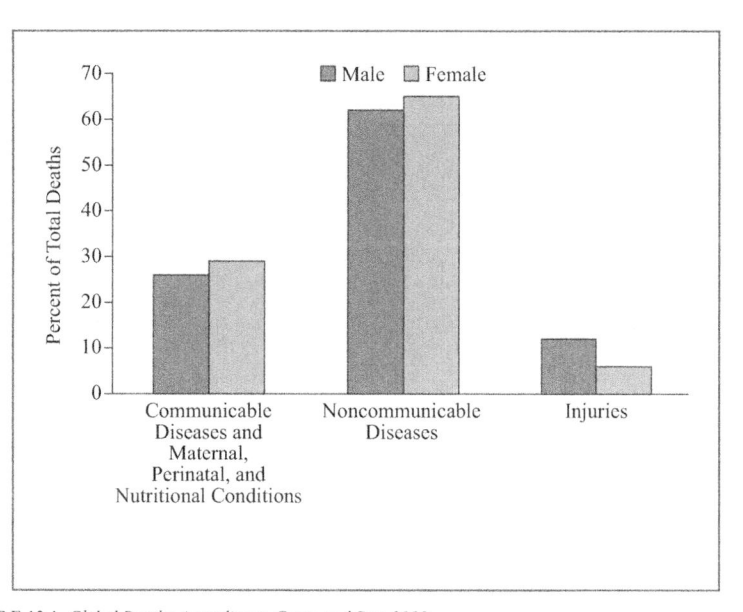

FIGURE 12.1 *Global Deaths According to Cause and Sex, 2008*
Adapted from the World Health Organization (WHO).[4]

Burden of Diseases, Injuries, and Risk Factors Study 2010 (GBD 2010) estimated that mortality due to noncommunicable diseases (with the use of a somewhat different definition of noncommunicable diseases than that used by the WHO) increased from 57% of total mortality in 1990 to 65% in 2010.[3,5] About 80% of deaths related to noncommunicable diseases occur in low- and middle-income countries, which also have a high proportion of deaths in middle age; such countries account for 90% of the 9 million noncommunicable disease–related deaths that occur before 60 years of age (Fig. 12.2).[6] This staggering toll of noncommunicable diseases and premature mortality in low- and middle-income countries sometimes surprises those who suppose that mortality in these countries is still dominated by maternal and child deaths and deaths due to infectious diseases.

Cardiovascular diseases account for the largest fraction of deaths related to noncommunicable diseases, followed by cancer, chronic obstructive pulmonary disease (COPD), and diabetes (Fig. 12.3A and interactive graphic, available at NEJM.org).[7] Proportional mortality from noncommunicable diseases is higher in high-income countries than in low- and middle-income countries, because high-income countries have a lower burden of maternal and child deaths and deaths due to infectious diseases. However, the absolute number of deaths due to noncommunicable diseases is higher in the low- and middle—income countries owing to their larger populations. Age-standardized rates of death due to noncommunicable diseases are also higher in these countries than in the high-income countries.[8]

The GBD 2010 also calculated disability-adjusted life-years (DALYs), which are the sum of years of life lost from premature death and years lived with

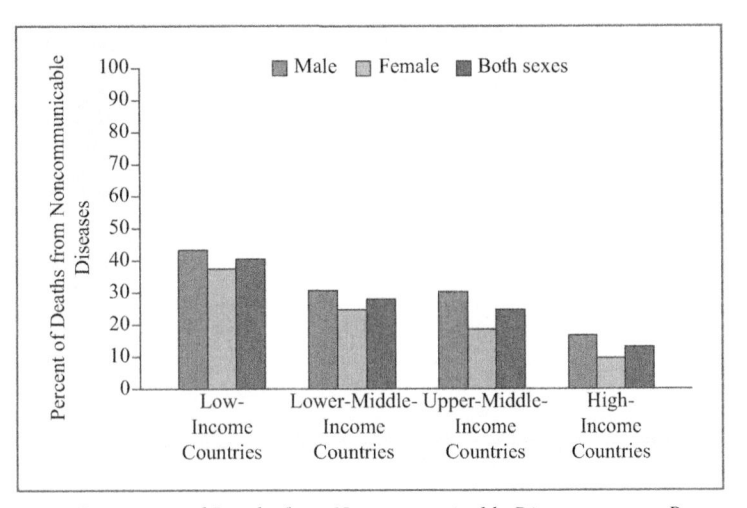

FIGURE 12.2 *Proportion of Deaths from Noncommunicable Diseases among Persons Younger than 60 Years of Age, According to Income Group of Countries*
Adapted from the WHO.[6]

disability, and estimated that 54% of DALYs worldwide in 2010 were due to non-communicable diseases, an increase from 43% in 1990.[7] Between 1990 and 2010, DALYs due to cardiovascular diseases, cancer, and diabetes mellitus increased by 22.6%, 27.3%, and 69.0%, respectively, whereas DALYs due to COPD decreased by 2.0% (Fig. 12.3B). In addition, a large share of the burden of disability is due to other noncommunicable diseases, such as asthma, digestive diseases, neurologic disorders, mental and behavioral disorders, kidney diseases, gynecologic disorders, hemoglobinopathies, musculoskeletal disorders, congenital anomalies, and skin, sense-organ, and oral disorders. Whereas these diseases were associated with only 19.6% of deaths in 2010, they accounted for 54.8% of DALYs.[7] For some of these diseases, the primary risk factors are similar to those for cardiovascular disease, cancer, COPD, and diabetes, but for many the risk factors are specific and unique—a reminder that not all aspects of control of noncommunicable diseases are addressed by strategies targeted to the four major groups of noncommunicable diseases.

The WHO projects that noncommunicable diseases will account for an increasing absolute number and proportion of worldwide deaths, rising to about 70% of deaths in 2030.[9] The increase in the absolute numbers of deaths is primarily due to the increase in the size and age of the world population.

ECONOMIC EFFECTS

The economic consequences of noncommunicable diseases are huge, because of the combined burden of health care costs and lost economic productivity due to illness and premature deaths. A study commissioned by the World Economic Forum concluded that the world will sustain a cumulative output loss of $47

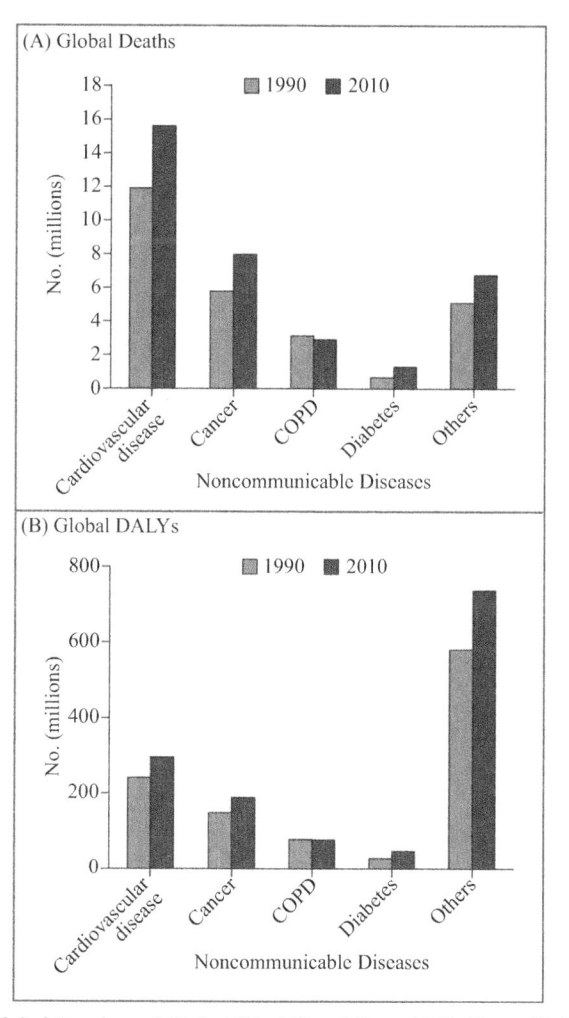

FIGURE 12.3 *Global Deaths and Global Disability-Adjusted Life-Years (DALYs) Due to Noncommunicable Diseases in 1990 and 2010*

DALYs are the sum of years of life lost from premature death and years lived with disability. COPD denotes chronic obstructive pulmonary disease. Adapted from Murray et al.[7]

trillion between 2011 and 2030 because of noncommunicable diseases and mental illness, about $30 trillion of which will be attributable to cardiovascular diseases, cancers, chronic pulmonary diseases, and diabetes.[10] Noncommunicable diseases are also a major cause of catastrophic health expenditure among the uninsured.[11]

PREVALENCE OF RISK FACTORS

Tobacco use, excessive alcohol consumption, poor diet, and lack of physical activity contribute to the development of noncommunicable diseases. Measurable phenotypes such as high blood pressure, hypercholesterolemia, and obesity mediate much of the relationship between these risk factors and the incidence of

noncommunicable disease. As summarized in the review by Ezzati and Riboli,[12] global trends in the prevalence of these behavioral risk factors and intermediate phenotypes portend substantial increases in most of the noncommunicable diseases worldwide, with the patterns of change in incidence varying between and within regions, depending on the level of economic development, the pace of the demographic transition from high birth and death rates to low birth and death rates, and the prevalence of risk factors.[12,13]

Ethnic variations in susceptibility to disease have also been described, such as an increased risk of stroke in East Asian populations and an increased risk of coronary heart disease in South Asians.[14,15] Risk factors vary across regions. For example, in South Asia, indoor air pollution due to burnt wood or biomass fuel at home is a major cause of COPD, and oral cancer is most often caused by chewed tobacco.

THE "UNFINISHED AGENDA" AND NONCOMMUNICABLE DISEASES

The term "unfinished agenda" is often used to refer to the health problems of less developed countries before the onset of the health transition—that is, mainly infectious diseases, malnutrition, and other diseases of poverty. In a cruel twist, some of the causes of noncommunicable diseases in these countries are due not to the behavioral risk factors listed above but rather to these "unfinished" problems. Heart disease due to rheumatic fever, for instance, is still a common cause of early-onset heart disease in low- and middle-income countries,[16] and the Barker hypothesis proposes that exposure to inadequate maternal nutrition in utero and during the first years of life increases the risk of noncommunicable diseases in adulthood.[17]

Trends in High-Income Countries

The rates of death due to noncommunicable diseases have peaked in some high-income countries, particularly with respect to cardiovascular diseases and some cancers, such as lung cancer. Figure 12.4 shows the 60-year trends in the United States, with age-adjusted rates of death from cardiovascular diseases decreasing by about 70% since the 1950s, rates of death from cerebrovascular disease decreasing by 78% since the 1950s, and rates of death from cancer down by 17% since 1980.[18] Similar reductions in the rate of death from cardiovascular diseases and, among men, the rate of death from lung cancer have been seen in many high-income countries.[13] The sobering news is that despite these falls in the age-adjusted rates, the decline in the absolute number of deaths per year is much less substantial because of the growth and aging of the population. Thus, even if countries with growing and aging populations can engineer decreases in mortality, they will need to prepare for substantial numbers of cases of noncommunicable diseases. Worldwide, the GBD 2010 estimates of age- and sex-specific rates

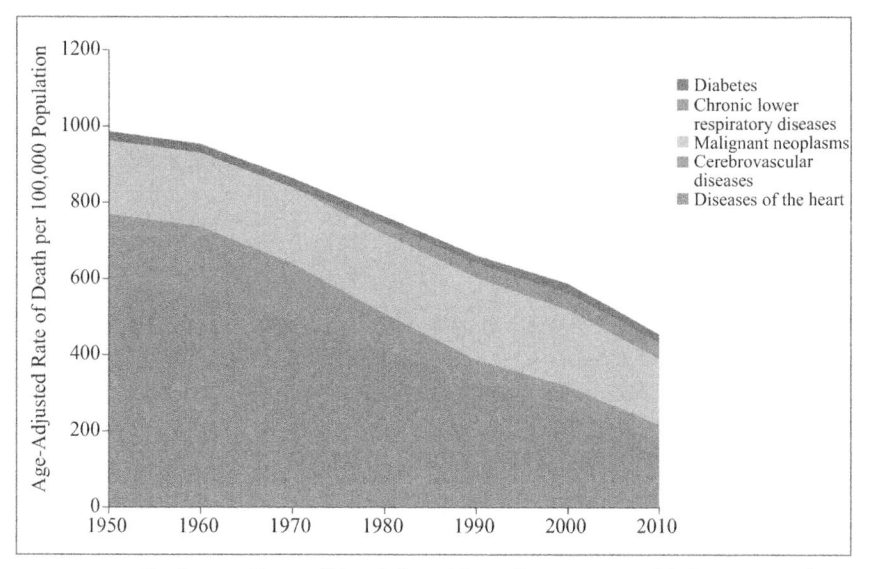

FIGURE 12.4 *Declines in Rates of Death from Major Noncommunicable Diseases in the United States, 1950 to 2010*

Adapted from the National Center for Health Statistics, Centers for Disease Control and Prevention.[18]

of deaths and DALYs due to noncommunicable diseases, as compared with rates in 1990, also show a substantial reduction in incidence rates, but these reductions are more than canceled out by increasing population size and population aging.[3,7]

Modeling suggests that risk-factor reduction explains approximately 44 to 76% of the decline in mortality from coronary heart disease in the United States and other high-income countries, and improvements in treatments and access to treatments explain 23 to 47%.[19] During the 20th century, mortality from cervical cancer decreased dramatically in high-income countries, mainly because organized cervical screening led to early detection and treatment.[20] Lung-cancer rates are dropping as a result of declines in the prevalence of smoking. Thus, trends in high-income countries suggest that the size of the epidemic of noncommunicable diseases is not predetermined, and the challenge for low- and middle-income countries is to intervene sufficiently early to mitigate the epidemic.

Strategies for Prevention and Control

To be comprehensive, a program for the prevention and control of noncommunicable diseases must integrate policies designed to foster a societal environment in which people are encouraged to make and maintain healthy living choices, promote health literacy so that people can protect and improve their health, and provide health services focused on early detection and cost-effective management of noncommunicable diseases and their risk factors (Table 12.1).

TABLE 12.1 Opportunities for Prevention, Detection, and Treatment of
Noncommunicable Diseases in Low- and Middle-Income Countries

Level of Approach	Prevention	Detection	Treatment
Government	Anti-tobacco policy; policies that promote reduction in salt intake; regulation and labeling of processed foods and high-sugar beverages; planning for safe, healthy environments that promote physical activity and limit the transition to a sedentary lifestyle; policies designed to mitigate the harmful effects of alcoholic beverages	Promotion of awareness of noncommunicable diseases, their signs and symptoms, and the need for early detection	Policies that ensure access to affordable essential medicines
Health care system	Intersectoral planning for health promotion; training of health personnel, including task shifting for detection and treatment of noncommunicable diseases (e.g., blood-pressure and glycemic control provided by nurses or ancillary health workers)	Surveillance to determine the prevalence of risk factors and noncommunicable diseases; facilities and equipment for low-cost detection of intermediate risk factors (e.g., high blood pressure)	Facilities and equipment for affordable treatments; recognition of the need for both short-term and long-term treatment of noncommunicable diseases
Clinicians	Counseling of patients in risk-factor reduction; treatment of tobacco addiction	Evaluation of intermediate risk factors, coupled with lifestyle and drug interventions to lower risk-factor profiles; appropriate screening (e.g., detection of human papillomavirus)	Evidence-based treatment with affordable essential medicines; procedural or surgical interventions, if appropriate

Population-based interventions include policy measures such as increasing taxation of tobacco and alcohol, reducing salt and saturated fat and eliminating trans fats in processed foods, and creating smoke-free and exercise-friendly public spaces. Among the risk factors identified as major causes of noncommunicable diseases,[13] dietary risk factors and physical inactivity are partially determined by individual preferences but are substantially influenced by the manufacturing and marketing practices of the food industry and by the built and social environments that permit or impede physical activity. Evidence is rapidly accumulating that the consumption of sugared beverages is an important cause of childhood obesity, and in randomized trials, the substitution of lower-calorie beverages is associated with weight loss.[21,22] Mass-media messaging as well as health promotion in specific settings (schools, workplaces, and community centers) may be

used to provide health education. Preventive interventions include risk-factor assessment and treatment with behavioral interventions and medication for persons at high risk. Although multidrug therapy for persons with established cardiovascular disease is required for secondary prevention, there is also a need to treat persons at high absolute risk for a first serious cardiovascular event. Some evidence-based therapies, such as the administration of generic antihypertensive agents and statins, are low-cost by the standards of high-income countries but are prescribed in low- and middle-income countries for only a small fraction of patients who are candidates for such treatment according to evidence-based guidelines, even though high blood pressure is the leading cause of deaths and DALYs.[13] Similarly, there is underutilization of therapies for secondary prevention of recurrent events—for example, after a myocardial infarction or cerebrovascular event. The development of combination pills (one form of which is called the "polypill") has now entered the clinical-trial phase and holds promise for a simplified regimen at even lower cost.[23,24]

Tobacco is the second largest cause of deaths and DALYs worldwide, and tobacco control could prevent about a third of all deaths from cancer in the United States[25] and could also rapidly reduce deaths from cardiovascular and chronic pulmonary diseases. The WHO Framework Convention on Tobacco Control provides proven tobacco-control strategies that need to be implemented within and between nations.[26,27] Public-interest litigation and changes in national laws such as the U.S. Tobacco Control Act[28] to provide greater government regulation of the tobacco industry are needed. Increasing obesity rates presage an increase in mortality from a wide variety of cancers[29]; thus, obesity prevention is a priority for cancer prevention, as well as for the prevention of cardiovascular disease and diabetes. In countries with infant vaccination against hepatitis B virus, chronic-carrier rates and rates of liver cancer have declined sharply.[30] The recent development of human papillomavirus vaccines for cervical-cancer prevention offers a new opportunity to control the fourth leading cause of cancer deaths in women worldwide.[31] Many cancers are highly treatable, if detected early, and the provision of evidence-based screening and treatment regimens in low- and middle-income countries is an important component of cancer control that requires larger investments in human and capital resources.[32]

Many of these interventions have been identified as cost-effective by the WHO.[33] A series of "best buys," determined on the basis of cost-effectiveness and the feasibility of implementation, have been suggested. For risk-factor reduction, these include tobacco and alcohol taxes, advertising bans and warnings, reductions in salt and trans fat intakes, promotion of physical activity, and hepatitis B vaccination. Health care "best buy" interventions include counseling regarding risk-factor reduction and multidrug therapy for persons at high risk for cardiovascular disease or diabetes, aspirin therapy for those with a history of acute myocardial infarction, and cervical-cancer screening and treatment. These interventions require a complex series of legislative actions, public-awareness campaigns, and public health interventions, as well as adequate numbers of clinical personnel, at least basic clinical facilities, and adequate supplies of drugs. Bloom

et al.[10] conclude, "Interventions in this area will undeniably be costly. But inaction is likely to be far more costly."

Challenges to Health Systems

The global epidemic of noncommunicable diseases poses challenges to the health systems of all countries, though the problems vary. High-income countries are confronted by the rising costs of technology-intensive health care for aging populations. The health systems of low- and middle-income countries must address the simultaneous challenges of multiple infectious diseases, undernutrition, and ongoing substandard maternal and child health, which vie with noncommunicable diseases for scarce financial and human resources. These problems are compounded by weak disease and risk-factor surveillance systems and lack of access to affordable drugs and laboratory and diagnostic tests.

In low- and middle-income countries, financial protection from the costs of treatment for noncommunicable diseases, in the form of public financing or insurance, is limited. The health care infrastructure is also limited, with inadequate facilities for advanced care and shortages of trained medical specialists, nurses, and allied health workers. Paradoxically, some low- and middle-income countries have highly advanced tertiary clinical care facilities in major cities, staffed by very skilled professionals. However, even in such countries, the diagnosis and treatment of noncommunicable diseases are usually very deficient at the primary and secondary care levels. In general, the health systems are configured to provide episodic care for acute illness and have not yet made the adaptations required to provide continuous care for chronic illness.

Access to essential drugs is not ensured in many countries, with inadequate supplies of cardiovascular drugs, anticancer agents, insulin and oral hypoglycemic agents, and bronchodilators.[34] An analysis of WHO data from 36 countries showed that the availability of cardiovascular drugs was poor (26.3% of public-sector facilities and 57.3% of private-sector facilities had such drugs),[35] and a survey of 6 countries by the WHO showed that the monthly cost of treatment with a single antihypertensive medication exceeded several days' wages in many countries.[36] When multiple drugs are used, the cost becomes unaffordable, and this problem is further compounded when more than one family member needs treatment.[36] In low- and middle-income countries, drug therapy for cardiovascular disease is a major contributor to high out-of-pocket health care expenditures, resulting in millions of people being pushed into poverty. Countries such as Thailand and India are resorting to compulsory licensing to domestically produce the more expensive cardiovascular or anticancer drugs. Lack of reform of national and international regulations on opiate production and export means that many patients with cancer are deprived of low-cost drugs such as morphine that could provide pain relief.[37]

At the same time, the reduced cost of care for many procedures, such as cardiac or cancer surgery, in developing countries is opening up markets in medical

tourism. Even as low- and middle-income countries can gain from access to technical expertise in high-income countries, the latter can learn from the highly cost-efficient and high-throughput models of surgery developed in some low- and middle-income countries[38] and new, lower-cost technologies developed under the rubric of "frugal innovation."[39]

In primary health care, there is a need to train and deploy nonphysician health care workers, ranging from community health workers to skilled nurses, while enhancing the ability of primary care physicians to provide appropriate care based on standard guidelines. The ability of nonphysician health workers to effectively detect and manage diabetes and high blood pressure has been shown in countries such as South Africa[40] and Iran.[41] The WHO Cardiovascular Risk Management Package has been shown to be useful for scaling up the management of cardiovascular diseases in primary health care settings in which physicians are not available.[42]

Cell phone–based "mHealth" tools have been successfully used by frontline health care workers for remote data collection, remote monitoring, and diagnostic and treatment support in several developing countries.[43] Further extending these applications with regard to noncommunicable diseases could also be promising, as shown in formative research on diabetes care in developed nations.[44] Information and communication technology can enable nonphysician health care providers to play an effective role in the diagnosis and management of noncommunicable diseases.

Progress toward the goal of a 25% reduction in the rate of premature death from noncommunicable diseases by 2025 will require both country-specific actions and global cooperation.[45] Country-specific actions require strong political leadership and the development of national action plans that mobilize a multisectoral response (e.g., multiple levels of government, the private sector, and nongovernmental organizations) and provide mechanisms to monitor progress and ensure accountability from the multiple sectors involved. Brazil, for instance, passed a new anti-tobacco law, signed agreements with the food industry to reduce salt consumption and eliminate trans fats from processed foods, and improved access to cardiovascular drugs.[45] Global cooperation is needed, given the globalization of tobacco exportation and agribusiness and multinational ownership of major food and soft-drink manufacturers.

The importance of addressing noncommunicable diseases at the global level has also become a major element of the ongoing discussion concerning the post-2015 development goals, which is being steered by the United Nations. Whereas noncommunicable diseases were omitted from the Millennium Development Goals in 2000, a consensus is emerging among the various United Nations agencies and other international organizations that a life-course perspective must be adopted, with an emphasis on noncommunicable diseases as part of the health goal to be included in the set of post-2015 Sustainable Development Goals. Whether the goal itself will be defined as "Gaining Health and Well-Being at All Stages of Life" or "Maximizing Healthy Life Expectancy" or "Universal Health Coverage"[46] (which are leading contenders

at present), it is clear that the prevention and control of noncommunicable diseases will be acknowledged as an integral part of the sustainable-development agenda. However, it remains to be seen whether the plan of action will address the many upstream determinants of noncommunicable diseases, going beyond the needed clinical services.[47]

Conclusions

Noncommunicable diseases will be the predominant global public health challenge of the 21st century. Prevention of premature deaths due to noncommunicable diseases and reduction of related health care costs will be the main goals of health policy. Improving the detection and treatment of noncommunicable diseases and preventing complications and catastrophic events will be the major goals of clinical medicine. A multilevel approach that integrates policy actions, regulations, health education, and efficient health systems to achieve these goals will be the mission of public health. All countries can benefit by sharing experience and pooling expertise for the prevention and control of noncommunicable diseases.

References

1. United Nations General Assembly. Political declaration of the High-level Meeting of the General Assembly on the Prevention and Control of Noncommunicable Diseases. September 16, 2011 (http://www.un.org/ga/search/view_doc.asp?symbol=A/66/L.1).
2. 65th World Health Assembly closes with new global health measures. Geneva: World Health Association,May26,2012 (http://www.who.int/mediacentre/news/releases/2012/wha 65_closes_20120526 /en /index.html).
3. Lozano R, Naghavi M, Foreman K, et al. Global and regional mortality from 235 causes of death for 20 age groups in 1990 and 2010: a systematic analysis for the Global Burden of Disease Study 2010. Lancet 2012;380:2095–128.
4. Cause-specific mortality, 2008: WHO region by country. Geneva: World Health Organization, 2011 (http://apps.who.int/gho/data/node.main.887?lang=en).
5. Murray CJL, Lopez AD. Measuring the global burden of disease. N Engl J Med 2013;369:448–57.
6. Noncommunicable diseases. Geneva: World Health Organization, 2013 (http://www.who.int/mediacentre/factsheets/fs355/en/).
7. Murray CJ, Vos T, Lozano R, et al. Disability-adjusted life years (DALYs) for 291 diseases and injuries in 21 regions, 1990-2010: a systematic analysis for the Global Burden of Disease Study 2010. Lancet 2012;380:2197–223.
8. Global status report on noncommunicable diseases. Geneva: World Health Organization, 2011 (http://www.who.int/nmh/publications/ncd_report2010/en).
9. Mathers CD, Loncar D. Projections of global mortality and burden of disease from 2002 to 2030. PLoS Med 2006;3(11):e442.

10. Bloom DE, Cafiero ET, Jané-Llopis E, et al. The global economic burden of non-communicable diseases. Geneva: World Economic Forum, 2011 (http://www.weforum.org/reports/global-economic-burden-non-communicable-diseases).

11. Heeley E, Anderson CS, Huang Y, et al. Role of health insurance in averting economic hardship in families after acute stroke in China. Stroke 2009;40:2149–56.

12. Ezzati M, Riboli E. Behavioral and dietary risk factors for noncommunicable diseases. N Engl J Med, 2013;369:954–64.

13. Ezzati M, Riboli E. Can noncommunicable diseases be prevented? Lessons from studies of populations and individuals. Science 2012;337:1482–87.

14. Lawes CMM, Rodgers A, Bennett DA, et al. Blood pressure and cardiovascular disease in the Asia Pacific region. J Hypertens 2003;21:707–16.

15. Joshi P, Islam S, Pais P, et al. Risk factors for early myocardial infarction in South Asians compared with individuals in other countries. JAMA 2007;297:286–94.

16. Seckeler MD, Hoke TR. The worldwide epidemiology of acute rheumatic fever and rheumatic heart disease. Clin Epidemiol 2011;3:67–84.

17. Barker DJP. Sir Richard Doll Lecture: developmental origins of chronic disease. Public Health 2012;126:185–89.

18. Health, United States, 2011: with special feature on socioeconomic status and health. Hyattsville, MD: National Center for Health Statistics, 2012 (http://www.cdc.gov/nchs/data/hus/hus11.pdf).

19. Ford ES, Capewell S. Proportion of the decline in cardiovascular mortality disease due to prevention versus treatment: public health versus clinical care. Annu Rev Public Health 2011;32:5–22.

20. Mathew A, George PS. Trends in incidence and mortality rates of squamous cell carcinoma and adenocarcinoma of cervix—worldwide. Asian Pac J Cancer Prev 2009;10:645–50.

21. de Ruyter JC, Olthof MR, Seidell JC, Katan MB. A trial of sugar-free or sugar-sweetened beverages and body weight in children. N Engl J Med 2012;367:1397–406.

22. Ebbeling CB, Feldman HA, Chomitz VR, et al. A randomized trial of sugar-sweetened beverages and adolescent body weight. N Engl J Med 2012;367:1407–16.

23. Yusuf S, Pais P, Afzal R, et al. Effects of a polypill (Polycap) on risk factors in middle-aged individuals without cardiovascular disease (TIPS): a phase II, double-blind, randomised trial. Lancet 2009;373:1341–51.

24. Wald NJ, Wald DS. The polypill concept. Postgrad Med J 2010;86:257–60.

25. Jemal A, Thun MJ, Ries LA, et al. Annual report to the nation on the status of cancer, 1975-2005, featuring trends in lung cancer, tobacco use, and tobacco control. J Natl Cancer Inst 2008;100:1672–94.

26. Myers ML. The FCTC's evidence-based policies remain a key to ending the tobacco epidemic. Tob Control 2013;22:Suppl 1:i45–46.

27. Glantz S, Gonzalez M. Effective tobacco control is key to rapid progress in reduction of non-communicable diseases. Lancet 2012;379:1269–71.

28. Husten CG, Deyton LR. Understanding the Tobacco Control Act: efforts by the US Food and Drug Administration to make tobacco-related morbidity and mortality part of the USA's past, not its future. Lancet 2013;381:1570–80.

29. Calle EE, Rodriguez C, Walker-Thurmond K, Thun MJ. Overweight, obesity, and mortality from cancer in a prospectively studied cohort of U.S. adults. N Engl J Med 2003;348:1625–38.

30. Plymoth A, Viviani S, Hainaut P. Control of hepatocellular carcinoma through hepatitis B vaccination in areas of high endemicity: perspectives for global liver cancer prevention. Cancer Lett 2009;286:15–21.

31. Jemal A, Bray F, Center MM, Ferlay J, Ward E, Forman D. Global cancer statistics. CA Cancer J Clin 2011;61:69–90. [Erratum, CA Cancer J Clin 2011;61:134.]

32. Farmer P, Frenk J, Knaul FM, et al. Expansion of cancer care and control in countries of low and middle income: a call to action. Lancet 2010;376:1186–93.

33. Bloom DE, Chisholm D, Jane-Llopis E, Prettner K, Stein A, Feigl A. From burden to "best buys": reducing the economic impact of non-communicable disease in low- and middle-income countries. Geneva: World Health Organization, 2011 (http://ideas.repec.org/p/gdm/wpaper/7511.html).

34. Kishore SP, Vedanthan R, Fuster V. Promoting global cardiovascular health ensuring access to essential cardiovascular medicines in low- and middle-income countries. J Am Coll Cardiol 2011;57:1980–87.

35. van Mourik MSM, Cameron A, Ewen M, Laing RO. Availability, price and affordability of cardiovascular medicines: a comparison across 36 countries using WHO/HAI data. BMC Cardiovasc Disord 2010;10:25.

36. Mendis S, Fukino K, Cameron A, et al. The availability and affordability of selected essential medicines for chronic diseases in six low- and middle-income countries. Bull World Health Organ 2007;85:279–88.

37. O'Brien M, Mwangi-Powell F, Adewole IF, et al. Improving access to analgesic drugs for patients with cancer in sub-Saharan Africa. Lancet Oncol 2013;14 (4):e176–82.

38. Venkatesh R, Muralikrishnan R, Balent LC, Prakash SK, Prajna NV. Outcomes of high volume cataract surgeries in a developing country. Br J Ophthalmol 2005;89:1079–83.

39. Emerging economies drive frugal innovation. Bull World Health Organ 2013;91:6–7.

40. Coleman R, Gill G, Wilkinson D. Noncommunicable disease management in resource-poor settings: a primary care model from rural South Africa. Bull World Health Organ 1998;76:633–40.

41. Farzadfar F, Murray CJL, Gakidou E, et al. Effectiveness of diabetes and hypertension management by rural primary health-care workers (Behvarz workers) in Iran: a nationally representative observational study. Lancet 2012;379:47–54.

42. Abegunde DO, Shengelia B, Luyten A, et al. Can non-physician health-care workers assess and manage cardiovascular risk in primary care? Bull World Health Organ 2007;85:432–40.

43. mHealth for development: the opportunity of mobile technology for healthcare in the developing world. Washington, DC, and Berkshire, United Kingdom: UN Foundation–Vodafone Foundation Partnership, 2009.

44. Krishna S, Boren SA, Balas EA. Healthcare via cell phones: a systematic review. Telemed J E Health 2009;15:231–40.

45. Bonita R, Magnusson R, Bovet P, et al. Country actions to meet UN commitments on non-communicable diseases: a stepwise approach. Lancet 2013;381:575–84.

46. Frenk J, de Ferranti D. Universal health coverage: good health, good economics. Lancet 2012;380:862–64.

47. Post-2015 consultation on health culminates in high-level dialogue. New York: International Institute for Sustainable Development, 2013 (http://post2015.iisd .org/news/post-2015-consultation-on-health-culminates-in-high-level-dialogue).

Mental Health and the Global Agenda

Anne E. Becker
and Arthur Kleinman

When the World Health Organization (WHO) European Ministerial Conference on Mental Health endorsed the statement "No health without mental health" in 2005,[1] it spoke to the intrinsic—and indispensable—role of mental health care in health care writ large. Yet mental health has long been treated in ways that reflect the opposite of that sentiment. This historical divide—in practice and in policy—between physical health and mental health has in turn perpetuated large gaps in resources across economic, social, and scientific domains. The upshot is a global tragedy: a legacy of the neglect and marginalization of mental health.[2] The scale of the global impact of mental illness is substantial, with mental illness constituting an estimated 7.4% of the world's measurable burden of disease.[3] The lack of access to mental health services of good quality is profound in populations with limited resources, for whom numerous social hazards exacerbate vulnerability to poor health. The human toll of mental disorders is further compounded by collateral adverse effects on health and social well-being, including exposure to stigma and human rights abuses, forestallment of educational and social opportunities, and entry into a pernicious cycle of social disenfranchisement and poverty.[4,5] Advances in efforts to alleviate the human and social costs of mental disorders have been both too slow and too few.

Recognizing the Mental Health Burden

The cumbrous and outsized global dimensions of mental illness remained largely unrecognized until the 1990s, when the population health metric disability-adjusted life years (DALYs), which encompassed both years of life lost from premature death and years lived with disability (YLDs), was introduced. The publication of these population health data in *Global Burden of Disease,*[6] which was regarded as a public health tour de force at the time, also

catalyzed a transformative narrative for global mental health. The DALY rubric, along with standardized diagnostic criteria for mental disorders, allowed comparability across disorders and nations and yielded estimates of the composite burden of mental disorders that were much higher than those recognized previously. In 1995, *World Mental Health*[7] outlined an agenda to redress the global crisis in mental health. These and other publications debunked lingering questions about the universality of mental disorders and illuminated the enormous suffering associated with these disorders in low- and middle-income countries, where health care resources devoted to neuropsychiatric illnesses were disproportionately low relative to the corresponding disease burden.[8] The scientific discourse, which had been largely theoretical and descriptive in nature, became one that encompassed an applied agenda with translational relevance.[9]

In 2013, further documentation renders an increasingly clear and troubling picture of the enormous global burden imposed by mental disorders. The economic burdens associated with mental disorders exceed those associated with each of four other major categories of noncommunicable disease: diabetes, cardiovascular diseases, chronic respiratory diseases, and cancer.[10] Major depressive disorder is the second leading cause of YLDs globally and ranks among the four largest contributors to YLDs in each of the socially diverse regions spanning the six continents assessed in the Global Burden of Disease Study 2010.[11] Anxiety disorders, drug-use disorders, alcohol-use disorders, schizophrenia, bipolar disorder, and dysthymia also rank among the 20 conditions contributing the largest global share of YLDs. The aggregate burden of YLDs resulting from mental and behavioral disorders (22.7%) continues to be higher than that resulting from any other disease category, with an estimated contribution to the proportion of burden in 2010 that was similar to that in 1990 (Fig. 13.1).[11] Yet the game-changing potential of these empirical data to increase global investments in mental health care in proportion to the size of the problem has not been realized. Instead, vast gaps in resources persist and seriously compromise access to care.

Closing Gaps in Treatment

More than 75% of persons with serious mental illness in less-developed countries do not receive treatment for it.[12] For the minority who do have access to mental health treatment in low- and middle-income countries, there are few data available to aid in the evaluation of the quality or effectiveness of the treatment. Major deficits in the provision of care include the size of the health care workforce and the training it receives; rigorous empirical evaluation of innovative, scalable models of care delivery; and the political will to support policy, research, training, and infrastructure as explicit priorities at the national, regional, and multinational levels. None of these deficits can be properly remedied without corresponding advances in the others, creating a Gordian knot familiar to global health advocates and practitioners.

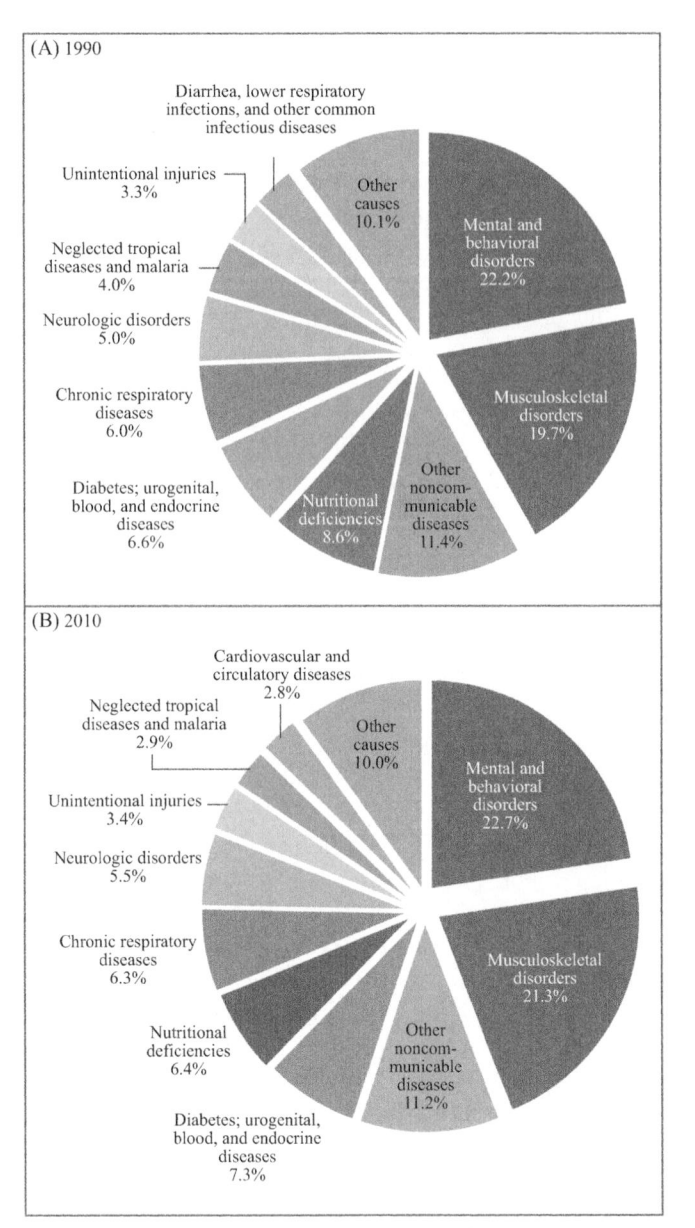

FIGURE 13.1 **Global Burden of Years Lived with Disability, 1990 and 2010** *Shown is the global burden of years lived with disability due to mental and behavioral disorders, as compared with disability due to other highest-ranked categories of disorders and conditions. For the year 1990, other causes include cardiovascular and circulatory diseases; transport injuries; neonatal disorders; HIV–AIDS and tuberculosis; other communicable, maternal, neonatal, and nutritional disorders; digestive diseases; cancer; intentional injuries; war and disaster; maternal disorders; and cirrhosis of the liver. For 2010, other causes include diarrhea, lower respiratory infections, and other common infectious diseases; transport injuries; HIV–AIDS and tuberculosis; neonatal disorders; digestive diseases; other communicable, maternal, neonatal, and nutritional disorders; cancer; war and disaster; intentional injuries; maternal disorders; and cirrhosis of the liver. The percentages corresponding to the individual sectors do not sum to 100% because of rounding. Categories and data are from Vos et al.[11]*

BUILDING CLINICAL CAPACITY

The shortage of clinicians with specialized training in assessing and managing the treatment of patients with mental disorders is a major barrier to providing adequate services in low- and middle-income countries.[2,8,13] Building the necessary mental health workforce will require political commitments to elevate mental health to the highest tier of the global health agenda and to develop corresponding national policies that will support the kind of multisectoral planning needed to align educational objectives and resource allocation with local priorities.[14,15] Partnerships among governments, nongovernmental organizations, multilateral agencies, and academia can also help to increase the capacity of the mental health workforce[16]—for instance, by developing institutional relationships, sometimes referred to as twinning, mirroring, or accompaniment, that would successfully integrate global expertise with local knowledge.[17]

Nonetheless, mere incremental augmentation of the workforce alone is unlikely to close the human resource gap—which is estimated to exceed 1 million mental health workers in low- and middle-income countries[13]—given the present capacities to recruit and train mental health professionals (Fig. 13.2)[15,18] and the prevailing models of mental health care delivery. In addition to training more mental health specialists, it is essential to make better use of their expertise by instituting enhancements and innovations that will increase the quality, relevance, and reach of clinical training.[14] Resolving the gaps in human resources, for example, will probably entail the use of nonspecialists to deliver mental health interventions.[19] This change will call for fresh approaches to training that anticipate the evolution of more prominent supervisory and consultative roles that can leverage the scarce supply of expertise in mental health specialties. The contribution of these specialists must go beyond that of direct service delivery alone. Specialists would be prepared to train and supervise peer nonspecialist professionals to deliver mental health treatment in primary care settings, and nonprofessional health workers would be trained in the tasks of basic case identification, monitoring, and treatment delivery. Novel pedagogic models are called for, as are rigorous evaluations of their effectiveness. The implementation of policy that supports the training, deployment, and decentralization of professionals who are qualified for assessing and delivering care for patients with mental illness—and are enabled to do so—will help to achieve meaningful, sustained progress.[20]

DEVELOPING NEW MODELS OF TREATMENT

The evidence base supporting the efficacy of various treatments for mental health is founded primarily on trials that were conducted in high-income countries. Because only a tiny fraction of published clinical trials have been conducted in low-income countries, the effectiveness of treatments across culturally diverse, low-income settings is largely unknown. In addition, the shortfall of health professionals with training to deliver mental health care in regions with limited resources diminishes the feasibility and relevance of these therapeutic

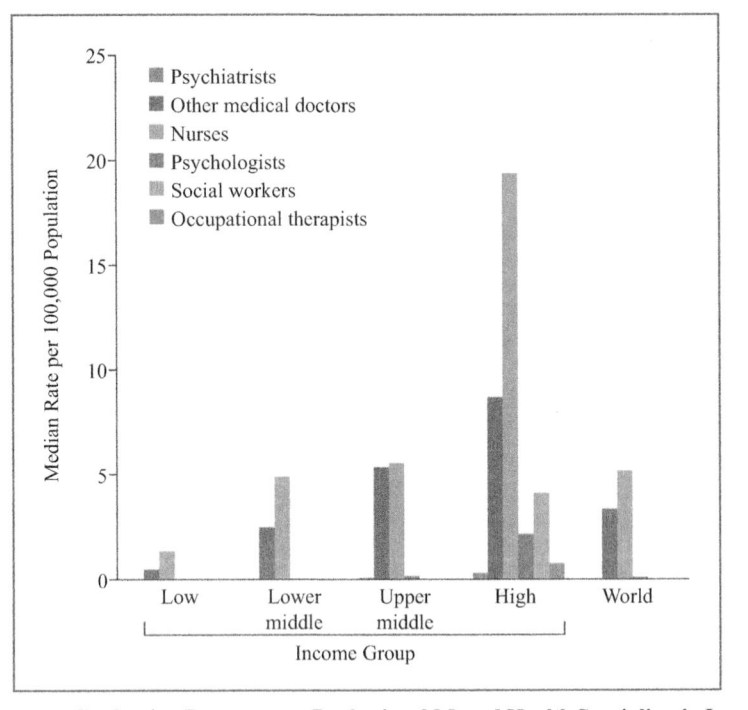

FIGURE 13.2 **Graduation Rates among Professional Mental Health Specialists in Low-, Middle-and High-Income Countries** *Income levels are in accordance with definitions from the World Bank. Data are from the World Health Organization Mental Health Atlas 2011 for the preceding academic year.[18]*

approaches, many of which would require radical adaptation if applied within the constraints of local health care resources. Critics have pointed out that current models that rely on mental health professionals to deliver care to patients are not only unsuitable for low- and middle-income countries[15] but are also impractical in high-income countries, where adequate numbers of mental health professionals are lacking.[21,22] In this respect, a shift to a collaborative model of care delivery has been proposed. This model reconfigures the role of the mental health specialist to emphasize training, supervision, and tertiary care while transferring the bulk of direct service delivery to community health workers or primary care professionals who would receive specific training and supervision in mental health.[22]

The success of this model of collaborative care is premised in part on the feasibility and effectiveness of shifting aspects of case identification and delivery of care from mental health professionals to community health workers who receive specialized training, periodic refresher training, and ongoing supervision by professionals. Similar models of "task shifting" in the delivery of health care (e.g., using community health workers in other clinical domains in low-income settings) have been successful, including in populations that are considered to

be especially difficult to treat.[23,24] Several landmark studies provide conceptual support for this model for the treatment of mental illness in resource-constrained settings, including trials evaluating the effectiveness of interpersonal psychotherapy and cognitive behavioral therapy.[25–29] These approaches hold undeniable promise for broadening access to effective treatments, but their potential to be scaled up and delivered in a sustained way remains untested and uncertain.

Several milestones mark substantive advances in the integration of mental health care into primary care in resource-constrained settings. Among these are the publication of the World Health Report in 2001,[30] which was devoted to mental health; the introduction in 2002 of the Mental Health Global Action Programme (mhGAP), a WHO-led multilateral initiative that encompassed a plan to equip primary care clinicians with training and skills in the care of patients with mental illness[31]; and a series of reviews published in 2009 that provided recommendations on incorporating primary and specialist health professionals as well as trained community health workers into a model of collaborative care that included case identification and management.[32,33] In 2010, the mhGAP Intervention Guide aimed to develop clinical capacities in mental health assessment and treatment among nonspecialists.[34] In 2012, the WHO released a training package designed to complement the guide and also encouraged field testing.[35]

These important achievements notwithstanding, there are scant data to allow evaluation of the large-scale feasibility and effectiveness of task shifting or its applicability across diverse settings[19,36]; the suite of recommendations in mhGAP likewise awaits rigorous empirical evaluation of implementation in low- and middle-income countries that can inform future iterations. Available data are also insufficient to evaluate and refine models for training lay health workers to deliver effective mental health care.[37] Serious efforts to incorporate local knowledge, moreover, can ensure that guidance regarding case identification and treatment continues to be refined and adjusted to the structure of a country's health system and the specific needs of its population. The perspectives of cultural psychiatrists, psychiatric epidemiologists, and medical anthropologists on the biosocial complexity of mental disorders and their presentation and course in specific cultural and social contexts will be invaluable in helping to create appropriate approaches to surveillance, diagnostic assessment, and therapeutic innovation. Although some mental health programs are noteworthy for their measure of early success (including those in Kenya[38] and Egypt[39]), other programs have failed as a result of daunting problems: attrition or reassignment of personnel with mental health training, disinclination to care for the mentally ill, and interruptions in supplies of essential psychotropic medicines.[40,41]

CREATING A FOCUSED AND RELEVANT RESEARCH AGENDA

Deficits in the global delivery of mental health services reflect, in part, substantial gaps in scientific knowledge about virtually all aspects of the delivery of such care in resource-poor settings.[42] Scientific publications relevant to global mental health lag behind those in other relatively well-researched and well-funded

clinical domains, such as the human immunodeficiency virus–acquired immune deficiency syndrome (HIV–AIDS), malaria, and tuberculosis (Fig. 13.3, and the Supplementary Appendix available at NEJM.org). At the same time, studies of mental health in populations living in regions outside high-income countries are underrepresented in the psychiatric literature,[43] a problem that both perpetuates global health inequities[44,45] and entails missed opportunities for important scientific research. A platform for scientific sharing and a research agenda honed to remediate deficits in the delivery of care are urgently required.[46] Finally, the augmentation of research capacity on mental health in low- and middle-income countries is vital to generating an evidence base that will guide strategic planning and implementation.[47]

Research is needed to refine diagnostic tools and algorithms for deployment in community and primary care settings, to identify mediators and modifiers of risk and resilience, and to measure the effectiveness of conventional and novel

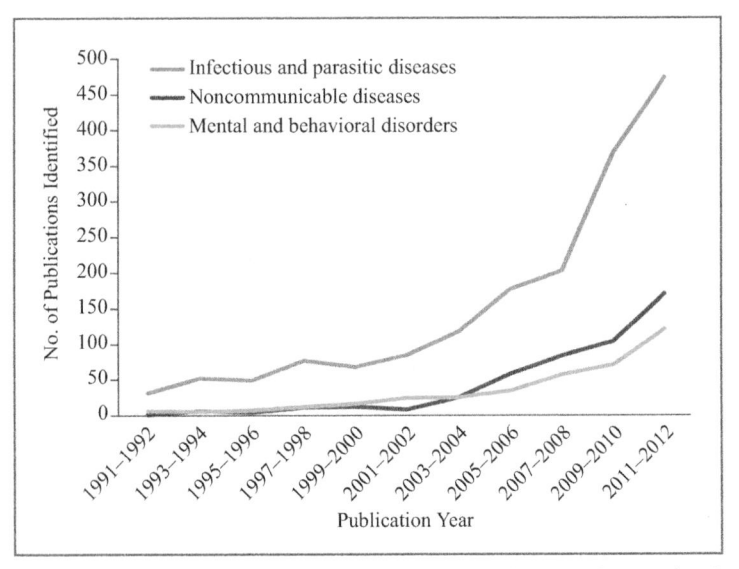

FIGURE 13.3 **Number of Scientific Publications Addressing Global or International Health, According to Broad Disease Category, 1991–2012** *The numbers of publications in the categories of infectious and parasitic diseases, noncommunicable diseases, and mental and behavioral disorders were determined by means of a customized search in the PubMed database for the terms international health, global health, or tropical medicine in combination with one of the three broad disease categories and selected diseases or conditions within them. The latter included terms—and selected common variants or closely related terms—referencing the top five causes of "All ages DALYs" (disability-adjusted life years among persons of all ages) reported for 2010 by Murray et al.[3] within each respective category, excluding birth complications, road injury, and self-harm. The noncommunicable diseases search included the top five categories, excluding mental and behavioral disorders. For more information on search procedures, see the Supplementary Appendix available at NEJM.org.*

treatment-delivery strategies in a variety of health systems. Implementation and health outcomes research are particularly exigent.[48] Analyses of the collateral, economic, and social effects of mental disorders may inform policymakers who are interested in understanding the relative cost-effectiveness of various mental health interventions as well as the costs of withholding them. Child and adolescent mental health is a neglected area that is of great concern given the strong evidence that mental disorders are predictors of adverse economic, social, and health outcomes in adulthood,[4] resulting in costs that are difficult to measure but easy to appreciate. Because adolescents with mental illness typically have difficulty accessing mental health care, interventions that effectively address the formidable barriers confronting them—and other vulnerable sectors of the population—are essential.[40] Another highly ranked research goal is the integration, to the greatest extent possible, of culturally informed screening for mental illness into primary care services.[46,48]

OVERCOMING BARRIERS TO EQUITABLE CARE

Even in regions in which mental health services are widely available, a sizable proportion of the population with mental illness does not receive care that is specific to the illness.[1,12] Cultural practices affect the ways in which people cope with social adversity, manifest emotional distress and mental disorders, and seek care. Economic and social vulnerabilities may make medicines, appointments with health care professionals, and transportation to a clinic unaffordable and time lost from work too costly. For example, even though most low-income countries include psychotropic agents on their list of essential medicines, in 85% of those countries these medications are not available at all primary health care facilities. Moreover, the high median cost of psychotropic medicines in these countries is often prohibitive (e.g., the cost of treatment with antipsychotic agents would equal 9% of the daily minimum wage, and antidepressants 7%) and together with the expenses of other necessary care may impose economically catastrophic costs on patients.[49] Social adversity is both a risk factor and an outcome of poor mental health, and it compounds the disenfranchisement that exacerbates social structural barriers to health care.

The most basic cultural and moral barrier to the amelioration of global mental health problems continues to be the enormously negative, destructive, and almost universal stigma that is attached to mental illnesses, to patients with a mental illness and their families, and to mental health caregivers. At its worst, this stigma nullifies personhood and constitutes an abuse of human rights. But other forms of discrimination are more subtle and more structural. Psychiatrists, psychologists, psychiatric nurses, and psychiatric social workers are not the only professionals who are targets of discrimination; it is our experience that health policy experts are also adversely affected by stigma, with the result that many shy away from making mental health care a priority. This situation may at last be undergoing positive change. The Ministry of Health in China has begun to advocate for patients with mental illness and to advance their interests, and similar agencies

in other countries have begun to do so as well. There is other evidence that the deeply institutionalized stigma surrounding the field of mental health is being challenged and overcome. This may be the most difficult barrier to quantify and yet the most important to address.

An example of how far we still have to go is the exclusion of the topic of mental health from a recent series of papers, policies, and actions advocating priority for four major noncommunicable diseases on the global health agenda. The very sound rationale for urgent and focused global attention to noncommunicable diseases includes the fact that they contribute to a high burden of disease and to poverty, that they impede economic development and the attainment of other Millennium Development Goals, and that there are evidence-based and cost-effective interventions available to address them[50]; these same arguments make an equally convincing case for the inclusion of mental health as a priority on the global agenda.[51-54]

The collective global investment in the HIV–AIDS pandemic led to the recognition that building clinical capacity, pursuing technological advances, providing training for health professionals and paraprofessionals, and engaging in other means of enhancing the health infrastructure in the service of a particular health intervention have the potential to strengthen health systems and accrue benefits across many clinical domains.[55] The distinct clinical and cultural challenges characterizing mental health care delivery notwithstanding, this sort of investment would also seem to be the preferred direction for mental health.

Conclusions

According to virtually any metric, grave concern is warranted with regard to the high global burden of mental disorders, the associated intransigent, unmet needs, and the unacceptable toll of human suffering. Compelling arguments have been made that investment in mental health services is a matter of cost-effectiveness, social justice, and even a smart development strategy.[5,56] Despite the dispiriting near-term forecast regarding improved quality and accessibility of mental health services in poor countries, important advances have been made in the requisite scientific knowledge base and political will to develop and implement policies that can upend these inequities and reset expectations for both the quality of global mental health care and the access to it. Closer alignment with the overarching agenda for global health is evident in the strengthened political commitment to mental health care and in the multilateral partnerships marshaling the resources to improve mental health in countries with limited resources. Several major initiatives have directed funding and attention toward addressing global mental health needs. These include the Mental Health and Poverty Project and the Programme for Improving Mental Health Care, both supported by the Department for International Development in the United Kingdom; the Grand Challenges Canada program; and Grand Challenges in Global Mental Health, led by the National Institute of Mental Health and the Global Alliance for Chronic

Disease, in partnership with others. In 2012, the report from the Sixty-fifth World Health Assembly urged member states and the WHO director-general to take bold corrective actions.[57] Mental health has arrived on the global health agenda; establishing it as a priority at the highest level is essential to match aspiration to need.

References

1. Mental health: facing the challenges, building solutions—report from the WHO European Ministerial Conference. Geneva: World Health Organization, 2005.
2. Saraceno B, Dua T. Global mental health: the role of psychiatry. Eur Arch Psychiatry Clin Neurosci 2009;259:Suppl:S109-S117.
3. Murray CJ, Vos T, Lozano R, et al. Disability-adjusted life years (DALYs) for 291 diseases and injuries in 21 regions, 1990-2010: a systematic analysis for the Global Burden of Disease Study 2010. Lancet 2012;380:2197-223.
4. Patel V, Flisher AJ, Hetrick S, McGorry P. Mental health of young people: a global public-health challenge. Lancet 2007;369:1302-13.
5. Mental health and development: targeting people with mental health conditions as a vulnerable group. Geneva: World Health Organization, 2010.
6. Murray CJL, Lopez AD, eds. The global burden of disease. Geneva: World Health Organization, 1996.
7. Desjarlais R, Eisenberg L, Good B, Kleinman A. World mental health. Oxford, United Kingdom: Oxford University Press, 1995.
8. Saxena S, Thornicroft G, Knapp M, Whiteford H. Resources for mental health: scarcity, inequity, and inefficiency. Lancet 2007;370:878-89.
9. Lancet Global Mental Health Group. Scale up services for global mental health: a call for action. Lancet 2007;370:1241-52.
10. Bloom DE, Cafiero ET, Jane-Llopis E, et al. The global economic burden of non-communicable diseases. Geneva: World Economic Forum, 2011.
11. Vos T, Flaxman AD, Naghavi M, et al. Years lived with disability (YLDs) for 1160 sequelae of 289 diseases and injuries 1990-2010: a systematic analysis for the Global Burden of Disease Study 2010. Lancet 2012;380:2163-96.
12. Demyttenaere K, Bruffaerts R, Posada-Villa J, et al. Prevalence, severity, and unmet need for treatment of mental disorders in the World Health Organization World Mental Health Surveys. JAMA 2004;291:2581-90.
13. Kakuma R, Minas H, van Ginneken N, et al. Human resources for mental health care: current situation and strategies for action. Lancet 2011;378:1654-63.
14. Celletti F, Reynolds TA, Wright A, Stoertz A, Dayrit M. Educating a new generation of doctors to improve the health of populations in low- and middle-income countries. PLoS Med 2011;8(10):e1001108.
15. Bruckner TA, Scheffler RM, Shen G, et al. The mental health workforce gap in low- and middle-income countries: a needs-based approach. Bull World Health Organ 2011;89:184-94.
16. Scaling up nursing & medical education: report on the WHO/PEPFAR planning meeting on scaling up nursing and medical education. Geneva: World Health Organization, 2009.

17. Fricchione GL, Borba CPC, Alem A, Shibre T, Carney JR, Henderson DC. Capacity building in global mental health: professional training. Harv Rev Psychiatry 2012;20:47–57.

18. Mental health atlas. Geneva: World Health Organization, 2011 (whqlibdoc.who.int/publications/2011/9799241564359_eng.pdf).

19. Eaton J, McCay L, Semrau M, et al. Scale up of services for mental health in low-income and middle-income countries. Lancet 2011;378:1592–603.

20. Saraceno B, van Ommeren M, Batniji R, et al. Barriers to improvement of the mental health services in low-income and middle-income countries. Lancet 2007;370:1164–74.

21. Muijen M. Challenges for psychiatry: delivering the Mental Health Declaration for Europe. World Psychiatry 2006;5:113–17.

22. Patel V. The future of psychiatry in low- and middle-income countries. Psychol Med 2009;39:1759–62.

23. Behforouz HL, Farmer PE, Mukherjee JS. From directly observed therapy to accompagnateurs: enhancing AIDS treatment outcomes in Haiti and in Boston. Clin Infect Dis 2004;38:S429-S436.

24. Ivers LC, Jerome J-G, Cullen KA, Lambert W, Celletti F, Samb B. Task-shifting in HIV care: a case study of nurse-centered community-based care in rural Haiti. PLoS One 2011;6(5):e19276.

25. Cohen A. The effectiveness of mental health services in primary care: the view from the developing world. Geneva: World Health Organization, 2001.

26. Bass J, Neugebauer R, Clougherty KF, et al. Group interpersonal psychotherapy for depression in rural Uganda: 6-month outcomes: randomised controlled trial. Br J Psychiatry 2006;188:567–73.

27. Rahman A, Malik A, Sikander S, Roberts C, Creed F. Cognitive behaviour therapy-based intervention by community health workers for mothers with depression and their infants in rural Pakistan: a cluster-randomised controlled trial. Lancet 2008;372:902–909.

28. Patel V, Weiss HA, Chowdhary N, et al. Lay health worker led intervention for depressive and anxiety disorders in India: impact on clinical and disability outcomes over 12 months. Br J Psychiatry 2011;199:459–66. [Erratum, Br J Psychiatry 2012;200:166.]

29. Petersen I, Bhana A, Baillie K. The feasibility of adapted group-based interpersonal therapy (IPT) for the treatment of depression by community health workers within the context of task shifting in South Africa. Community Ment Health J 2012;48:336–41.

30. The world health report 2001—mental health: new understanding, new hope. Geneva: World Health Organization, 2001.

31. Mental Health Global Action Programme: mhGAP. Geneva: World Health Organization, 2002.

32. Patel V, Thornicroft G. Packages of care for mental, neurological, and substance use disorders in low- and middle-income countries. PLoS Med 2009;6(10): e1000160.

33. Patel V, Simon G, Chowdhary N, Kaaya S, Araya R. Packages of care for depression in low- and middle-income countries. PLoS Med 2009;6(10):e1000159.

34. WHO mhGAP intervention guide for mental, neurological, and substance use disorders in non-specialized health settings. Geneva: World Health Organization,

2010,(http://www.who.int/mental_health/publications/mhGAP_intervention_guide/en/index.html).

35. WHO mhGAP newsletter, June 2012 (http://www.who.int/mental_health/mhgap/en).

36. Patel V, Cohen A. Mental health services in primary care in 'developing' countries. World Psychiatry 2003;2:163–64.

37. Lewin SA, Dick J, Pond P, et al. Lay health workers in primary and community health care. Cochrane Database Syst Rev 2005;1:CD004015.

38. Kiima D, Jenkins R. Mental health policy in Kenya—an integrated approach to scaling up equitable care for poor populations. Int J Ment Health Syst 2010;4:19.

39. Jenkins R, Heshmat A, Loza N, Siekkonen I, Sorour E. Mental health policy and development in Egypt—integrating mental health into health sector reforms 2001-9. Int J Ment Health Syst 2010;4:17.

40. Thara R, Padmavati R, Aynkran JR, John S. Community mental health in India: a rethink. Int J Ment Health Syst 2008;2:11.

41. Olugbile O, Zachariah MP, Coker O, Kuyinu O, Isichei B. Provision of mental health services in Nigeria. Integr Psychiatry 2008;5:32–34.

42. Razzouk D, Sharan P, Gallo C, et al. Scarcity and inequity of mental health research resources in low- and middle- income countries: a global survey. Health Policy 2010;94:211–20.

43. Patel V, Kim Y-R. Contribution of low- and middle-income countries to research published in leading psychiatry journals, 2002-2004. Br J Psychiatry 2007;190:77–78.

44. Horton R. Medical journals: evidence of bias against the diseases of poverty. Lancet 2003;361:712–13.

45. Tyrer P. Combating editorial racism in psychiatric publications. Br J Psychiatry 2005;186:1–3.

46. Tomlinson M, Rudan I, Saxena S, Swartz L, Tsai AC, Patel V. Setting priorities for global mental health research. Bull World Health Organ 2009;87:438–46.

47. Thornicroft G, Cooper S, Van Bortel T, Kakuma R, Lund C. Capacity building in global mental health research. Harv Rev Psychiatry 2012;20:13–24.

48. Collins PY, Patel V, Joestl SS, March D, Insel TR, Daar AS. Grand challenges in global mental health. Nature 2011;475:27–30.

49. Mental health systems in selected low- and middle-income countries: a WHO-AIMS cross-national analysis. Geneva: World Health Organization, 2009.

50. Beaglehole R, Bonita R, Horton R, et al. Priority actions for non-communicable disease crisis. Lancet 2011;377:1438–47.

51. Lee PT, Henderson M, Patel V. A UN summit on global mental health. Lancet 2010;376:516.

52. Raviola G, Becker AE, Farmer PE. A global scope for global health—including mental health. Lancet 2011;378:1613–15.

53. Humayun Q, Mirza S. Priority actions for the non-communicable disease crisis. Lancet 2011;378:565.

54. Bass JK, Bornemann TH, Burkey M, et al. A United Nations General Assembly Special Session for mental, neurological, and substance use disorders: the time has come. PLoS Med 2012;9(1):e1001159.

55. The Global Fund strategic approach to health systems strengthening: report from WHO to the Global Fund Secretariat. Geneva: World Health Organization, 2007.

56. Lund C, De Silva M, Plagerson S, et al. Poverty and mental disorders: breaking the cycle in low-income and middle-income countries. Lancet 2011;378:1502–514.

57. World Health Assembly. The global burden of mental disorders and the need for a comprehensive, coordinated response from health and social sectors at the country level. Presented at the Sixty-fifth World Health Assembly, Geneva, May 21–26, 2012 (http://www.who.int/mental_health/WHA65.4_resolution.pdf).

Injuries

Robyn Norton and Olive Kobusingye

Injuries have traditionally been defined as physical damage to a person caused by an acute transfer of energy (mechanical, thermal, electrical, chemical, or radiation energy) or by the sudden absence of heat or oxygen. This definition has been broadened to include damage that results in psychological harm, maldevelopment, or deprivation.[1] Injuries are most commonly categorized with reference to the presumed underlying intent: injuries considered to be unintentional include those caused by road-traffic incidents, falls, drowning, burns, and poisonings, and injuries considered to be intentional include those caused by self-harm, interpersonal violence, and war and conflict.[2,3]

The subject of injuries has received relatively scant attention from the medical community, as evidenced by the absence of this topic in the curricula of most medical schools, and even schools of public health, and by the limited coverage of the topic in most medical journals. The Global Burden of Disease (GBD) study has at least placed injuries on the global health agenda by categorizing the major causes of death and disability worldwide into three main groups: group I includes communicable, maternal, perinatal, and nutritional conditions; group II includes noncommunicable diseases; and group III includes injuries.[2,3] Concurrent with the recognition of the burden of injuries has been the growing acknowledgment that an evidence-based approach to the prevention and management of injuries can and should be adopted, as has been done in the case of other major global causes of death and disability.[4,5]

Burden of Injuries

In 2010, there were 5.1 million deaths from injuries—almost 1 out of every 10 deaths in the world—and the total number of deaths from injuries was greater than the number of deaths from infection with the human immunodeficiency

virus–acquired immune deficiency syndrome (HIV–AIDS), tuberculosis, and malaria combined (3.8 million).[3] Persons in low- and middle-income countries sustained a disproportionate number of injury-related deaths: 89% of the total number of deaths due to injury, as compared with 84% of deaths from all causes, occurred in these countries.[2] Whereas injuries accounted for 6% of deaths in high-income countries, they caused 12% of deaths in low-income countries in the Americas and 11% of deaths in low-income countries in Southeast Asia.[2] The burden of injury is even greater in some individual countries, such as South Africa, where injuries are the second leading cause of both death and disability-adjusted life-years (DALYs).[6]

A disproportionate number of injuries are sustained by males, who accounted for about 68% of all injury-related deaths in 2010 (Table 14.1).[3] Although injuries are sustained across the life cycle, they affect young people (persons between 10 and 24 years of age) in particular, accounting for more than 40% of deaths in this age group.[3,7] More than half of all deaths (52%) occurring in males 10 to 24 years of age are caused by injuries.[3]

UNINTENTIONAL INJURIES

In 2010, unintentional injuries were the cause of the majority of injury-related deaths (69%),[3] as well as the majority of DALYs (72%).[8] Transportation-related

TABLE 14.1 Deaths from Cause-Specific Injuries in 2010[*]

Cause of Death	No. of Deaths/ 100,000 Persons	% of All Deaths	% of Injury- Related Deaths	% Involving Males
All causes	52,770	100.0	—	54.8
All injuries	5,073	9.6	100.0	68.2
Unintentional injuries	3,520	6.7	69.4	67.4
Transportation-related injuries	1,397	2.6	27.5	75.1
Falls	541	1.0	10.7	59.0
Drowning	349	0.7	6.9	70.5
Injuries from fires, heat, and hot substances	338	0.6	6.7	47.5
Poisonings	180	0.3	3.5	65.6
Other	715	1.4	14.1	66.9
Intentional injuries	1,340	2.5	26.4	70.7
Self-harm	884	1.7	17.4	65.5
Interpersonal violence	456	0.9	9.0	80.7
Forces of nature, war, and legal intervention[†]	214	0.4	4.2	65.4
Exposure to forces of nature	196	0.4	3.9	65.3
Collective violence and legal interventions	18	<0.1	0.4	63.9

[*]Data are from Lozano et al.[3]

[†]Deaths from legal intervention include, among others, those that result from death penalties imposed by governments.

injuries (including injuries from both road-traffic incidents and non–road-traffic causes, such as incidents on the water or in the air) were the leading cause of injury-related deaths in 2010 and were responsible for 1.4 million deaths.[3] Injuries from road-traffic incidents were the eighth leading cause of death overall[3] and the leading cause of death among persons 10 to 24 years of age and were responsible for 17% of all deaths among males in this age group.[3]

Although injuries from road-traffic incidents impose a substantial burden across all regions of the world, the burden is greatest in low- and middle-income countries (Table 14.2). In 2004, injuries from road-traffic incidents were the sixth leading cause of death and the fourth leading cause of DALYs in middle-income countries.[9] The highest death rates, however, occurred in low- and middle-income countries in Africa and in the Eastern Mediterranean and Western Pacific regions. Notably, Africa currently has the lowest motorization rate (i.e., the number of registered vehicles per person) of all the world's regions, but its fatality rates are already similar to those in regions that have considerably higher motorization rates.[10]

Falls are the next most common cause of deaths related to unintentional injuries globally, followed by drowning, burns, and poisonings (Table 14.1). The rates of death from falls and from poisonings are generally higher in high-income

TABLE 14.2 Estimates of the Rate of Death per 100,000 Persons Associated with Cause-Specific Injuries, According to Income Level and Region, in 2008.*

Cause of Death	High-Income Countries	Low-Income and Middle-Income Countries					
		Africa	The Americas	Eastern Mediterranean Region	Europe	Southeast Asia	Western Pacific Region
		rate per 100,000 persons					
Unintentional injuries							
Road-traffic injuries	10.3	20.9	17.6	21.6	17.2	17.6	21.2
Falls	7.8	2.4	3.7	4.1	5.7	12.0	8.2
Drowning	1.8	5.2	2.8	3.9	5.5	5.5	5.7
Fires	0.9	4.9	0.7	5.2	4.2	4.8	0.9
Poisoning	4.1	4.9	0.7	2.8	18.1	1.8	2.9
Other	10.9	16.9	11.8	13.6	30.6	22.8	14.4
Intentional injuries							
Self-harm	13.4	6.3	5.8	5.5	16.9	15.6	11.4
Interpersonal violence	2.7	20.1	24.1	3.9	9.9	5.8	2.9
War and conflict	0.1	3.6	1.2	17.7	1.2	2.3	0.2

*Data are from the World Health Organization.[2]

countries than in low- and middle-income countries combined[2]; however, the rate of death from falls is highest in the low- and middle-income countries of Southeast Asia, whereas the rate of death from poisoning is highest in the low- and middle-income countries of Europe (Table 14.2). More than 90% of deaths from drowning and from fires occur in low- and middle-income countries.[2] Males account for more than 50% of all injury-related, cause-specific deaths, other than deaths from burns (Table 14.1).

INTENTIONAL INJURIES

Deaths from self-harm and from interpersonal violence are, respectively, the second and fourth leading causes of injury-related deaths (Table 14.1) and of DALYs.[8] Self-harm is the cause of disproportionately more deaths among persons in high-income countries than among those in low- and middle-income countries,[2] although the rates of death from self-harm are highest in the low- and middle-income countries of Europe and Southeast Asia (Table 14.2). Almost 95% of deaths and DALYs due to interpersonal violence and almost all deaths and DALYs due to war and conflict occur among persons in low- and middle-income countries.[2] The rates of death from interpersonal violence are substantially higher in low- and middle-income countries in both Africa and the Americas than in other regions of the world, and the rates of death from war and conflict are highest in the low- and middle-income countries of the Eastern Mediterranean region (Table 14.2). In South Africa, almost 50% of all injury-related deaths result from interpersonal violence.[6]

OTHER HEALTH OUTCOMES

The data reported above clearly identify injuries as major causes of death and DALYs. However, the importance of injuries as a contributor to other health outcomes is not captured in these statistics. It has been shown, for example, that victims of childhood maltreatment suffer long-term psychological sequelae, such as low self-esteem, anxiety, and depression,[11–13] and survivors of sexual abuse during childhood are more likely to engage in high-risk sexual behaviors, have multiple sex partners, become pregnant as teenagers, and be the victims of sexual assault as adults.[14–16]

FUTURE BURDEN OF INJURIES

The global burden of injuries is expected to increase over the next 20 years; it is projected that by 2030, injuries from road-traffic accidents will be the 5th leading cause of death worldwide, and deaths from self-harm will be the 12th leading cause of death.[9] Overall, the number of deaths from injuries increased by 24% between 1990 and 2010. The increases in deaths from transportation-related injuries, self-harm, falls, burns, and interpersonal violence during this period suggest that further increases in these categories might be observed over the next

20 years. In contrast, deaths from drowning and poisonings ranked lower in 2010 than in 1990.[3]

The burden of injuries is likely to diminish over the next 20 years in high-income countries, whereas injuries are projected to continue to be a major burden in middle-income countries and to become increasingly important in low-income countries.[9] These projections probably reflect the increasing exposure to risks in the low- and middle-income countries (e.g., increasing motorization) combined with the increasing implementation of effective prevention strategies in the high-income countries.[3,17,18] If these projected increases in injuries are to be thwarted, efforts aimed at prevention, especially in low- and middle-income countries, must become a priority.

Prevention of Injuries

The prevention of injuries, which should be the first priority, is achievable, as evidenced by the halving of rates of death from road-traffic injuries over the past three decades in countries such as Australia, Canada, and the United States.[18] These achievements have required a multisectoral response, focused not only on road users, but also on vehicles, roads, and to a lesser degree the broader transportation system (i.e., the ways in which transportation systems are organized and planned). Rigorous methodologic approaches to assessing the effectiveness of these prevention efforts have been limited, and interventions have been adopted largely on the basis of before-and-after comparisons of their effects on a range of noninjury-related outcomes, such as changes in behavior or increases in knowledge.[5,18]

UNINTENTIONAL INJURIES

In 2004, the World Health Organization (WHO) and the World Bank published the World Report on Road Traffic Injury Prevention.[18] The report provided a comprehensive summary of the best available evidence on the prevention of injuries from road-traffic incidents and also highlighted the paucity of research data from low- and middle-income countries. Since then, the WHO, in partnership with governments around the world, especially those in low- and middle-income countries, has taken the lead in facilitating campaigns to implement legislation aimed at further reducing injuries from road-traffic incidents globally.[19,20] These campaigns have focused on efforts to reduce the rates of speeding and drinking while driving and to increase the use of motorcycle helmets, seat belts, and child safety restraints—interventions that have been shown in data from high-income countries to be effective in reducing injuries[18,21,22] and for which appropriate legislation in many low- and middle-income countries has been lacking.[19] Concurrently, the WHO has supported research in countries such as Vietnam that has shown that the introduction of legislation requiring the use of helmets by motorcyclists, accompanied by education and enforcement, has had a substantial

effect both on increasing the use of motorcycle helmets (from about 40% to >90%) and on decreasing the numbers of deaths (by 18%) and head injuries (by 16%).[23,24]

A multisectoral and legislative approach toward prevention has been extended to most other cause-specific unintentional injuries[25] (Table 14.3)— in part because the majority of preventive strategies lie outside the traditional health sector (e.g., the installation of isolation fencing around swimming pools to prevent drowning[26] or the setting and enforcing of standards for playground equipment to prevent falls and injuries from falls[27]) and in part because there is still little evidence to support the effectiveness of educational strategies. For example, programs to promote (but not require by law) the installation of smoke alarms to prevent household fires have had only modest beneficial effects with respect to ownership of alarms and the presence in the house of functioning alarms and no proven beneficial effects with respect to the prevention of fires or fire-related injuries.[28]

The health sector, and especially the primary care sector, can play a potentially important role in the prevention of injuries to children and the prevention of falls among the elderly. Although it is possible that these sectors can also play a role in the prevention of injuries in other age groups, evidence to support this is lacking.[29] Promising interventions include those that focus on counseling and educating parents regarding the prevention of childhood injuries[30] and those that are aimed at reducing the risks of falling among older populations through the use of individually prescribed home-based exercise programs or programs to review and modify medication regimens. [31]

Much of the evidence regarding effective strategies for the prevention of unintentional injuries is derived from research conducted in high-income countries and thus may have limited direct applicability for the prevention of injuries in low- and middle-income countries.[5,32] However, it is highly likely that strategies that are effective in high-income countries can be suitably adapted to low- and middle-income settings—as was shown in the case of the prevention of injuries from road-traffic incidents. For example, the required use of isolation fencing or covers to prevent access to open water in low- and middle-income countries will probably reduce deaths from drowning in much the same way that the enactment and enforcement of legislation relating to isolation fencing around swimming pools has in high-income settings.

INTENTIONAL INJURIES

The best available evidence regarding the prevention of self-harm suggests that the medical sector has an important role to play (Table 14.3). Specifically, there is increasingly strong evidence of the effectiveness of educating clinicians in the appropriate identification and treatment of persons with mood disorders.[33] In addition, there is good evidence to suggest that restricting access to the means of suicide, including the access to pesticides, guns, and unprotected heights, is an effective preventive strategy, although it is one that is traditionally outside the realm of the health sector.[33]

TABLE 14.3 Evidence-Based Strategies Involving Legislative and Nonlegislative Approaches for Primary Prevention of Cause-Specific Injuries.*

Cause of Injury	Legislative Approaches	Nonlegislative Approaches
Road-traffic injuries	Implementing and enforcing speed limits; implementing and enforcing legislation regarding driving under the influence of alcohol, the use of motorcycle helmets, the use of seat belts and child safety restraints, and the addition of daytime running lights on motorcycles; implementing graduated driver licensing systems for novice drivers	Developing safer roadway infrastructure, including separating four-wheeled vehicles from pedestrians, bicyclists, and sometimes motorcyclists; introducing traffic calming (engineering and other measures put in place on roads with a goal of slowing down or reducing traffic) to reduce speeds in urban areas; implementing vehicle and safety-equipment standards
Falls	Implementing and enforcing window-guard laws for tall buildings	Redesigning furniture and other products; implementing and enforcing standards for playground equipment; implementing home-based exercise programs for older persons
Drowning	Implementing and enforcing legislation related to isolation fencing around swimming pools	Removing or covering water hazards; promoting the use of personal flotation devices
Burns	Implementing and enforcing laws on smoke alarms and on hot tap water temperatures	Implementing and enforcing standards for child-resistant lighters
Poisoning	Implementing and enforcing laws for child-resistant packaging of medicines and poisons	Removing toxic products from homes and other environments where they might be accessed easily
Self-harm		Ensuring early detection and effective treatment of mood disorders and behavioral therapy for persons with suicidal thoughts and behaviors; restricting access to the means of self-harm (including pesticides, guns, and unprotected heights)
Interpersonal violence		Developing safe, stable, and nurturing relationships between children and their caregivers; developing life skills in children and adolescents; reducing the availability and harmful use of alcohol; reducing access to guns and knives; promoting sex equality to prevent violence against women; changing cultural and social norms that support violence

*Data are from Norton et al.[5] and the World Health Organization.[25]

Evidence regarding effective interventions to prevent interpersonal violence is not strong but is accumulating (Table 14.3). Two U.S.-based programs, the Nurse–Family Partnership home visiting program[34] and the Positive Parenting Program (Triple P),[35] have been shown to be successful in reducing the incidence of child maltreatment. In contrast, the best evidence regarding the prevention of violence against women is emerging from low- and middle-income regions. The Intervention with Microfinance for AIDS and Gender Equity (IMAGE) initiative in South Africa[36] combines the provision of small loans with sex-equity training, and the Stepping Stones programs in Africa and Asia[37] use life-skills training focused on sex-based violence, relationship skills, assertiveness training, and communication about HIV infection.

Improving the Management of Injuries

Although prevention is likely to have the greatest effect on reducing the global burden of injuries, safe, effective, and affordable prehospital and hospital management, as well as appropriate rehabilitation services, are essential to reducing this burden. However, on a global level, the financial and human resources available to deliver these services vary widely. In most high-income countries, care of injured persons is characterized by sophisticated trauma systems. These organized and coordinated services within defined geographic areas deliver the full range of care to injured persons by integrating prehospital, transport, and trauma-center components within the local public health system.[38,39] Emergency medical technicians, emergency department physicians, and trauma surgeons are typically central to the management of severe injuries. Such systems contrast sharply with the care available in the majority of low-income settings where, except for urban centers, trauma care is dependent mostly on lay first responders, unplanned and often inconsistently available transportation for the injured, and health facilities with varying capabilities for managing severe injuries.[40]

PREHOSPITAL MANAGEMENT

There continues to be debate regarding the level of training that should be required for health care providers in the prehospital care setting and the interventions that can be safely undertaken in the field without causing undue delay in the transfer to a hospital.[41,42] Much of the evidence relies on the results of before-and-after studies.[43] Randomized trials need to be conducted in light of the diversity of prehospital care services that are proliferating despite limited evidence to support their effectiveness.[44]

A range of low-cost strategies to improve access to prehospital care, especially in low- and middle-income countries, has been outlined in detail; these strategies include the use of trained lay first responders, access to essential equipment and supplies, improved communications, and provision of appropriate transportation

systems.[40] Although there is evidence to show that trained lay first responders do improve trauma outcomes,[45] other strategies still need to be examined.

HOSPITAL MANAGEMENT

In the past decade, large-scale, randomized, controlled trials conducted in emergency departments and intensive care units, including research focused specifically on the care of injured patients, have set new benchmarks for the provision of evidence-based, in-hospital trauma care.[46–49] These trials provide evidence regarding effective treatments, such as the use of tranexamic acid to reduce the risk of death in patients with trauma-related bleeding (as shown in the Clinical Randomisation of an Antifibrinolytic in Significant Hemorrhage 2 [CRASH 2] study[46]). They also provide evidence of useless and potentially harmful practices, such as the administration of glucocorticoids[47] and the use of albumin for fluid resuscitation in the treatment of patients with major head injuries.[48]

In low-resource settings, where surgeons are not readily available, evidence indicates that outcomes can be improved if nonspecialist physicians or nonphysician clinicians can be trained in certain skills that would normally be carried out by emergency physicians or trauma surgeons in centers with better resources.[50–54] Although such task shifting is likely to be widespread, particularly in low-income countries, there is scant information on exactly how it is done, and rigorous evaluations are needed to inform practice. Many important issues remain unresolved, even in high-income countries, such as which system (e.g., specialist pediatric trauma center, adult trauma center, or adult trauma center with pediatric specialists) offers severely injured children the best odds for recovery[55] and how best to evaluate the effectiveness of trauma systems.[56]

REHABILITATION

In June 2011, the WHO and the World Bank issued the World Report on Disability, the first-ever global report on disabilities.[57] The report comprehensively outlined the scope of rehabilitation services available worldwide and the range of services that might be provided, especially in low- and middle-income countries, where few such services currently exist. However, the report also made it clear that although some rehabilitation services are supported by an evidence base, the majority are not, and the field is almost totally lacking in large, randomized, controlled trials. The Physiotherapy Evidence Database,[58] for example, which records information on more than 20,000 trials, shows that many of these trials were poorly designed, involved small numbers of patients, and did not provide evidence of effectiveness with regard to major health outcomes. Not surprisingly, the World Report calls for more research to ensure the development of rehabilitation guidelines that are based on strong evidence.[55]

The Way Forward

Given the uncertainties about the quality of current data on injuries in some countries[59] and the absence of data in others,[60] there remains a need to more accurately define the burden of injuries. Yet, there can be no doubt that injuries are already a major global health issue and require the same attention as that afforded HIV–AIDS, malaria, and tuberculosis.

Increasing economic development in low- and middle-income countries, accompanied by increasing levels of motorization, almost ensures that the projected increases in the global burden of injury will be realized. These increases can be mitigated only if the evidence-based strategies for prevention and management that have been developed are adopted worldwide and if innovative and cost-effective approaches continue to be identified. To achieve the latter, we must ensure that the medical and public health communities, particularly in low- and middle-income countries, become "injury-literate." In addition to capacity-building initiatives such as those offered by the TEACH-VIP[61] and MENTOR-VIP[62] programs of the WHO—both of which aim to introduce those in public health to the topic of injury prevention, with the latter focusing particularly on those committed to working in the injury field—and the capacity-building activities offered by the Road Traffic Injuries Research Network,[63] medical schools, schools of public health, and programs associated with the training of allied health professionals will need to be at the forefront of providing such education.

References

1. Krug E, Dahlberg LL, Mercy JA, Zwi AB, Lozano R, eds. World report on violence and health. Geneva: World Health Organization; 2002.
2. Cause-specific mortality: regional estimates for 2008. Geneva: World Health Organization (http://www.who.int/healthinfo/global_burden_disease/estimates_regional/en/index.html).
3. Lozano R, Naghavi M, Foreman K, et al. Global and regional mortality from 235 causes of death for 20 age groups in 1990 and 2010: a systematic analysis for the Global Burden of Disease Study 2010. Lancet 2012;380:2095–128.
4. Rivara FP, Grossman DC, Cummings P. Injury prevention. N Engl J Med 1997;337:543–48.
5. Norton R, Hyder AA, Butchart A. Unintentional injuries and violence. In: Merson MH, Black RE, Mills AJ, eds. Global health: diseases, programs, systems, and policies. 3rd ed. Burlington, MA: Jones & Bartlett Learning, 2011:407–44.
6. Seedat M, Van Niekerk A, Jewkes R, Suffla S, Ratele K. Violence and injuries in South Africa: prioritizing an agenda for prevention. Lancet 2009;374:1011–22. [Erratum, Lancet 2009;374:978.]
7. Patton GC, Coffey C, Sawyer SM, et al. Global patterns of mortality in young people: a systematic analysis of population health data. Lancet 2009;374:881–92.

8. Murray CJL, Vos T, Lozano R, et al. Disability-adjusted life years (DALYs) for 291 diseases and injuries in 21 regions, 1990–2010: a systematic analysis for the Global Burden of Disease Study 2010. Lancet 2012;380:2197–223.

9. The global burden of disease: 2004 update. Geneva: World Health Organization, 2008.

10. Status report on road safety in countries of the WHO African Region, 2009. Brazzaville, Republic of the Congo: World Health Organization Regional Office for Africa, 2010.

11. Arias I. The legacy of child maltreatment: long-term health consequences for women. J Womens Health (Larchmt) 2004;13:468–73.

12. Turner HA, Finkelhor D, Ormrod R. The effect of lifetime victimization on the mental health of children and adolescents. Soc Sci Med 2006;62:13–27.

13. Briere J, Jordan CE. Childhood maltreatment, intervening variables, and adult psychological difficulties in women: an overview. Trauma Violence Abuse 2009;10:375–88.

14. Andrews G, Corry J, Slade T, Issakidis C, Swanston H. Child sexual abuse. In: Ezzati M, Lopez AD, Rodgers A, Murray CJL, eds. Comparative quantification of health risks: global and regional burden of disease attributable to selected major risk factors. Vol. 2. Geneva: World Health Organization, 2004.

15. Brown DW, Riley L, Butchart A, Meddings D, Kann L, Harvey A. Exposure to physical and sexual violence among African youth and associations with adverse health behaviors: results from the Global School-based Student Health Survey. Bull World Health Organ 2009;87:447–55.

16. Lalor K, McElvaney R. Child sexual abuse, links to later sexual exploitation/ high-risk sexual behavior, and prevention/treatment programs. Trauma Violence Abuse 2010;11:159–77.

17. Kopits E, Cropper M. Traffic fatalities and economic growth. Washington, DC: World Bank, 2003. (Policy Research Working Paper 3035.)

18. Peden M, Scurfield R, Sleet D, et al., eds. World report on road traffic injury prevention. Geneva: World Health Organization, 2004.

19. Global status report on road safety: time for action. Geneva: World Health Organization, 2009.

20. Global plan for the decade of action for road safety 2011–2020. Geneva: World Health Organization, 2011 (http://www.who.int/roadsafety/decade_of_action/en/index.html).

21. Liu BC, Ivers R, Norton R, Boufous S, Blows S, Lo SK. Helmets for preventing injury in motorcycle riders. Cochrane Database Syst Rev 2008;1:CD004333.

22. Seat-belts and child restraints: a road safety manual for decision-makers and practitioners. London: FIA Foundation for the Automobile and Society, 2009.

23. Pervin A, Passmore J, Sidik M, McKinley T, Nguyen TH, Nguyen PN. Viet Nam's mandatory motorcycle helmet law and its impact on children. Bull World Health Organ 2009;87:369–73.

24. Passmore J, Tu NT, Luong MA, Chinh ND, Nam NP. Impact of mandatory motorcycle helmet wearing legislation on head injuries in Viet Nam: results of a preliminary analysis. Traffic Inj Prev 2010;11:202–206.

25. Injuries and violence: the facts. Geneva: World Health Organization, 2010 (http://whqlibdoc.who.int/publications/2010/9789241599375_eng.pdf).

26. Thompson DC, Rivara FP. Pool fencing for preventing drowning in children. Cochrane Database Syst Rev 2000;2:CD001047.

27. Peden M, Oyebite K, Ozanne-Smith J, Hyder AA, Branche C. Rahman, et al., eds. World report on child injury prevention. Geneva: World Health Organization, 2008.

28. DiGuiseppi C, Higgins JPT. Interventions for promoting smoke alarm ownership and function. Cochrane Database Syst Rev 2001;2:CD002246.

29. Ship AN. The most primary of care—talking about driving and distraction. N Engl J Med 2010;362:2145–47.

30. Kendrick D, Barlow J, Hampshire A, Stewart-Brown S, Polnay L. Parenting interventions and the prevention of unintentional injuries in childhood: systematic review and meta-analysis. Child Care Health Dev 2008;34:682–95.

31. Gillespie LD, Robertson MC, Gillespie WJ, et al. Interventions for preventing falls in older people living in the community. Cochrane Database Syst Rev 2009;2:CD007146.

32. Ameratunga S, Hijar M, Norton R. Road traffic injuries: confronting disparities to address a global health problem. Lancet 2006;367:1533–40.

33. Mann JJ, Apter A, Bertolote J, et al. Suicide prevention strategies: a systematic review. JAMA 2005;294:2064–74.

34. Olds DL, Sadler L, Kitzman H. Programs for parents of infants and toddlers: recent evidence from randomized trials. J Child Psychol Psychiatry 2007;48:355–91.

35. Prinz RJ, Sanders MR, Shapiro CJ, Whitaker DJ, Lutzker JR. Population-based prevention of child maltreatment: the U.S. Triple P System Population Trial. Prev Sci 2009;10:1–12.

36. Pronyk PM, Hargreaves JR, Kim JC, et al. Effect of a structural intervention for the prevention of intimate-partner violence and HIV in rural South Africa: a cluster randomized trial. Lancet 2006;368:1973–83.

37. Jewkes R, Nduna M, Levin J, et al. Impact of Stepping Stones on incidence of HIV, HSV-2 and sexual behavior in rural South Africa: cluster randomized controlled trial. BMJ 2008;337:a506.

38. Liberman M, Mulder DS, Lavoie A, Sampalis JS. Implementation of a trauma care system: evolution through evaluation. J Trauma 2004;56:1330–35.

39. Kristiansen T, Søreide K, Ringdal KG, et al. Trauma systems and early management of severe injuries in Scandinavia: review of the current state. Injury 2010;41:444–52.

40. Kobusingye OC, Hyder AA, Bishai D, et al. Emergency medical services. In: Jamison DT, Breman JG, Measham AR, et al., eds. Disease control priorities in developing countries. 2nd ed. New York: Oxford University Press, 2006:1261–79.

41. Liberman M, Roudsari BS. Prehospital trauma care: what do we really know? Curr Opin Crit Care 2007;13:691–96.

42. Timmermann A, Russo SG, Hollmann MW. Paramedic versus emergency physician emergency medical service: role of the anaesthesiologist and the European versus the Anglo-American concept. Curr Opin Anaesthesiol 2008;21:222–27.

43. Cochrane Injuries Group (CIG) home page (http://injuries.cochrane.org).

44. Global forum on trauma care: meeting report, 2009. Geneva: World Health Organization (www.who.int/entity/violence_injury_prevention/services/traumacare/global_forum_meeting_report.pdf).

45. Murad MK, Husum H. Trained lay first responders reduce trauma mortality: a controlled study of rural trauma in Iraq. Prehosp Disaster Med 2010;25:533–39.

46. The CRASH-2 Trial Collaborators. Effects of tranexamic acid on death, vascular occlusive events, and blood transfusion in trauma patients with significant haemorrhage (CRASH-2): a randomised, placebo-controlled trial. Lancet 2010;376:23–32.

47. Edwards P, Arango M, Balica L, et al. Final results of MRC CRASH, a randomised placebo-controlled trial of intravenous corticosteroid in adults with head injury-outcomes at 6 months. Lancet 2005;365:1957–59.

48. The SAFE Study Investigators. Saline or albumin for fluid resuscitation in patients with traumatic brain injury. N Engl J Med 2007;357:874–84.

49. Cooper DJ, Rosenfeld JV, Murray L, et al. Decompressive craniectomy in diffuse traumatic brain injury. N Engl J Med 2011;364:1493–502. [Erratum, N Engl J Med 2011;365:2040.]

50. Van Heng Y, Davoung C, Husum H. Non-doctors as trauma surgeons? A controlled study of trauma training for non-graduate surgeons in rural Cambodia. Prehosp Disaster Med 2008;23483–89.

51. Chu K, Rosseel P, Gielis P, Ford N. Surgical task shifting in Sub-Saharan Africa. PLoS Med 2009;6(5):e1000078.

52. Luboga S, Macfarlane SB, von Schreeb J, et al. Increasing access to surgical services in sub-Saharan Africa: priorities for national and international agencies recommended by the Bellagio Essential Surgery Group. PLoS Med 2009;6(12):e1000200.

53. Atiyeh BS, Gunn SW, Hayek SN. Provision of essential surgery in remote and rural areas of developed as well as low and middle-income countries. Int J Surg 2010;8:581–85.

54. Chu KM, Ford NP, Trelles M. Providing surgical care in Somalia: a model of task shifting. Confl Health 2011;5:12.

55. Petrosyan M, Guner YS, Emami CN, Ford HR. Disparities in the delivery of pediatric trauma care. J Trauma 2009;67:Suppl:S114–19.

56. Evans C, Howes D, Pickett W, Dagnone L. Audit filters for improving processes of care and clinical outcomes in trauma systems. Cochrane Database Syst Rev 2009;4:CD007590.

57. World report on disability. Geneva: World Health Organization/World Bank, 2011 (http://www.who.int/disabilities/world_report/2011/en/index.html).

58. Physiotherapy Evidence Database (PEDro) home page (http://www.pedro.org.au/).

59. Hu G, Baker T, Baker SP. Comparing road traffic mortality rates from police-reported data and death registration date in China. Bull World Health Organ 2011;89:41–45.

60. Bhalla K, Harrison JE, Fingerhut LA, Shahraz S, Abraham J, Yeh PH. The global injury mortality data collection of the Global Burden of Disease Injury Expert Group: a publicly accessible research tool. Int J Inj Contr Saf Promot 2011;18:249–53.

61. Meddings DR. WHO launches TEACH–VIP E-learning. Inj Prev 2010;16:143.

62. *Idem.* MENTOR-VIP—a global mentoring program for violence and injury prevention. Inj Prev 2007;13:69.

63. The Road Traffic Injuries Research Network (RTIRN) home page (http://www.rtirn.net).

{ PART IV }

Health System Responses

INTRODUCTION

Whether under the rubric of *health policy, health services administration*, or *health care management*, public health has a long tradition of training the personnel needed to design and operate health care systems. In more recent times the broad architecture of health care delivery and disease prevention has been described as the analysis of *health systems*, recognizing in the name that these are highly complex, multidimensional entities that should be thought of more as a whole (including response to the environment) rather than as a skeleton that merely supports other functions. Health systems are politically, socially, and culturally determined.

It should thus be no surprise that the design of health systems often reflects the socioeconomic circumstances and mores of the specific time and place of the society served. It should also come as no surprise that countries that are in a position to influence the health systems of other countries, particularly by providing advice or resources, may be likely to recommend solutions that are more compatible with the needs and traditions of the donor country rather than those the recipient.

Policies and ideologies, in faraway locations like Washington, Brussels, or Geneva may influence the architecture of health systems in a quite different country. During the era of "structural adjustment" policies at the World Bank, for example, government-managed and financed health systems in many developing countries were starved of resources, sometimes owing to externally imposed policies, such as the requirement to exact "user fees" from patients. Individual loans and support were also caught up in larger debates about the merits of public versus private provision of government services in general. Thus decisions about how the health system should provide services, to whom, and at what cost often reflects a range of influences

other than the questions of what populations need and how to efficiently deliver services tailored to these needs.

A major focus of the global health movement has been the needs of mothers and children, addressed here by Zulfiqar Bhutta and Robert Black. The rationale is clear: women and children are often the most vulnerable members of society with the least financial and political agency to take care of their needs. They have quite specific medical requirements—family planning, care during pregnancy and childbirth, nutrition, immunizations, and growth monitoring. The coordination of this care in maternal and child health clinics may enable multiple needs to be met in a single visit and takes advantage of the potential for synergy between promoting the health of both mother and child, since a child is at high risk of being sick if the mother is sick. As Bhutta and Black remind us, despite immense progress in child survival, much remains to be done. In many countries, particularly in Sub-Saharan Africa and South Asia, reaching the millennium development goals[1] (MDGs) for reducing the under-age-5 mortality rate by 2015 (MDG 4) has not been achieved. MDG 5 called for reducing maternal mortality by three-quarters by 2015. Although it has been close to halved since 1990, over 200,000 women still die in childbirth every year, and the lifetime probability of a women dying in childbirth in some countries is still 1 in 20, compared with 1 in 14,900 in Norway.[2]

Anne Mills discusses approaches to the design and financing of health systems in low- and middle-income countries. The percent of gross domestic product (GDP) spent on health from both public and private sources is about 10% globally, with a range from less than 2% (in several developing countries) to 18% (in the United States). Thus, on a global basis, the health sector is one of the largest components of the world economy and is predicted to increase in size as populations age and countries become more economically developed. The report of the Commission on Macroeconomics and Health of the WHO in 2001 emphasized the two-way links between level of development and health status, providing the economic rationale for increased spending in the health sector in developing countries.[3] The subsequent movement toward universal health care coverage inevitably leads to the question of "coverage for what" and whether coverage should be monitored by the provision of health services or broader indicators of population health.

Finally, Leaning and Guha-Sapir review a highly visible example of health system functioning—the response to disasters. In high-income countries, unexpected mass casualty events strain health systems, but good communications, transport, and prior planning mean that a large-scale response is possible. However, the chaos induced in New Orleans by Hurricane Katrina is a reminder that a robust government-led response capacity cannot be taken for granted even in the country with the world's largest economy and military. When calamities strike in areas with poor communications and transport, far from the infrastructure

and supply hubs, help may arrive too little and too late. Better satellite imagery and communications in the age of cellphones and Twitter have vastly decreased the time it takes to broadcast information when disaster strikes, yet these cannot replace the "boots on the ground" needed for both acute and chronic responses. Human-made disasters such as civil wars pose increasing problems for humanitarian responders, with large populations living in refugee camps for decades, along with moral dilemmas when the humanitarian response may be used to aid and abet warring parties or punish foes by denying access to services. Instability anywhere threatens health everywhere; the outbreak of polio in Syria in 2013 imperiled the global campaign to eradicate the disease, as do the assassinations of polio vaccinators in Afghanistan, Pakistan, and Nigeria.

In sum, the operation of health systems is emblematic of one of the basic aspirations of public health—the ability to influence the health of populations through organizational design. The comparative analysis of health systems allows some potentially generalizable observations to be made, some of which may be testable experimentally but most of which represent judgments on complex matters of institutional and individual behavior. The design of health systems should reflect both the goals of health care itself and our most basic ethical and community values. The design of health systems cannot be left to bureaucrats and technocrats. It also requires a wide range of inputs from those who work in the system and those whom the system is designed to serve.

References

1. United Nations (2015). Millennium development goals and beyond 2015. Available at: http://www.un.org/millenniumgoals/
2. World Health Organization, UNICEF, UNFPA, The World Bank, and the United Nations Population Division (2014). *Trends in maternal mortality: 1990 to 2013*. Geneva: World Health Organization. Available at: http://data.worldbank.org/indicator/SH.MMR.RISK
3. World Health Organization (2001). Macroeconomics and health: investing in health for economic development. *Report of the commission on macroeconomics and health*. Geneva: World Health Organization. Available at: http://whqlibdoc.who.int/publications/2001/924154550x.pdf

Global Maternal, Newborn, and Child Health

SO NEAR AND YET SO FAR

Zulfiqar A. Bhutta and Robert E. Black

In September 2000, world leaders assembled in New York to sign the Millennium Declaration to address some of the greatest moral dilemmas of our times—unequal global health, poverty, and inequities in development—and to establish a set of interrelated goals and targets to be met by 2015. Key goals included the Millennium Development Goal (MDG) 4 targeting a reduction in mortality among children younger than 5 years of age by two thirds and MDG 5 targeting a reduction in maternal mortality by three quarters, both from 1990 base figures. Despite overall global progress, these two MDGs are seriously off target for many countries.[1]

Recent assessment of global statistics suggests that despite major gains, among the 75 so-called Countdown countries that have 98% of all maternal deaths and deaths among children younger than 5 years of age, only 17 are on track to reach the MDG 4 target for child mortality and only 9 are on track to reach the MDG 5 target for maternal mortality.[2] However, estimates from the Institute for Health Metrics and Evaluation suggest that 31 countries will achieve MDG 4, 13 countries will achieve MDG 5, and only 9 countries will achieve both targets.[3] As we celebrate the fact that the annual number of deaths among children younger than 5 years of age has fallen to 6.6 million (uncertainty range, 6.3 to 7.0 million), which is a 48% reduction from the 12.6 million deaths (uncertainty range, 12.4 to 12.9 million) in 1990, despite an increased number of births in many high-burden countries during the same time period,[4] the sobering realization is that even in countries that will reach their MDG 4 and 5 targets, many will still have high numbers of deaths, with much scope for improvement.

Global Burden and Mortality Trends

The largest numbers and highest rates of maternal, neonatal, and child deaths are in countries of sub-Saharan Africa and South Asia (Fig. 15.1).[3–5] A total of 10

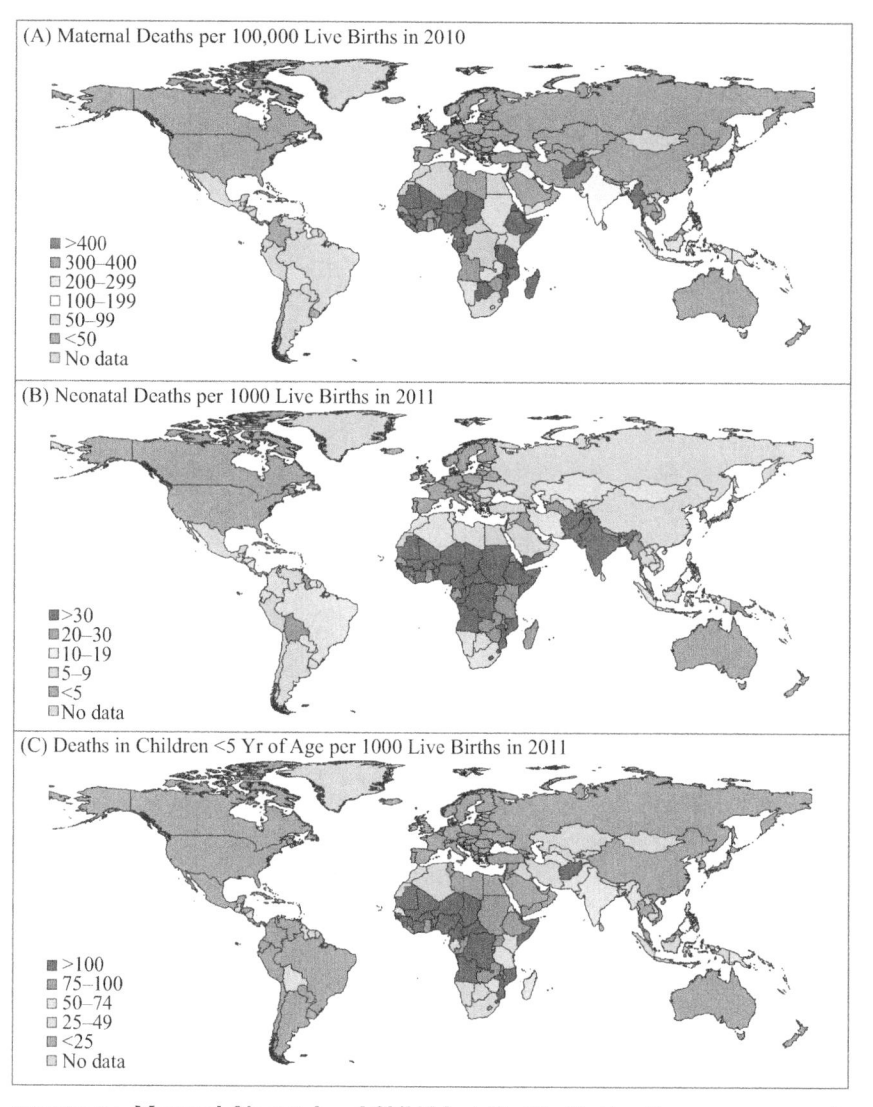

FIGURE 15.1 **Maternal, Neonatal, and Child Mortality Worldwide** *Maps were generated with data from Lozano et al.,[3] the United Nations Children's Fund,[4] and the United Nations Population Fund.[5]*

countries have almost two thirds of the global burden of maternal and newborn deaths, as well as stillbirths.[6] Lozano et al.[3] compared the rates of decline from 1990 through 2000 with the rates of decline from 2000 through 2011 and found that the majority of countries (106 of 193 countries) had accelerated declines in child mortality in the period from 2000 through 2011. Much of the decline was related to a reduction in postneonatal mortality, whereas the reduction in neonatal mortality was much lower. Lozano et al. also reported an estimated decline in maternal mortality, from 409,100 deaths worldwide in 1990 (uncertainty range,

382,900 to 437,900) to 273,500 deaths in 2011 (uncertainty range, 256,300 to 291,700), which was broadly consistent with the estimate calculated by a United Nations interagency group.[5]

As has been underscored recently,[7] the bulk of the reduction in child mortality occurred in the decade after the MDG targets were set in 2000 (a 3.2% reduction per year between 2000 and 2011 vs. a 1.8% reduction per year between 1990 and 2000). To reach the global MDG target for child survival by 2015, countries would need to accelerate their efforts and achieve at least an annual rate of reduction of 5.5% to reach a projected mortality target for children younger than 5 years of age of 35 deaths per 1000 live births by 2020.[7,8] Much of the reduction would need to result from a reduction in newborn mortality, which currently accounts for 30 to 50% of all deaths among children younger than 5 years of age in sub-Saharan Africa and South Asia.[3,4,8]

Causes of Death

Our knowledge of major causes of maternal, newborn, and child death has increased in parallel with improved global statistics on mortality burden and trends and improved methods for allocating cause of death, although methods and estimates vary considerably. The Child Health Epidemiology Reference Group estimated that 40.3% of 7.6 million deaths among children younger than 5 years of age in 2010 (3.1 million deaths) occurred in neonates.[8] Major causes of death in newborns included complications of premature birth (14.1% of deaths among children younger than 5 years of age [1.1 million deaths; uncertainty range, 0.9 to 1.3 million]); intrapartum-related complications, previously labeled as birth asphyxia (9.4% [0.7 million deaths; uncertainty range, 0.6 to 0.9 million]); and sepsis or meningitis (5.2% [0.4 million deaths; uncertainty range, 0.3 to 0.6 million]). Other leading causes of death among children younger than 5 years of age included pneumonia (18.4% of deaths [1.4 million deaths; uncertainty range, 1.2 to 1.6 million]), diarrhea (10.4% [0.8 million deaths; uncertainty range, 0.6 to 1.2 million]), and malaria (7.4% [0.6 million deaths; uncertainty range, 0.4 to 0.8 million]) (Fig. 15.2A).

It must be noted that much of the data are derived from oral autopsies (which are based on questioning family members regarding the mode of death and the events preceding it in circumstances in which medical certification of causes of death and pathological autopsies are not possible) and that in 2010 only 2.7% of the deaths among children younger than 5 years of age (0.2 million deaths) were medically certified. Recent estimates from the Global Burden of Disease (GBD2010) study[9] suggested broadly similar figures for deaths among children younger than 5 years of age, although some categories were clearly different—notably, a higher proportion of deaths from malaria among children younger than 5 years of age in the GBD2010 estimates and lower numbers of death from pneumonia.

Understanding the causes of deaths allows for improved planning and targeting of interventions. Between 2000 and 2010, most of the reduction in mortality

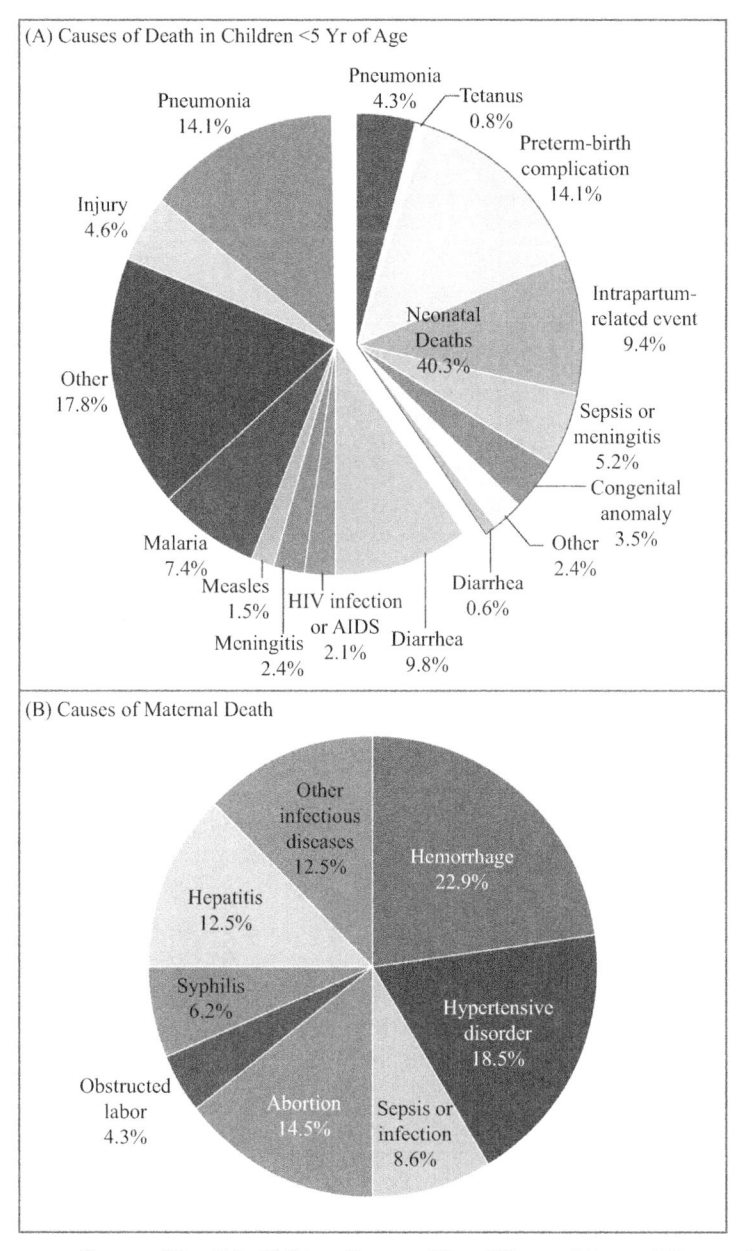

FIGURE 15.2 **Causes of Death in Children Younger Than 5 Years of Age and Causes of Maternal Death** *The causes of death in children younger than 5 years of age are shown separately for neonates and for children 1 to 4 years of age. Data for causes of death in children younger than 5 years of age are from Liu et al.[8] Data for causes of maternal death are from Lozano et al.[9] Percentages do not sum to 100 owing to rounding.*

among children younger than 5 years of age was related to decreases in the rates of death from pneumonia (decrease of 0.5 million deaths; uncertainty range, 0.3 to 0.5 million), measles (decrease of 0.4 million deaths; uncertainty range, 0.3 to 0.4 million), and diarrhea (decrease of 0.4 million deaths; uncertainty range, 0.2 to 0.5 million). The reductions in neonatal deaths during that period from causes other than tetanus, notably those associated with prematurity and intrapartum complications, were minimal. Targeting interventions toward major causes of death and risk factors is a critical step toward achieving MDG 4.

Stillbirth is an unrecognized and unaddressed burden globally. It is not included in the GBD2010 estimates but has been reported separately. An estimated 2.6 million stillbirths (uncertainty range, 2.1 to 3.8 million) occurred worldwide in 2009, of which 76.2% occurred in South Asia and sub-Saharan Africa, mostly among rural populations.[10] An estimated 45% of these stillbirths (1.2 million stillbirths; uncertainty range, 0.8 to 2.0 million) occur during the intrapartum period, which reflects a clear extension of the category of neonatal deaths related to intrapartum events, previously labeled as deaths due to birth asphyxia.[10] This combined burden of stillbirth and early newborn death related to intrapartum events (1.9 million deaths) is similar to the combined number of deaths among children younger than 5 years of age that are related to diarrhea or pneumonia; however, as yet, the burden of stillbirths has not received adequate policy attention.

The information on major causes of maternal death globally is more limited than data on causes of death in children. The last effort to define major categories of maternal death in various regions of the world involved available databases from 1997 through 2002 and was based largely on a review of the literature rather than on registration data on births and deaths.[11] Since then, there have been substantial changes in the reporting hierarchy, and recent estimates of causes of maternal death in the GBD2010 analysis (Fig. 15.2B)[9] exclude 18,970 deaths related to human immunodeficiency virus (HIV) infection, which are reported separately. As a reflection of the ways in which the diagnostic hierarchies of the *International Classification of Diseases, 10th Revision*, and methods of analysis affect global estimates, the same group reported in 2011 that there were an estimated 56,100 deaths due to HIV infection among pregnant women.[3]

Causes of the Causes

No discussion of global maternal, newborn, and child health is complete without addressing basic issues of social determinants.[12] Marmot notes that, according to the World Health Organization, "Social determinants of health are the conditions in which people are born, grow, live, work, and age; these circumstances are shaped by the distribution of money, power and resources at global, national, and local levels."[13] Much of the burden of maternal and child mortality and ill health is concentrated among the poorest populations in countries of sub-Saharan Africa and South Asia. In many of these countries, the highest mortality is observed

among the marginalized and poor, who frequently reside in remote and rural areas with limited access to health care services.

However, a sizable proportion of deaths occurs among the urban poor, who live in slum conditions with limited social-support networks and abysmal living conditions. It has been noted that environmental health factors such as over-crowding, poor air quality, and poor sanitary conditions may be much worse in urban slums than in many rural areas and can adversely affect women and children.[14,15] This clustering of deaths also reflects the lack of access to quality health services in both rural and urban settings for a number of reasons, including the paucity of trained medical personnel and transportation facilities in rural populations and the lack of knowledge about health services among marginalized, socially isolated migrant families in urban slums.[16]

The close link between poverty and under-nutrition is also well recognized. It has been estimated that 45% of all deaths among children younger than 5 years of age may be associated with undernutrition, as manifested by fetal growth restriction, stunting, wasting, deficiencies of vitamin A and zinc, and subopti-mal breast-feeding (e.g., partial or no breast-feeding and early weaning).[17] Recent analyses of trends in the global burden of stunting suggest that the reductions in rates of stunting in Africa and Asia remain very slow, although there have been improvements elsewhere in the world.[18,19] The concern regarding undernutri-tion has also been heightened because of economic crises and an unprecedented increase in food prices.[20] The global food-price indexes are at their highest in decades, with the greatest increases occurring in the prices of cereals, dairy products, and oils.[21]

The relationship of excess child mortality with armed conflict and popula-tion displacement is well recognized, although it is not adequately highlighted in global dialogues.[22] Not only are women and children much more vulnerable to excess risks than men are, but more than one third (36%) of the total global burden of maternal death, child death, and stillbirth exists in countries that have ongoing national or subnational armed conflict.

For example, it has been estimated that among the 24,853 civilian deaths in the Iraq conflict (among persons of known age) between 2003 and 2008, a total of 15% of the civilian deaths were among women and children, according to the so-called Dirty War Index.[23] The Dirty War Index is calculated as the ratio of undesirable or prohibited cases (defined as civilian death and child death, tor-ture, or injury) as a proportion of total documented cases and deaths, including those in combatants.[24] As is evident from the lamentable use of chemical weap-ons against women and children in Syria,[25] the targeting of innocent women and children in conflict zones has become a weapon of war and frequently takes place concomitantly with disrupted and dysfunctional health services. Interventions and approaches to care in such contexts have received inadequate attention.

The disproportionate effect of poverty on the lives of women and children is intertwined with issues of female empowerment and gender equity. The contribu-tion of maternal education to a reduction in child mortality is well described.[26] Closely linked with female-empowerment and sociocultural factors are issues of

fertility and population growth. These important determinants of maternal and child health have been adversely affected by the lack of attention and funding for reproductive health care and family planning globally.[27]

Implementing Evidence-Based Interventions

A series of rigorous studies during the previous decade has underscored the fact that there is a host of evidence-based interventions that can potentially reduce child mortality. A decade ago, a systematic review of the evidence regarding key interventions suggested that a number of evidence-based interventions had the potential to reduce child mortality by nearly two thirds.[28] Since then, much progress has been made in refining the evidence base for interventions. Table S1 in the Supplementary Appendix, available at NEJM.org, highlights the consensus across a range of United Nations agencies, academic bodies, and professional groups regarding the key essential evidence-based interventions that should be implemented and scaled up within health systems.

Despite wide recognition of evidence-based interventions and the availability of information and guidelines, major gaps remain in implementation. Figure 3 shows the current median coverage of key interventions across the major Countdown countries (the 75 countries with more than 98% of the current burden of maternal and child mortality) and highlights the wide disparities in coverage.[1] It is clear that interventions that have a relatively narrow delivery channel and separate management, such as immunizations, do achieve high coverage, whereas those that require functional health systems and facilities, such as skilled birth attendance and postnatal care, reach barely half the population in need. Current coverage rates for other interventions, such as the appropriate use of zinc supplements, oral rehydration solutions, and antibiotic agents for the treatment of childhood diarrhea or pneumonia, are abysmally low.

In addition to the challenge of promoting changes in behavior at the level of persons and families, there are two additional challenges with regard to scaling up key interventions. One pertains to the need to provide appropriate delivery platforms for scaling up coverage, especially in circumstances in which there is a widespread shortage of health workers.[29] The other pertains to the removal of financial barriers that preclude the seeking of care and access to health services in areas in which such care is not freely available within the public health system.[30]

The global shortage of a skilled health workforce has been a key barrier to effective coverage, especially among rural and difficult-to-reach populations. In many instances, policymakers and planners are making use of community health workers who are provided with basic training in preventive and therapeutic strategies. Such task shifting to health workers with lesser training has been shown to yield beneficial results in diverse contexts, such as the management of maternal, newborn, and child conditions, malaria, HIV infection, and the acquired immunodeficiency syndrome (AIDS).[29]

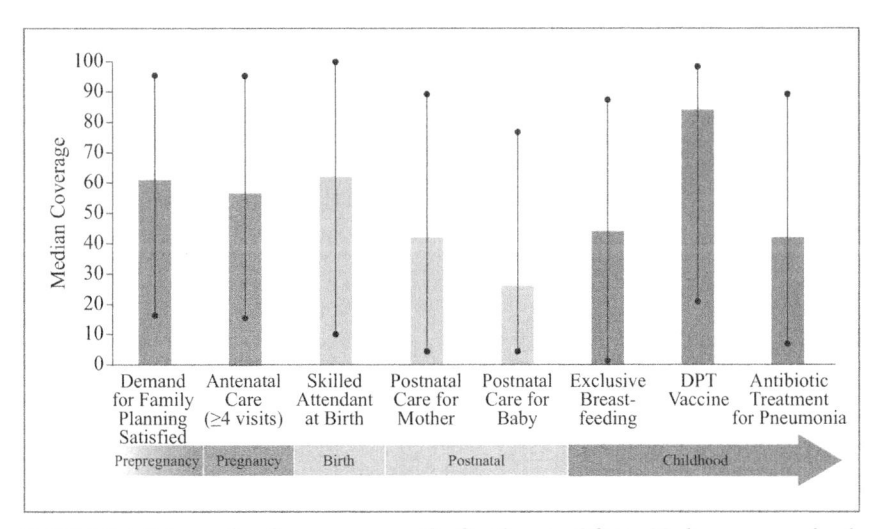

FIGURE 15.3 **Intervention Coverage across the Continuum of Care** *Median coverage levels are shown for selected World Health Organization (WHO) Commission for Information and Accountability indicators of intervention coverage for Countdown countries (i.e., the 75 countries that account for more than 95% of all maternal deaths and deaths among children younger than 5 years of age) with data for the -period from 2007 through 2012. Vertical bars indicate the range of coverage estimates across the 75 countries with available data. Data on diphtheria, pertussis, and tetanus (DPT) are from the WHO and the United Nations Children's Fund (UNICEF) global database for immunization coverage (www.childinfo.org/immunization.html) and the UNICEF 2012 State of the World's Children report (www.unicef.org/sowc2012/fullreport.php). Data on postnatal care for mothers and postnatal care for babies are from a special compilation by Saving Newborn Lives that was based on Demographic and Health Survey data available for the 75 countries (www.measuredhs.com). Data on all other indicators are from UNICEF global databases, which include data from major household surveys such as the UNICEF Multiple Indicator Cluster Surveys (www.unicef.org/statistics/index_24302.html), Demographic and Health Surveys, and national surveys (www.childinfo.org).*

Recent systematic reviews convincingly show improvements in household practices, care seeking, and perinatal and newborn outcomes in community settings when community health workers deliver packages of care for maternal and newborn care.[31,32] Others have highlighted the role of participatory women's groups in inducing changes in practices and outcomes.[33] The effect of community-based approaches to addressing childhood diarrhea and pneumonia[34] and undernutrition[35] among the poorest populations has been well recognized and could be an important foundation for reducing morbidity and mortality.

Community-health-worker programs depend not only on training but also on the provision of basic toolkits and a steady and reliable supply of key commodities. A lack of adequate supplies and frequent depletion of necessary stock are major impediments to effective programs and implementation in primary care settings. The United Nations Commission on Life-Saving Commodities for

Women and Children has recently finalized a global strategy for the procurement and availability of key commodities for family planning, as well as for the prevention and treatment of major causes of maternal, newborn, and child death.[36] It should be recognized, however, that the mere provision and availability of human resources and commodities are insufficient; to ensure effective coverage and effect, these must be coupled with sound governance, assurance of the supply chain, and attention to quality-of-care issues.[2]

Challenges and the Way Ahead

Despite myriad challenges, innovations such as the deployment of community health workers and the use of mobile phones to reach hitherto difficult-to-reach populations and households have enormous potential to improve access to care. These innovations also include improved ways of delivering interventions, the use of low-cost technology and tools to screen for biomarkers, and improved methods of drug and vaccine delivery.

Using the Lives Saved Tool[37] (see the Supplementary Appendix available at NEJM.org), we estimated the potential effect on maternal and child survival of various packages of care when implemented singly and when expanded to target 90% coverage. Table 15.1 shows the potential evidence-based packages of care, with possible innovations that could be used to scale up coverage to 90%, as well as the estimated global maternal and child deaths that could be averted by the year 2020, as assessed by means of the Lives Saved Tool. The model indicates that many lives can be saved with packages for maternal preventive care and child care, packages for newborn resuscitation and care, and packages related to community-based case detection and management.

The effect of several intervention packages is considerably enhanced by innovations for scaling up coverage. The majority of innovations relate to low-cost interventions and diagnostic tools in the hands of health workers and to communication and information-technology platforms. In particular, targeting interventions to reach the rural and urban poor would also reduce the enormous inequalities that favor the rich and that pose a huge human-rights challenge across the developing world.

It is possible to reduce the excess mortality among the poorest and marginalized sections of the population and to accomplish this reduction rapidly—as has been shown in two recent global simulations that used targeted preventive and therapeutic strategies for addressing childhood pneumonia and diarrhea[34] and maternal and childhood undernutrition.[35] This is not just a theoretical possibility. A recent analysis of sequential household surveys in 35 countries with equity data showed clearly that a rapid scale-up generally favors the poor and reduces inequities.[40] Accelerating the global rate of reduction of maternal and child mortality would require rapid scale-up of interventions and focused attention on maternal and child health well beyond the MDG target date of 2015.

TABLE 15.1 Packages of Care, Innovations for Delivery, and Effect on Lives Saved among Mothers, Newborns, and Children.*

Care Package	Interventions	Innovations to Increase Access and Reduce Inequity	Estimated Lives Saved by 2020[†]	Applicable Deaths[‡]	Total Maternal and Child Deaths Averted
			no.	%	%
Improvement of maternal nutrition during pregnancy	Increasing minimum age at marriage and age at the birth of the first child to 18 years and limiting family size; periconception folic acid supplementation or fortification; calcium supplementation in at-risk populations; multiple micronutrient supplementation during pregnancy; balanced energy supplementation during pregnancy	Use of women's groups and financial support programs, including microcredit programs; communication innovations and maternal-health platforms for monitoring	105,569	3.3	1.4
Maternal emergency obstetrical care and postpartum hemorrhage prevention and treatment	Management of preeclampsia with magnesium sulfate; induction of labor to prevent birth at ≥41 wk of gestation; labor and delivery management; basic emergency obstetrical care in an appropriate facility; comprehensive emergency obstetrical care; safe abortion services; case management after abortion; active management of the third stage of labor	Outreach community health workers and community midwives; safe-childbirth checklists; community use of misoprostol; use of Odon device for facilitating safe birth[38]; improved training and simulation devices	345,744	10.9	4.7
Expanded antenatal care, including prevention of stillbirth and premature birth	Antibiotic agents for preterm premature rupture of membranes; screening for and appropriate management of fetal growth restriction; antenatal glucocorticoids in preterm labor to promote fetal lung development; diabetes screening and management; tetanus toxoid vaccination; malaria prevention in pregnant women by means of intermittent preventive treatment during pregnancy or by use of an insecticide-treated bed net or protection of household by means of indoor residual spraying; syphilis detection and treatment	Improved bedside and low-cost diagnostics for infections; intrauterine growth monitoring; social-franchising models for use of antimalarial commodities	482,666	15.2	6.6

Emergency neonatal resuscitation and immediate newborn care	Clean practices and immediate essential newborn care in the home; clean postnatal practices; thermal care; Kangaroo Mother Care (skin-to-skin care); full supportive care; immediate assessment and stimulation; neonatal resuscitation	Scaled-up use of clean delivery kits; use of 4% chlorhexidine for cleaning the umbilical cord; emollient use for newborns; low-cost training materials and standardized training manuals and equipment (e.g., mannequins and resuscitation bags); thermal-care materials and low-cost heated cots	688,089	21.6	9.4
Improvement of nutrition for infants and young children	Promotion of breast-feeding (early initiation, exclusive breast-feeding for 6 mo, and continuation there-after); appropriate complementary feeding between 6 and 24 mo of age; vitamin A supplementation; preventive zinc supplementation	Maternal-health platforms; use of ready-to-use supplementary foods	558,751	7.9	7.7
Detection and management of serious maternal and neonatal infections	Detection and case management of maternal sepsis; case management of neonatal infection, including oral or injectable antibiotics with the use of a simplified regimen	Bedside diagnostics; injectable anti-biotics for primary care use (e.g., Uniject system [Becton Dickinson])	360,749	12.4	4.9
Detection and management of severe childhood illness (diarrhea, pneumonia, meningitis, and malaria)	Oral rehydration solution for diarrhea treatment; zinc for diarrhea treatment; antibiotics for dysentery treatment; oral antibiotics for case management of pneumonia; antimalarial agents (e.g., artemisinin compounds)	Simplified low-cost commodities (e.g., dispersible amoxicillin); community delivery platforms; social marketing	570,244	8.1	7.8

(continued)

TABLE 15.1 Continued

Care Package	Interventions	Innovations to Increase Access and Reduce Inequity	Estimated Lives Saved by 2020 (no.)	Applicable Deaths[†] (%)	Total Maternal and Child Deaths Averted (%)
Management of severe acute malnutrition	Therapeutic feeding for severe acute malnutrition	Community use of RUTF; improved case-management protocols	72,962	1.8	1.0
Vaccination during childhood	Vaccines (e.g., rotavirus, Hib, pneumococcus, measles, and DPT vaccines)	New pricing and procurement systems and improved vaccines (especially combination vaccines)	546,742	13.3	7.5
Water, sanitation, and hygiene interventions	Improved water source; water connection in the home; hygienic disposal of children's stools; hand washing with soap; improved sanitation and use of latrines or toilets	Water purification with solar-powered devices; point-of-use systems for water purification; hand sanitizers; low-cost latrines	467,489	11.3	6.4

*DPT denotes diphtheria, pertussis, and tetanus, Hib *Haemophilus influenzae* type b, and RUTF ready-to-use therapeutic food (usually a fortified spread consisting of a lipid paste made from peanuts, chickpeas, or other local resources, milk powder, oil, sugar, and a micronutrient supplement).

†The estimates of lives saved were calculated with the use of the Lives Saved Tool.[37,39]

‡The denominator for calculating the percentage was the number of current deaths for which that care package would have been applicable.

Clearly, countries need to tackle multiple priorities, and many countries struggle with the growing demands for addressing the increasing burden of noncommunicable diseases as well as the challenges of maternal, newborn, and child health and infectious disease. Thus, there are enormous challenges regarding integration into generally fragmented health systems. The integration of new maternal and child health interventions with existing programs for maternal, newborn, and child health has been limited and has occurred only relatively recently at a global policy level. The situation is much worse with regard to integration across other, disease-specific programs and the management of various diseases. This lack of integration is most notable in large-scale vertical programs such as those addressing initiatives in HIV infection, AIDS, tuberculosis, and malaria, which have largely failed to link up with essential interventions for maternal, newborn, and child health and nutrition.

Despite the efforts with respect to reproductive health and initiatives for the prevention of HIV infection and AIDS and programs such as the President's Emergency Plan for AIDS Relief, there has been little focus on general issues related to adolescent health and nutrition and virtually no programs dealing with preconception care.[41] Given the critical importance of family planning in reducing maternal mortality,[42] family-planning interventions may also have a robust effect on birth spacing and fertility regulation and intergenerational effects on the health and nutrition of populations.

Although the focus during the past decade has been on the saving of lives, it is also important to look beyond survival to issues of reducing morbidity and disability and improving long-term outcomes of relevance to human development. The close links among poverty, inequity, undernutrition, and human deprivation are well known, and all these factors have been shown to reduce the potential for human development considerably.[43] There are promising interventions that can benefit survival as well as human development,[44,45] and there is a huge public health need to integrate the two issues. Linking the agenda for maternal and child health and nutrition with the emerging issues of long-term development, human capital, and economic growth may well be the most appropriate strategy to ensure that we stay the course in solving one of the most important moral dilemmas of our times. Although the MDG target dates are in 2015, the need to keep a sustained focus on maternal and child health will remain.

References

1. Countdown to 2015 for maternal, newborn and child survival: accountability for maternal, newborn and child survival. Geneva: World Health Organization, 2013 (http://www.countdown2015mnch.org/documents/2013Report/Countdown_2013-Update_noprofiles.pdf).
2. Independent Expert Review Group. Every woman every child: strengthening equity and dignity through health (http://www.childhealthnow.org/vi/node/14126).
3. Lozano R, Wang H, Foreman KJ, et al. Progress towards Millennium Development Goals 4 and 5 on maternal and child mortality: an updated systematic analysis. Lancet 2011;378:1139–65.

4. UN Inter-agency Group for Child Mortality Estimation (IGME). Levels and trends in child mortality. Report 2013 (http://www.unicef.org/media/files/2013 _IGME_ child_mortality_Report.pdf).

5. Trends in maternal mortality: 1990-2010—estimates developed by WHO, UNICEF, UNFPA and the World Bank. 2012 (http://www.unfpa.org/public/home/publications/ pid/10728).

6. Cousens S, Blencowe H, Stanton C, et al. National, regional, and worldwide estimates of stillbirth rates in 2009 with trends since 1995: a systematic analysis. Lancet 2011;377:1319–30.

7. UNICEF. Committing to child survival: a promise renewed—progress report, 2012 (http://www.apromiserenewed.org/files/APR_Progress_Report_2012_final_ web.pdf).

8. Liu L, Johnson HL, Cousens S, et al. Global, regional, and national causes of child mortality: an updated systematic analysis for 2010 with time trends since 2000. Lancet 2012;379:2151–61. [Erratum, Lancet 2012;380:1308.]

9. Lozano R, Naghavi M, Foreman K, et al. Global and regional mortality from 235 causes of death for 20 age groups in 1990 and 2010: a systematic analysis for the Global Burden of Disease Study 2010. Lancet 2012;380:2095–128.

10. Lawn JE, Blencowe H, Pattinson R, et al. Stillbirths: Where? When? Why? How to make the data count? Lancet 2011;377: 1448–63.

11. Khan KS, Wojdyla D, Say L, Gülmezoglu AM, Van Look PF. WHO analysis of causes of maternal death: a systematic review. Lancet 2006;367:1066–74.

12. Commission on Social Determinants of Health. Closing the gap in a generation: health equity through action on the social determinants of health. Final report of the Commission on Social Determinants of Health. Geneva: World Health Organization,2008 (http://www.who.int/social_determinants/thecommission/final-report/en/index.html).

13. Marmot M. Closing the health gap in a generation: the work of the Commission on Social Determinants of Health and its recommendations. Glob Health Promot 2009;16:Suppl 1:23–27.

14. Awasthi S, Agarwal S. Determinants of childhood mortality and morbidity in urban slums in India. Indian Pediatr 2003;40:1145–61.

15. Matthews Z, Channon A, Neal S, Osrin D, Madise N, Stones W. Examining the "urban advantage" in maternal health care in developing countries. PLoS Med 2010;7(9):e1000327.

16. Bocquier P, Beguy D, Zulu EM, Muindi K, Konseiga A, Yé Y. Do migrant children face greater health hazards in slum settlements? Evidence from Nairobi, Kenya. J Urban Health 2011;88:Suppl 2:S266-S281.

17. Black RE, Victora CG, Walker SP, et al. Maternal and child undernutrition and overweight in low-income and middle—income countries. Lancet 2013;382:427–51. [Erratum, Lancet 2013;382:396.]

18. Stevens GA, Finucane MM, Paciorek CJ, et al. Trends in mild, moderate, and severe stunting and underweight, and progress towards MDG 1 in 141 developing countries: a systematic analysis of population representative data. Lancet 2012;380:824–34.

19. de Onis M, Blössner M, Borghi E. Prevalence and trends of stunting among pre-school children, 1990-2020. Public Health Nutr 2012;15:142–48.

20. Bhutta ZA, Bawany FA, Feroz A, Rizvi A, Thapa SJ, Patel M. Effects of the crises on child nutrition and health in East Asia and the Pacific. Global Social Policy 2009;9:Suppl:119–43.

21. Food and Agriculture Organization of the United Nations. World food situation: FAO Food Price Index. 2013 (http://www.fao.org/worldfoodsituation/wfs-home/foodpricesindex/en).

22. Southall D. Armed conflict women and girls who are pregnant, infants and children; a neglected public health challenge. What can health professionals do? Early Hum Dev 2011;87:735–42.

23. Hicks MH-R, Dardagan H, Guerrero Serdán G, Bagnall PM, Sloboda JA, Spagat M. Violent deaths of Iraqi civilians, 2003-2008: analysis by perpetrator, weapon, time, and location. PLoS Med 2011;8(2):e1000415.

24. Chulov M, Mahmood M, Sample I. Syria conflict: chemical weapons blamed as hundreds reported killed. The Guardian. August 21, 2013 (http://www.theguardian.com/world/2013/aug/21/syria-conflcit-chemical-weapons-hundreds-killed).

25. Hicks MH, Spagat M. The dirty war index: a public health and human rights tool for examining and monitoring armed conflict outcomes. PLoS Med 2008;5(12):e243.

26. Gakidou E, Cowling K, Lozano R, Murray CJ. Increased educational attainment and its effect on child mortality in 175 countries between 1970 and 2009: a systematic analysis. Lancet 2010;376:959–74.

27. Financing the ICPD Programme of Action: data for 2009, estimates for 2010/2011. New York: United Nations Population Fund, 2009 (http://www.unfpa.org/webdav/site/global/shared/documents/publications/2011/Advocacy%20Brochure%202010-1.pdf).

28. Jones G, Steketee RW, Black RE, Bhutta ZA, Morris SS. How many child deaths can we prevent this year? Lancet 2003;362:65–71.

29. Bhutta ZA, Lassi ZS, Pariyo G, Huicho L. Global experience of community health workers for delivery of health related millennium development goals: a systematic review, country case studies, and recommendations for integration into national health systems. Geneva: World Health Organization, 2010.

30. Bassani DG, Arora P, Wazny K, Gaffey MF, Lenters L, Bhutta ZA. Financial incentives and coverage of child health interventions: a systematic review and meta-analysis. BMC Public Health 2013;13:Suppl 3:S30.

31. Lassi ZS, Haider BA, Bhutta ZA. Community-based intervention packages for reducing maternal and neonatal morbidity and mortality and improving neonatal outcomes. Cochrane Database Syst Rev 2010;11:CD007754.

32. Lewin S, Munabi-Babigumira S, Glenton C, et al. Lay health workers in primary and community health care for maternal and child health and the management of infectious diseases. Cochrane Database Syst Rev 2010;3:CD004015.

33. Prost A, Colbourn T, Seward N, et al. Women's groups practising participatory learning and action to improve maternal and newborn health in low-resource settings: a systematic review and meta-analysis. Lancet 2013;381:1736–46.

34. Bhutta ZA, Das JK, Walker N, et al. Interventions to address deaths from childhood pneumonia and diarrhoea equitably: what works and at what cost? Lancet 2013;381:1417–29.

35. Bhutta ZA, Das JK, Rizvi A, et al. Evidence-based interventions for improvement of maternal and child nutrition: what can be done and at what cost? Lancet 2013;382:452–77.

36. UN Commission on Life-Saving Commodities for Women and Children. Commissioner's report. September 2012 (http://www.unicef.org/media/files/UN_ Commission_Report_September_2012_Final.pdf).

37. Fox MJ, Martorell R, van den Broek N, Walker N. Assumptions and methods in the Lives Saved Tool (LiST): introduction. BMC Public Health 2011;11:Suppl 3:I1.

38. Requejo JH, Belizán JM. Odon device: a promising tool to facilitate vaginal delivery and increase access to emergency care. Reprod Health 2013;10:42.

39. Walker N, Yenokyan G, Friberg IK, Bryce J. Patterns in coverage of maternal, newborn, and child health interventions: projections of neonatal and under-5 mortality to 2035. Lancet 2013;382:1029–38.

40. Victora CG, Barros AJ, Axelson H, et al. How changes in coverage affect equity in maternal and child health interventions in 35 Countdown to 2015 countries: an analysis of national surveys. Lancet 2012;380:1149–56.

41. Dean SV, Imam AM, Lassi ZS, Bhutta ZA. Importance of intervening in the preconception period to impact pregnancy outcomes. Nestle Nutr Inst Workshop Ser 2013;74:63–73.

42. Ahmed S, Li Q, Liu L, Tsui AO. Maternal deaths averted by contraceptive use: an analysis of 172 countries. Lancet 2012;380:111–25.

43. Walker SP, Wachs TD, Gardner JM, et al. Child development: risk factors for adverse outcomes in developing countries. Lancet 2007;369:145–57.

44. Engle PL, Fernald LC, Alderman H, et al. Strategies for reducing inequalities and improving developmental outcomes for young children in low-income and middle-income countries. Lancet 2011;378:1339–53.

45. Shonkoff JP, Richter L, van der Gaag J, Bhutta ZA. An integrated scientific framework for child survival and early childhood development. Pediatrics 2012; 129(2):e460–72.

Health Care Systems in Low- and Middle-Income Countries

Anne Mills

Over the past 10 years, debates on global health have paid increasing attention to the importance of health care systems, which encompass the institutions, organizations, and resources (physical, financial, and human) assembled to deliver health care services that meet population needs. It has become especially important to emphasize health care systems in low- and middle-income countries because of the substantial external funding provided for disease-specific programs, especially for drugs and medical supplies, and the relative underfunding of the broader health care infrastructures in these countries.[1] A functioning health care system is fundamental to the achievement of universal coverage for health care, which has been the focus of recent statements by advocacy groups and other organizations around the globe, including a declaration by the United Nations in 2012.[2]

Recent analyses have drawn attention to the weaknesses of health care systems in low- and middle-income countries. For example, in the 75 countries that account for more than 95% of maternal and child deaths, the median proportion of births attended by a skilled health worker is only 62% (range, 10 to 100%), and women without money or coverage for this service are much less likely to receive it than are women with the means to pay for it.[3] Lack of financial protection for the costs of health care means that approximately 100 million people are pushed below the poverty line each year by payments for health care,[4] and many more will not seek care because they lack the necessary funds.

In response to such deficiencies in the health care system, a number of countries and their partners in development have been introducing new approaches to financing, organizing, and delivering health care. This article briefly reviews the main weaknesses of health care systems in low- and middle-income countries, lists the most common responses to those weaknesses, and then presents three of the most popular responses for further review. These responses, which have attracted considerable controversy, involve the questions of whether to pay for health care

through general taxation or contributory insurance funds to improve financial protection for specific sections of the population, whether to use financial incentives to increase health care utilization and improve health care quality, and whether to make use of private entities to extend the reach of the health care system.

This review draws on what is now quite an extensive literature on the deficiencies of health care systems[1] and on the Health Systems Evidence database.[5] However, the poor quality and uneven coverage of evidence on the strengthening of health care systems means that evidence of deficiencies is stronger than evidence of remedies. Moreover, the specific circumstances of individual countries strongly influence both decisions about which approaches might be relevant and their success, so any generalizations made from health systems research in particular countries must be carefully considered.[6] It is unlikely that there is one single blueprint for an ideal health care system design or a magic bullet that will automatically remedy deficiencies. The strengthening of health care systems in low- and middle-income countries must be seen as a long-term developmental process.

Health Care System Constraints and Responses

A framework for categorizing the constraints on health care systems[7] was originally developed in 2001 for the Commission on Macroeconomics and Health of the World Health Organization and has been widely applied since then. This framework has the merit of looking at systems both horizontally (e.g., assessing each level to determine all the elements needed for effective service delivery) and vertically (e.g., accounting for the support functions of the higher levels in a system). Table 16.1 lists six levels that exist within any health care system, from the community level to the global level; the main constraints of the system at each level; and the main responses to these constraints. Three issues drawn from these responses have been selected for detailed consideration below.

These issues have been selected for several reasons. They involve critical functions of the health care system (i.e., financing and health care delivery), receive considerable prominence in international debates on how to strengthen the health care system, and have been evaluated somewhat more rigorously than other issues.

GENERAL TAXATION VS. CONTRIBUTORY INSURANCE

As indicated in Table 16.1, a major problem in low- and middle-income countries is lack of financial support for those who need health care, deterring service use and burdening household budgets. Figure 16.1 shows the sources of health care financing according to country income. On average, almost 50% of health care financing in low-income countries comes from out-of-pocket payments, as compared with 30% in middle-income countries and 14% in high-income countries. When payments from general government expenditures, social (public) health insurance, and prepaid private insurance are combined, only 38% of health care

TABLE 16.1 Health Care System Constraints and Responses*

Level of Health Care System	Constraints[†]	Responses[‡]
Community and household	Lack of demand for effective interventions	Provide financial incentives to encourage use of services, mobilize communities (e.g., by supporting creation of women's groups to spread information about antenatal and delivery services)
	Barriers to use of effective interventions (physical, financial, social)	Expand "close-to-client" services (e.g., those provided by village health workers and trained drug sellers), remove financial barriers at point of service through increased prepayment, increase responsiveness of providers (e.g., through pay-for-performance approaches)
Service delivery	Shortage and poor distribution of appropriately qualified staff, especially at primary care level	Increase numbers of health workers, implement task shifting (e.g., by training community health workers to treat common illnesses), increase allowances for work in remote areas
	Low staff pay and poor motivation	Increase pay, improve supervision
	Weak technical guidance, program management, and supervision	Strengthen training and supervision, contract management
	Inadequate drugs and medical supplies	Strengthen public systems of supply, make use of private retail system
	Lack of equipment and infrastructure, including poor accessibility of health services	Renovate, upgrade, and expand public facilities, contract nongovernmental organizations to provide services
Policy and strategic management in the health sector	Weak and overly centralized systems for planning and management	Decentralize planning and management
	Weak drug policies and supply systems	Introduce new supply mechanisms
	Inadequate regulation of pharmaceutical industry and other segments of the private sector, improper industry practices	Strengthen regulation through legal mechanisms and incentives
	Lack of cooperative action and partnership for health between government and civic organizations	Require engagement of civic organizations in planning and service oversight
	Weak incentives to use inputs efficiently and to respond to user needs and preferences	Use output-based payments and external assistance programs
	Fragmented donor funding, which reduces flexibility and ownership; low priority given to systems support	Implement reforms to aid management and delivery (e.g., SWAPS, IHP+), provide increased financing for systems support

(continued)

TABLE 16.1 Continued

Level of Health Care System	Constraints[†]	Responses[‡]
Government policy	Bureaucracy (e.g., civil service rules and remuneration, centralized management systems)	Make greater use of private sector in financing, management, and service delivery; move health management into autonomous agencies
	Limited communication and transport infrastructure	Not seen as health care issue
Political and physical environment	Governance and overall policy framework (e.g., corruption, weak government, weak rule of law and enforceability of contracts, political instability and insecurity, social sectors not given priority in funding decisions, weak structure for public accountability, lack of free press)	Encourage improved stewardship and accountability mechanisms by encouraging growth in civic organizations and supporting an active and informed media
	Climatic and geographic predisposition to disease, physical environment unfavorable for service delivery	Not amenable to change
Global	Fragmented governance and management structures for global health	Improve global coordination (e.g., the Paris Declaration, Accra Agenda for Action)
	Emigration of doctors and nurses to high-income countries	Seek voluntary agreements on migration of doctors and nurses

*IHP+ denotes International Health Partnership Plus, and SWAPS sectorwide approaches.

[†]Information is adapted from Hanson et al.[7]

[‡]Information is adapted from Mills and Ranson,[8] Mills et al.,[9] and the Taskforce on Innovative International Financing for Health Systems.[1]

financing in low-income countries is combined in funding pools, which allow the risks of health care costs to be shared across population groups, as compared with approximately 60% in middle-income countries and 80% in high-income countries.

Thus, the key financing issue for low- and middle-income countries is how to provide increased financial protection for households. That part of the population in the formal sector of employment, in which payroll taxes can be levied, could be included in social insurance arrangements. It is also commonly accepted that the poorest people require complete subsidization for health care costs from general taxation, and those with low incomes need at least partial subsidization. The key question is whether the rest of the population—those who are outside the formal sector of the economy but who are not the very poorest—should be covered by funds raised through general taxation or encouraged to enroll in contributory insurance programs.

This issue has been at the core of debates on the financing of universal coverage in South and Southeast Asia.[11] The Philippines and Vietnam, for instance,

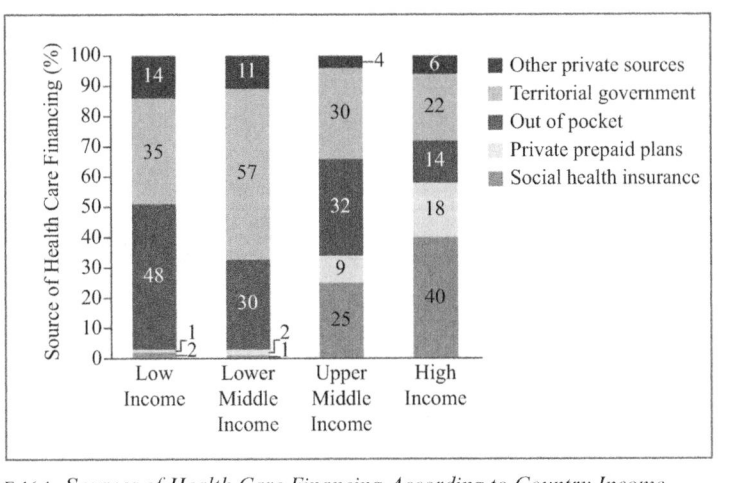

FIGURE 16.1 *Sources of Health Care Financing According to Country Income*
Data are from the World Health Organization.[10]

have sought to expand financial protection by encouraging voluntary enrollment in social health insurance programs, whereas other countries, such as Thailand, have used funds from general taxation that are channeled to ministries of health or local health authorities. The recent report from the High Level Expert Group on Universal Health Coverage, which was charged by the Indian Planning Commission to develop a blueprint for achieving universal coverage in India by 2020, recommended channeling considerably increased funding from general tax revenue to largely public providers through a public purchaser at the state level. The report is clear in its rejection of contributory insurance arrangements.[12]

In Africa, Rwanda is frequently referred to as a country that has achieved remarkably high voluntary insurance coverage,[13] although the depth of coverage (i.e., the number of services covered) is limited and there is still insufficient financial protection for the poorest groups. Ghana, another African country cited for its efforts to expand health care coverage, introduced a national health insurance program in which enrollment is compulsory for the formal sector and voluntary for the informal sector and in which coverage is free for the poorest members of the population. However, problems in making premiums affordable and in maintaining voluntary enrollment led the ruling party to propose one-time payment rather than annual payment from those outside the formal sector.[14] General taxation (through a value-added tax) is already the main financing source for Ghana's national health insurance, but the introduction of a one-time payment would clearly signal a decrease in the importance attached to contributory insurance.

Given the limited tax base in low- and middle-income countries and the limited ability of many households to pay for health care, whether directly or through contributory insurance, progress toward improved financial protection will inevitably be gradual. Countries need to and do draw on a mix of financing sources, but their key concern should be to determine which

financing arrangements, given their particular economic, social, and political environment, will best protect the most vulnerable segment of the population and ensure both breadth of coverage (the number of people protected) and reasonable depth of coverage.

FINANCIAL INCENTIVES FOR HOUSEHOLDS AND PROVIDERS

A second key issue in efforts to strengthen health systems has been whether to deploy financial incentives as a way of encouraging households to use services and encouraging providers to deliver services of good quality. Such strategies form part of a wider approach known as results-based financing, "pay for performance," or output-based aid,[15] which is intended to address the problems of lack of demand for effective interventions and poor responsiveness and motivation on the part of providers. Incentives can be targeted to the recipients of health care (e.g., through vouchers or cash payments conditional on the use of services) or to individual health care workers or health care facilities.

An overview[16] of systematic reviews of the effectiveness of such financial incentives suggests some successes in the short run for incentives targeting recipients of health care and individual health care workers and seeking to achieve distinct, well-defined behavioral goals related to the provision and use of fairly simple services. For example, in Latin America, the use of conditional cash transfers has been associated with increased use of preventive services,[17] and in Rwanda, performance-based payment of primary care providers has increased the number of babies delivered in hospitals or other facilities and preventive care visits by young children.[18] But the limited evidence base provides little guidance on how well such programs may work in other countries. There is concern as to whether the programs can be difficult to implement in countries with limited resources where the governments lack the staff, skills, and systems to manage and monitor services, payments, and performance. This was the case with a maternity incentive payment in Nepal,[19] where the "less poor" benefited more than the poor.[20] Further concerns are whether changes will be sustained over time and whether incentives are also useful for more complex services.

Financial incentives are powerful, and undesirable responses, though rarely investigated, are likely to occur. For instance, a recent analysis of what is probably the world's largest demand-side incentive program promoting hospital births, India's Janani Suraksha Yojana, indicated that although the provision of cash incentives increased women's access to services, it was also associated with an increase in fertility.[21]

Financial incentives represent just one means of improving levels of health care utilization and the quality of services, but virtually no studies in low- and middle-income countries have compared the use of financial incentives with alternative ways of achieving these outcomes,[16] such as nonfinancial approaches to changing professional behavior.[22,23] This lack of information on alternative approaches makes it difficult to develop clear policy recommendations.

USE OF PRIVATE ENTITIES TO EXTEND COVERAGE

There is extensive private participation in the health care systems of low- and middle-income countries, especially in service delivery. The private sector ranges from a limited number of formal not-for-profit and for-profit providers to numerous informal providers, including itinerant drug sellers. There has been an increase in the number of private providers, driven both by rising incomes and the failure of public services to meet expectations. This situation has led to the pragmatic argument that since such private providers are available, they should be harnessed to address the physical inaccessibility of services, the shortage and maldistribution of staff, and inadequate stocks of drugs and supplies (Table 16.1).

There is indeed evidence that introducing shopkeeper training, drug packaging, and franchising can improve the quality of private services used by the poor, especially services provided at retail drug outlets.[24] The training of drug sellers on the Kenyan coast, for instance, has increased the proportion of sales of antimalarial drugs that contain an adequate dose,[25] and the channeling of artemisinin-based combination therapies through private-sector outlets (by means of the Affordable Medicines Facility–Malaria initiative) has helped to increase the availability of quality-assured drugs in six pilot countries.[26] However, private retail markets appear to vary greatly from one country to another, and the evidence base is too limited to draw general conclusions.

It has been argued that given the failure or capacity limitations of public-sector efforts, the more formal private sector can be contracted to manage services such as primary care and hospital facilities on behalf of the public sector. A number of studies of contractual arrangements suggest that nongovernmental organizations working under contract to manage district services have increased service delivery in previously underserved areas in some countries.[27] There is much less evidence of the value of contracting for-profit providers, although studies from South Africa suggest that the state must have the capacity to design and manage the contracts.[28]

The engagement of the private sector remains a topic of considerable controversy, seen by some as inviting the privatization of health care and making it a commodity.[29] However, when the capacity of the public sector is limited and there is a concentration of human resources in the private sector, seeking a mix of public and private provision of services can be seen as a pragmatic response. For example, current proposals for national health insurance in South Africa call for a system in which public financing is used to purchase a comprehensive package of services from accredited public and private providers.[30]

A Long-Term Process of Development

On the basis of the evidence presented above, few clear-cut conclusions can be drawn with regard to the best strategies for strengthening countries' health care systems. An approach that works well in one country may work less well in another, and not all approaches are equally acceptable to all governments or their multiple

BOX 16.1 Characteristics of Successful Health Systems

Have vision and long-term strategies

Take into account the constraints imposed by history and previous decisions (path dependency)

Build consensus at the societal level

Allow flexibility and autonomy in decision-making

Are resilient and learn from experience, feeding back into the policy cycle

Receive support from the broader governance and socioeconomic context and are in harmony with the culture and population preferences

Achieve synergies among sectors and actors

Demonstrate openness to dialogue and collaboration between public and private sectors, with effective government oversight

Adapted from Balabanova et al.[32]

---

constituencies. There is no one blueprint for an ideal health care system, nor are there any magic bullets that will automatically elicit improved performance. This is hardly surprising: health care systems are complex social systems,[31] and the success of any one approach will depend on the system into which it is intended to fit as well as on its consistency with local values and ideologies.

A recent historical study of the contribution of the health care system to improved health in five countries identified a number of characteristics of successful health care systems (see Box 16.1).[32] Such systems were able to develop the capacity to select promising strategies and to learn from the efforts of other countries as well as from their own experimentation. The strengthening of a health care system requires a focus not only on specific strategies, such as those considered above, but also on the creation of an environment that supports innovation. Health care strengthening must thus be seen as a long-term process that involves complex systems and requires carefully orchestrated action on a number of fronts. The global community can help by supporting country-led processes of reform and by helping to create a stronger evidence base that contributes to cross-country learning.

References

1. Taskforce on Innovative International Financing for Health Systems. Constraints to scaling up and costs. Geneva: World Health Organization, 2009.

2. World Health Organization. Universal health coverage (http://www.who.int/universal_health_coverage/un_resolution/en/index.html).

3. Countdown to 2015: accountability for maternal, newborn and child survival: the 2013 update. World Health Organization and UNICEF, 2013 (http://www.countdown2015mnch.org/documents/2013Report/Countdown_2013-Update_noprofiles.pdf).

4. Health systems financing: the path to universal coverage. Geneva: World Health Organization, 2010.

5. Health systems evidence. Hamilton, ON, Canada: McMaster University (http://www.mcmasterhealthforum.org).

6. Gilson L, Hanson K, Sheikh K, Agyepong IA, Ssengooba F, Bennett S. Building the field of health policy and systems research: social science matters. PLoS Med 2011;8(8):e1001079.

7. Hanson K, Ranson K, Oliveira-Cruz V, Mills A. Expanding access to priority health interventions: a framework for understanding the constraints to scaling-up. J Int Dev 2003;15:1–14.

8. Mills A, Ranson MK. The design of health systems. In: Merson M, Black R, Mills A, eds. Global health: diseases, programs, systems and policies. 3rd ed. Boston: Jones and Bartlett, 2011:615–51.

9. Mills A, Tollman S, Rasheed F. Improving health systems. In: Jamison D, Breman J, Measham A, et al., eds. Disease control priorities in developing countries. Washington DC: World Bank, 2006:87–102.

10. Global health expenditure database. Geneva: World Health Organization (http://apps.who.int/nha/database/CompositionReportPage.aspx).

11. Tangcharoensathien V, Patcharanarumol W, Ir P, et al. Health-financing reforms in southeast Asia: challenges in achieving universal coverage. Lancet 2011;377:863–73.

12. High Level Expert Group. Report on universal health coverage for India: submitted to the Planning Commission of India. New Delhi: Planning Commission of India, 2011.

13. Lu C, Chin B, Lewandowski JL, et al. Towards universal health coverage: an evaluation of Rwanda *Mutuelles* in its first eight years. PLoS One 2012;7(6):e39282.

14. Abotisem Abiiro G, McIntyre D. Universal financial protection through National Health Insurance: a stakeholder analysis of the proposed one-time premium payment policy in Ghana. Health Policy Plan 2013;28:263–78.

15. Savedoff W. Incentive proliferation? Making sense of a new wave of development programs. Washington, DC: Center for Global Development, 2011.

16. Oxman AD, Fretheim A. Can paying for results help to achieve the Millennium Development Goals? Overview of the effectiveness of results-based financing. J Evid Based Med 2009;2:70–83.

17. Lagarde M, Haines A, Palmer N. Conditional cash transfers for improving uptake of health interventions in low- and middle-income countries: a systematic review. JAMA 2007;298:1900–10.

18. Basinga P, Gertler PJ, Binagwaho A, Soucat ALB, Sturdy J, Vermeersch CMJ. Effect on maternal and child health services in Rwanda of payment to primary health-care providers for performance: an impact evaluation. Lancet 2011;377:1421–28.

19. Powell-Jackson T, Morrison J, Tiwari S, Neupane BD, Costello AM. The experiences of districts in implementing a national incentive programme to promote safe delivery in Nepal. BMC Health Serv Res 2009;9:97.

20. Powell-Jackson T, Neupane BD, Tiwari S, Tumbahangphe K, Manandhar D, Costello AM. The impact of Nepal's national incentive programme to promote safe delivery in the district of Makwanpur. Adv Health Econ Health Serv Res 2009;21:221–49.

21. Powell-Jackson T. Financial incentives in health: new evidence from India's Janani Suraksha Yojana. London: London School of Hygiene and Tropical Medicine, 2011 (http://ssrn.com/abstract=1935442).

22. Siddiqi K, Newell J, Robinson M. Getting evidence into practice: what works in developing countries? Int J Qual Health Care 2005;17:447–54.

23. Bosch-Capblanch X, Liaqat S, Garner P. Managerial supervision to improve primary health care in low- and middle-income countries. Cochrane Database Syst Rev 2011;9:CD006413.

24. Patouillard E, Goodman CA, Hanson KG, Mills AJ. Can working with the private for-profit sector improve utilization of quality health services by the poor? A systematic review of the literature. Int J Equity Health 2007;6:17.

25. Marsh VM, Mutemi WM, Willetts A, et al. Improving malaria home treatment by training drug retailers in rural Kenya. Trop Med Int Health 2004;9:451–60.

26. Tougher S, Ye Y, Amuasi JH, et al. Effect of the Affordable Medicines Facility—malaria (AMFm) on the availability, price, and market share of quality-assured artemisinin-based combination therapies in seven countries: a before-and-after analysis of outlet survey data. Lancet 2012;380:1916–26.

27. Lagarde M, Palmer N. The impact of contracting out on health outcomes and use of health services in low and middle-income countries. Cochrane Database Syst Rev 2009;4:CD008133.

28. Broomberg J, Masobe P, Mills A. To purchase or to provide? The relative efficiency of contracting out versus direct public provision of hospital services in South Africa. In: Bennett S, McPake B, Mills A, eds. Private health providers in developing countries: serving the public interest? London: Zed Press, 1997.

29. Unger J-P, Van Dessel P, Sen K, De Paepe P. International health policy and stagnating maternal mortality: is there a causal link? Reprod Health Matters 2009;17:91–104.

30. National Department of Health. Green Paper on national health insurance in South Africa. Pretoria: National Department of Health, Republic of South Africa, 2011.

31. Gilson L. Health systems and institutions. In: Smith RD, Hanson K, eds. Health systems in low- and middle-income countries: an economic and policy perspective. Oxford, England: Oxford University Press, 2011.

32. Balabanova D, Mills A, Conteh L, et al. Good Health at Low Cost 25 years on: lessons for the future of health systems strengthening. Lancet 2013;381:2118–33.

{ 17 }

Natural Disasters, Armed Conflict, and Public Health

Jennifer Leaning
and Debarati Guha-Sapir

Natural disasters and armed conflict have marked human existence throughout history and have always caused peaks in mortality and morbidity. But in recent times, the scale and scope of these events have increased markedly. Since 1990, natural disasters have affected about 217 million people every year,[1] and about 300 million people now live amidst violent insecurity around the world.[2] The immediate and longer-term effects of these disruptions on large populations constitute humanitarian crises. In recent decades, public health interventions in the humanitarian response have made gains in the equity and quality of emergency assistance.

Natural disasters are broadly classified as biologic, climate-related (hydro-meteorologic), or geophysical (Box 17.1). (Biologic events are not considered in this article because they require very specific analytic approaches and are often not directly connected to geophysical and climate-related disasters.) There were three times as many natural disasters from 2000 through 2009 as there were from 1980 through 1989 (Fig. 17.1 and interactive graphic, available at NEJM.org). Although better communications may play a role in the trend, the growth is mainly in climate-related events, accounting for nearly 80% of the increase, whereas trends in geophysical events have remained stable. During recent decades, the scale of disasters has expanded owing to increased rates of urbanization, deforestation, and environmental degradation and to intensifying climate variables such as higher temperatures, extreme precipitation, and more violent wind and water storms. The effects of disasters on populations include immediate death and disabilities and disease outbreaks caused by ecologic shifts. For example, the 2010 earthquake in Haiti and Cyclone Nargis, which hit Myanmar in 2008, killed 225,000 and 80,000 people, respectively, in a matter of minutes; destroyed health care facilities; and left many homeless.

BOX 17.1 Classification of Natural Disasters.*

Biologic

Epidemic infectious disease: viral, bacterial, parasitic, fungal, prion
Insect infestation
Animal stampede

Geophysical

Earthquake
Volcano
Mass movement (dry): rockfall, landslide, avalanche, subsidence

Climate-related

Hydrologic
Flood: general flood, flash flood, storm surge or coastal flood
Mass movement (wet): rockfall, landslide, avalanche, subsidence

Meteorologic

Storm: tropical cyclone, extratropical cyclone, local storm
Extreme temperature: heat wave, cold wave, extreme winter condition
Drought
Wildfire: forest fire, land fire

*The classification is from the Center for Research on the Epidemiology of Disasters, University of Louvain.

In contrast, armed conflicts have decreased globally, although some persist, with entrenched internal violence lasting for years, such as in Darfur (in Sudan) and in the eastern Democratic Republic of Congo. Advances in small-arms technology and struggles over natural resources of international value (oil and rare minerals) make conflict resolution challenging. Civilians bear the burden. Families are forced to move from their homes to escape internecine violence. Refugees cross national borders and are legally entitled to assistance in United Nations (UN)–managed camps. But increasingly since the mid-1980s, people have been unable to cross international frontiers and so remain internally displaced (Fig. 17.2). They are often at higher risk for malnutrition and disease than residents or refugees.[3]

Advances in Humanitarian Public Health Response since 1970

The early 1970s were watershed years for public health in emergencies. The Biafran War (in Nigeria), the 1970 cyclone in Bangladesh, and the sweeping famines in Africa deeply engaged the public health community in trying to meet the need for impartial and effective medical aid. The use of epidemiologic methods to reduce civilian morbidity and mortality in mass emergencies began in earnest at this time.[4,5] This period also saw the engagement of health care practitioners in the elaboration of international norms on ethics, human rights, and humanitarian law in emergency settings.[6–8]

Public health is a major component of the larger operational framework of international relief. It includes disease control, reproductive health and maternal

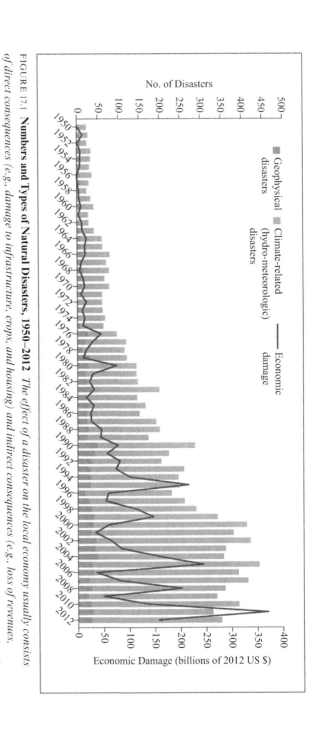

FIGURE 17.1 **Numbers and Types of Natural Disasters, 1950–2012** *The effect of a disaster on the local economy usually consists of direct consequences (e.g., damage to infrastructure, crops, and housing) and indirect consequences (e.g., loss of revenues, unemployment, and market destabilization). The estimated economic damage is for the year in which the disasters occurred and is given in billions of 2012 U.S. dollars. Data are from the EM-DAT International Disaster Database, Center for Research on the Epidemiology of Disasters, University of Louvain (www.emdat.be/). Although this database tracks biologic events, such events are not shown here because they require very specific analytic approaches and are often not directly connected to geophysical and climate-related disasters.*

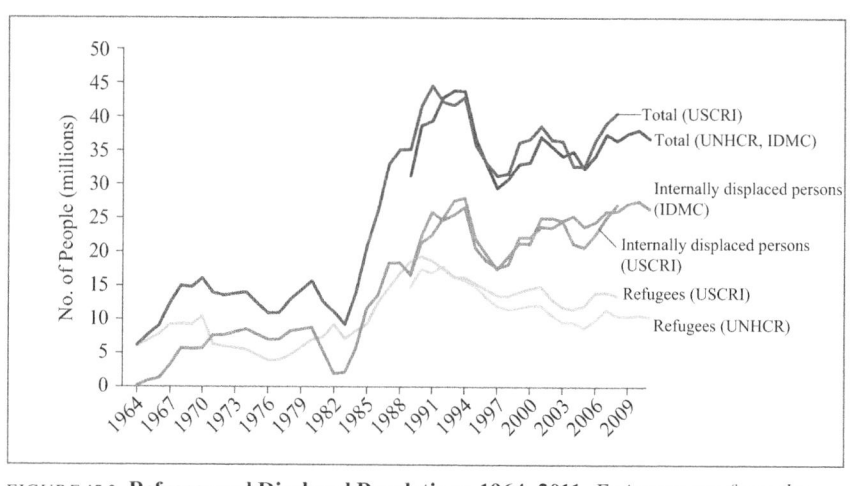

FIGURE 17.2 **Refugees and Displaced Populations, 1964–2011** *Estimates are from the Office of the United Nations High Commissioner for Refugees (UNHCR), the U.S. Committee for Refugees and Immigrants (USCRI), and the Internal Displacement Monitoring Centre (IDMC).*

care, psychosocial support, short-term or emergency medical and surgical interventions, and sanitation and nutritional services. Although the health needs during and after natural disasters and armed conflicts are similar, the differences arise from the political complexities of the latter, in which civilian populations serve as targets of war and human rights abuses aggravate health and protection needs.

The main health consequences of internal armed conflicts are not combat-related injuries and deaths. Mortality is driven by many direct and indirect factors (Fig. 17.3); severe malnutrition, malaria, and other common childhood diseases are the main factors.[10] Typically, health status deteriorates as violence and insecurity lead to population displacements and the breakdown of health care systems and supply chains; this breakdown, in turn, degrades essential services such as vaccination programs, maternal care, and therapeutic feeding.

The main relief needs in natural disasters are water, food, sanitation, and shelter. Poor countries require more extensive assistance than wealthier ones, although severe natural disasters in wealthy regions, such as the 2011 tsunami in Japan, create needs that challenge nation-based responses. In disasters, unlike armed conflicts, the need for emergency relief is comparatively short-lived. However, in some under-resourced regions hit by recurrent natural disasters, such as South Asia and Haiti, there is now increasing evidence of longer-term health effects, such as chronic malnutrition, mediated through intensifying food insecurity.[11,12]

In acute disasters, such as earthquakes and cyclones, physical trauma may require specialized interventions. The probability of survival from serious injury decreases substantially 12 to 24 hours after the disaster strikes, and good outcomes in most cases are thus highly dependent on the rapidity of appropriate medical and surgical responses.[13] Advance preparedness of local health care

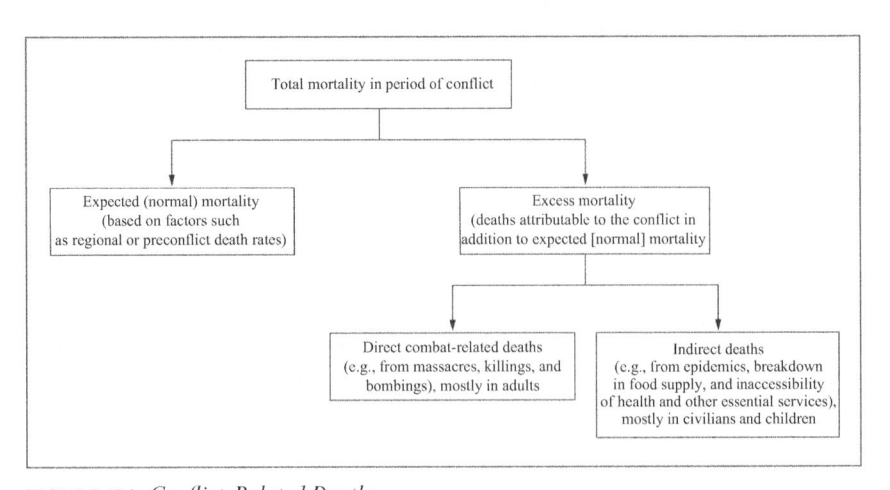

FIGURE 17.3 *Conflict-Related Deaths*
Adapted from Guha-Sapir and van Panhuis.[9]

personnel in search-and-rescue capacities and immediate emergency care are crucial for improving victim survival. An additional requirement that is less widely recognized is for adequate local follow-up nursing care and infection control in postoperative settings and rehabilitation services.

Expanding Use of Epidemiologic Methods in Crises

The critical role of epidemiologic methods in natural disasters was recognized in the 1970s and 1980s in studies after a series of massive catastrophes,[14,15] including the Bangladesh cyclone,[16] Guatemala[17] and Naples[18] earthquakes, and African Sahel famines.[19] These population-based quantitative assessments identified determinants of mortality that helped improve future preparedness and the response of medical teams. Innovative approaches for rapid medical assessment among refugees from the Pol Pot mass killings in the Thai border camps in 1979 and 1980 also drew attention to the importance of conducting an early and accurate evaluation of needs.[20]

During humanitarian responses to the subsequent wave of African famines and postcolonial civil wars in the 1980s, these epidemiologic methods were widely applied. Health analysts were thus able to describe how mortality and morbidity differed across population groups and over time, providing crucial insights for improving response and preparedness.[21] But high population mobility, the breakdown of vital registration or surveillance systems, homelessness, and insecurity posed serious methodologic barriers to generalizing from epidemiologic or risk analyses conducted with small samples. Emergency health assessments also suffered from the lack of baselines against which to calculate excess deaths (Fig. 17.3) and calibrate the criticality of a situation.[22]

In response to growing concerns regarding equity and needs-based response, public health analysts within the humanitarian aid community worked to

identify thresholds of key indicators of mortality and malnutrition in order to classify situations as critical and establish triggers for the provision of emergency relief.[23] Recognizing the major implications of using such thresholds,[24] a group of academics, nongovernmental organizations, and UN agencies developed Standardized Monitoring and Assessment of Relief and Transitions (SMART), a rapid cluster-sampling method that divides the population into groups, or clusters, and randomly selects a sample among these clusters for data collection, in order to provide statistically sound estimates of mortality and malnutrition.[25] Now widely used by relief agencies,[26] this method generates comparable epidemiologic data to quantify crisis thresholds and monitor the effectiveness of the relief,[27] strengthening the evidence-based response.

Collecting reliable epidemiologic information still presents unique challenges in these disrupted field contexts.[28] Because the SMART method does not require household listing, it has advantages over random sampling.[29] However, the relative uncertainties of cluster sampling (lower levels of precision and constraints on extrapolation of key variables such as mortality) can prove problematic, because risks are highly variable across small areas.[30] Given the importance of correctly measuring malnutrition and mortality, on the one hand, and the shortcomings of cluster sampling in transient settings, on the other, alternative methods, such as lot quality assurance sampling (which involves taking a large number of unusually small random samples from each set in the population to determine whether they meet an established standard) or collection of data from key informants, are increasingly used.[31] For insecure settings (e.g., in a zone of conflict), these alternatives show promising advantages because of ease of implementation and the provision of nearly real-time estimates of mortality.

Although these advances have contributed to a greatly improved understanding of the determinants of mortality and morbidity and the effectiveness of aid, the Haiti earthquake response (2010) revealed persistent weaknesses in international emergency relief, particularly with regard to initial assessment and coordination. An authoritative evaluation has noted the long delay in obtaining a "rapid" health assessment (reported on day 45 vs. day 12, which is the standard[32]), owing to the widespread initial chaos but also explicitly to the bureaucratic complexity of the UN Health Cluster system.[33] Trauma response by foreign field hospitals in a recent review was found to be completely uncoordinated and poorly documented. The field units arrived in unprecedented numbers (44 total vs. 41 for the 2005 Pakistan earthquake) but much later than recommended for clinical efficacy (a mean of 10.2 days after the earthquake rather than the standard of 1 to 5 days) and left scant and scattered information on surgical outcomes and patient follow-up.[34]

EVOLVING NORMS AND PRACTICE GUIDELINES
FOR PUBLIC HEALTH RESPONSE

Much of the progress described above has been driven by the ethical imperatives of medical and public health interventions in humanitarian emergencies.

Ensuring unimpeded access to all victims of a disaster or conflict, providing relief according to need rather than political expediency, and documenting or sounding the alert on grave human rights abuses are central to the engagement of health care professionals in responding to humanitarian emergencies. The global health community has made major advances on these issues by working within the international humanitarian framework of law and practice.[35,36] Normative and operational guidance for health care responders within the humanitarian community has been codified in a number of key publications (see the Supplementary Appendix available at NEJM.org).

Medical responders[37] in disaster or conflict zones face stressful situations that demand experience and seasoned judgment beyond medical skills. For example, impartial provision of medical care to victims requires negotiating humanitarian space to prevent hostile interference from local authorities and armed combatants who are the perpetrators of the violence. Delivering food or medical aid to vulnerable or high-risk persons or groups may require population-based triage decisions that can be technically complex and morally challenging.[38]

The collection of data on sensitive topics such as mortality estimates, combat injuries, or witnessed human rights violations requires adherence to standards of informed consent, confidentiality, and informant protection. In oppressive and hostile settings, these standards are difficult to maintain because of risks to those who provide information and to those who collect it.[39]

Norms of equity, particularly in areas of severe need, dictate that the provision of emergency health care cannot be restricted to the survivors but must extend to the surrounding poor communities that help take them in.[40] Broader societal issues related to humanitarian response are often neglected, such as the need to maintain respect for cultural practices regarding death and grief.[41] On occasion, mass emergency interventions may still violate human rights norms of mutual respect and cause discontent in local communities whose cooperation with external assistance is vital. Experiences from massive earthquakes have shown that the longer-term, social consequences of such oversights can be severe.[42] For instance, the citizens of Soviet Armenia (sensitive to the historical echoes of genocide) were incensed at the Soviet Union for offering to take orphans in the immediate aftermath of the December 1988 earthquake that killed at least 25,000 people—an affront that lingers to this day[43] and that foreshadowed the controversy about post-disaster international child adoption that surfaced with the earthquakes in Haiti[44] and Japan.[45]

Challenges

Much has been learned in the past few decades, but some important issues need urgent attention. The rapidity of emergency health care intervention has greatly improved, with teams on the ground within days, but coordination of health needs assessments performed by multiple groups is weak. Although coordination of health data has been widely recognized as an ongoing problem through

in-depth evaluations of the Rwanda genocide and Haiti earthquake, little progress has been made in addressing this problem.

Bridging the transition from emergency health response to local health systems has not been adequately addressed in most post-conflict or post-disaster settings and especially in poor regions afflicted by recurrent conflicts or natural disasters. Sudden infusions of outside aid and expertise can compromise existing community public health operations by setting up parallel systems with different norms and resources. Abrupt departures of emergency teams may also leave patients without locally viable follow-up nursing care. Resolving such transitional issues by reducing vulnerabilities and strengthening the resilience of local systems will inform the strategies needed to address root causes of these crises.

Finally, humanitarian health care personnel regularly face political and military barriers to providing humane and appropriate care for those most in need.[46] These crises often uncover deep fissures in societies. In particular, humanitarian health care providers confront the need to maintain silence about witnessed violations of international humanitarian and human rights law in order to maintain access to stigmatized or oppressed populations.[47] These ethical dilemmas have provoked sustained controversy and require health care personnel to possess not only medical and public health expertise but also a practical understanding of when to negotiate or speak out on the basis of applicable humanitarian norms and legal principles.[48] Health care personnel need adequate training in these aspects of the humanitarian response as situations become increasingly politicized and neutral space constricts.[49]

Conclusions

The effects of armed conflict and natural disasters on global public health are widespread. Much progress has been made in the technical quality, normative coherence, and efficiency of the health care response. But action after the fact remains insufficient. In the years ahead, the international community must address the root causes of these crises. Natural disasters, particularly floods and storms, will become more frequent and severe because of climate change. Organized deadly onslaughts against civilian populations will continue, fueled by the availability of small arms, persistent social and political inequities, and, increasingly, by a struggle for natural resources. These events affect the mortality, morbidity, and well-being of large populations. Humanitarian relief will always be required, and there is a demonstrable need, as in other areas of global health, to place greater emphasis on prevention and mitigation.

We thank Peter Louis Heudtlass, Ph.D. candidate, World Health Organization Collaborating Center for Research on the Epidemiology of Disasters, Institute of Health and Society, University of Louvain, Brussels, and Bonnie Shnayerson and Angela Murray, François-Xavier Bagnoud Center for Health and Human Rights, Harvard School of Public Health, Boston, for their help in the preparation of the manuscript.

References

1. Guha-Sapir D, Vos F, Below R. Annual disaster statistical review 2011: the numbers and trends. Brussels: Center for Research on the Epidemiology of Disasters, 2012.

2. Guha-Sapir D, D'aoust O. Demographic and health consequences of civil conflict: background paper. In: World development report 2011: conflict, security, and development. Washington, DC: World Bank, 2011.

3. Feikin DR, Adazu K, Obor D, et al. Mortality and health among internally displaced persons in western Kenya following post-election violence, 2008: novel use of demographic surveillance. Bull World Health Organ 2010;88:601–608.

4. Waldman RJ, Kruk ME. Conflict, health, and health systems: a global perspective. In: Parker R, Sommer M, eds. Routledge handbook of global public health. Abingdon, Oxfordshire, United Kingdom: Routledge, 2011:229–35.

5. Noji EK, Toole MJ. The historical development of public health responses to disaster. Disasters 1997;21:366–76.

6. Universal declaration of human rights. United Nations General Assembly resolution 217A (III) on 10 December 1948 (http://www.un.org/cyberschoolbus/human-rights/resources/universal.asp).

7. The Fourth Geneva Convention of 1949. Geneva: International Committee of the Red Cross, August 1949.

8. Brown RE, Mayer J. Famine and disease in Biafra: an assessment. Trop Geogr Med 1969;21:348–52.

9. Guha-Sapir D, Panhuis WG. Conflict-related mortality: an analysis of 37 datasets. Disasters 2004;28:418–28.

10. Salama P, Spiegel P, Talley L, Waldman R. Lessons learned from complex emergencies over past decade. Lancet 2004;364:1801–13.

11. Rodriguez-Llanes JM, Ranjan-Dash S, Degomme O, Mukhopadhyay A, Guha-Sapir D. Child malnutrition and recurrent flooding in rural eastern India: a community-based survey. BMJ Open 2011;1(2):e000109.

12. Ferris E, Petz D, Stark C. The year of recurring disasters. Washington, DC: Brookings Institution, March 2013 (http://www.brookings.edu/research/reports/2013/03/natural-disaster-chapter-1-ferris).

13. Roces MC, White ME, Dayrit MM, Durkin ME. Risk factors for injuries due to the 1990 earthquake in Luzon, Philippines. Bull World Health Organ 1992;70:509–14.

14. Western KA. The epidemiology of natural and man-made disasters: the present state of the art. (DTPH dissertation. London: London School of Hygiene and Tropical Medicine, University of London, June 1, 1972; http://cidbimena.desastres.hn/docum/crid/Agosto2004/pdf/eng/doc3610.htm.)

15. Lechat MF. The epidemiology of disasters. Proc R Soc Med 1976;69:421–26.

16. Sommer A, Mosley WH. East Bengal cyclone of November, 1970: epidemiological approach to disaster assessment. Lancet 1972;1:1029–36.

17. Glass RI, Urrutia JJ, Sibony S, Smith H, Garcia B, Rizzo L. Earthquake injuries related to housing in a Guatemalan village. Science 1977;197:638–43.

18. De Bruycker M, Greco D, Lechat MF, Annino I, De Ruggiero N, Triassi M. The 1980 earthquake in Southern Italy—morbidity and mortality. Int J Epidemiol 1985;14:113–17.

19. Rivers JPW, Holt JFJ, Seaman JA, Bowden MR. Lessons for epidemiology from the Ethiopian famines. Ann Soc Belg Med Trop 1976;56:345–60.

20. Glass RI, Cates W Jr, Nieburg P, et al. Rapid assessment of health status and preventive-medicine needs of newly arrived Kampuchean refugees, Sa Kaeo, Thailand. Lancet 1980;1:868–72.

21. Famine-affected, refugee, and displaced populations: recommendations for public health issues. MMWR Recomm Rep 1992;41(RR-13):1–76.

22. Byass P. Person, place and time—but who, where, and when? Scand J Public Health 2001;29:84–86.

23. The Sphere handbook: humanitarian charter and minimum standards in humanitarian response. Geneva: Sphere Project, 2011:311.

24. Boss LP, Toole MJ, Yip R. Assessments of mortality, morbidity, and nutritional status in Somalia during the 1991-1992 famine: recommendations for standardization of methods. JAMA 1994;272:371–76.

25. Katz J. Sample-size implications for population-based cluster surveys of nutritional status. Am J Clin Nutr 1995;61:155–60.

26. Standard Monitoring and Assessment of Relief and Transitions (SMART). Measuring mortality, nutritional status, and food security in crisis situations, version I. 2006 (http://smartmethodology.org/documents/manual/SMART_Methodology_08-07-2006.pdf).

27. Reed HE, Keely CB, eds. Forced migration and mortality. National Research Council. Washington, DC: National Academy Press, 2001.

28. Guha-Sapir D, van Panhuis WG, Degomme O, Teran V. Civil conflicts in four African countries: a five-year review of trends in nutrition and mortality. Epidemiol Rev 2005;27:67–77.

29. Checchi F, Roberts L. Interpreting and using mortality data in humanitarian emergencies: a primer for non-epidemiologists. Humanitarian practice network paper 52. London: Overseas Development Institute, 2005.

30. Degomme O, Guha-Sapir D. Patterns of mortality rates in Darfur conflict. Lancet 2010;375:294–300.

31. Deitchler M, Deconinck H, Bergeron G. Precision, time, and cost: a comparison of three sampling designs in an emergency setting. Emerg Themes Epidemiol 2008;5:6 (http://www.ete-online.com/content/5/1/6).

32. Inter-Agency Standing Committee (IASC). Initial Rapid Assessment (IRA): guidance notes. June 2000:3 (http://www.who.int/hac/network/global_health_cluster/ira_guidance_note_june2009.pdf).

33. de Ville de Goyet C, Sarmiento JP, Grunewald F. Health response to the earthquake in Haiti January 2010: lessons to be learned for the next massive sudden onset disaster. Washington, DC: Pan American Health Organization, 2011:112–13.

34. Gerdin M, Wladis A, von Schreeb J. Foreign field hospitals after the 2010 Haiti earthquake: how good were we? Emerg Med J 2012;30(1):e8.

35. Thurer D. Dunant's pyramid: thoughts on the "humanitarian space." Intl Rev Red Cross 2007;89:47–61.

36. The Sphere Project. The Sphere handbook: humanitarian charter and minimum standards in humanitarian response (http://www.sphereproject.org/handbook/).

37. Coupland RM. Epidemiological approach to surgical management of the casualties of war. BMJ 1994;308:1693–97.

38. Iserson KV, Moskop JC. Triage in medicine. I. Concept, history, and types. Ann Emerg Med 2007;49:275–81.

39. Ford N, Mills EJ, Zachariah R, Upshur R. Ethics of conducting research in conflict settings. Confl Health 2009;3:7.

40. United Nations High Commissioner for Refugees. Public health equity in refugee and other displaced persons settings. Public Health and HIV section, DPSM. Policy Development and Evaluation Service. April 2010 (http://www.unhcr.org/4bdfe1699. pdf).

41. Management of dead bodies in disaster situations. Disaster manuals and guidelines series. No. 5. Washington, DC: Pan American Health Organization, 2004:85–128.

42. Batniji R, Van Ommeren M, Saraceno B. Mental and social health in disasters: relating qualitative social science research and the Sphere standard. Soc Sci Med 2006;62:1853–64.

43. Libaridian GJ. Armenian earthquakes and Soviet tremors. Society 1989;26:59–63.

44. Thompson G. After Haiti quake, the chaos of US adoptions. New York Times. August 4, 2010:A1 (http://www.nytimes.com/2010/08/04/world/americas/04adoption. html?pagewanted=all).

45. Macedo D. Foreigners looking to adopt Japanese earthquake orphans need not apply. Fox News Network. March 22, 2011 (http://www.foxnews.com/world/2011/03/21/ foreigners-looking-adopt-japanese-earthquake-orphans-need-apply/).

46. Weissman F. Liberia: can relief organizations cope with the warlords? In: Médecins sans Frontières. World in crisis: the politics of survival at the end of the twentieth century. London: Rutledge, 1997:100–21.

47. Bruderlein C, Leaning J. New challenges for humanitarian protection. BMJ 1999;319:430–35.

48. Leaning J, Briggs SM, Chen L, eds. Humanitarian crises: the medical and public health response. Cambridge, MA: Harvard University Press, 1999.

49. Leaning J. The dilemma of neutrality. Prehosp Disaster Med 2007;22:418–21.

Global Institutional Responses

INTRODUCTION

Many global health threats require a coordinated global response. As discussed in the Introduction, the institutions involved and their interrelationships have changed substantially in recent decades. Global health is now a stage crowded with many actors. This heightened interest is mainly to the good, but it does raise questions about competition for resources, control of agendas, duplication of effort, and the potential for the imposition of political and moral frameworks by stronger countries and agencies on weaker countries.

Health is primarily a responsibility of sovereign nations; in some countries such as India, states within the nation are the major loci of responsibility for health. In rare cases of failed states or war, the international system may take on responsibility for the health of local populations, but the norm is that global health institutions operate within the framework of national laws and customs. This implies a necessity for adaptation and flexibility in global health activities in order to accommodate multiple ethical, cultural, legal, and political frameworks as well as very diverse health needs and infrastructures.

A reality for global health is that multiple agencies, not normally thought of as related to health, have potentially immense influence over the health of nations. Activities of the World Trade Organization for instance, govern aspects of intellectual property and patent agreements that may facilitate or deny access to pharmaceutical drugs. Agreements made to combat international trafficking of illegal narcotics have influence over the supply and distribution of medical narcotics for pain relief. The consequences of the failure of multiple conferences to agree on robust international responses to climate change will have increasing effects on the health of any populations

in low-lying coastal areas and for those exposed to weather-related disasters and deleterious changes in agricultural production.

The article by Frenk and Moon reviews the many institutions that now participate in global health governance, noting that many of these are relatively recent creations and new models for funding and service delivery are constantly emerging. They point out the relative weakness of many of these institutions in the face of the threats we face consequent to globalization, both with respect to the international transfer of risks (e.g., toxic wastes, counterfeit drugs, the tobacco industry) and the large-scale threats of pandemics and climate change. Gostin and Sridhar review global health law, a system of "soft" laws, treaties, and norms. Within countries, the legal system has been used by public health advocates to advance access or change policies; examples include the constitutional court decision in South Africa in 2002 to mandate the government to provide nevirapine in public hospitals for the prevention of maternal-infant HIV transmission and the decision by the Supreme Court of India in 1998 to direct the Delhi local government to develop a program to switch taxis and buses to lower-emission fuels. Apart from some trade, patent, and human rights issues, the ability of public health advocates to find international solutions through a legal system is far more limited owing to the absence of courts with transnational legal jurisdiction.

A final issue in great need of better global institutional approaches is the development and maintenance of the health workforce. The world is not training enough health professionals, and there is marked maldistribution geographically. Within many countries, there are too many doctors in cities and too few in rural areas; some countries are magnets for doctors from other countries that cannot afford to lose them. Many health professionals wish to migrate to make more money and others seek to avoid working in inadequate, even dangerous health facilities. Chen and Crisp discuss the huge disparities in the distribution of the health workforce globally as well as the movement to address migration issues and larger issues of how training health professionals in the 21st century should not simply be an extension of 20th-century practices.[1]

Reference

1. Bhutta ZA, Chen L, Cohen J, et al. Education of health professionals for the 21st century: a global independent Commission. *Lancet* 2010;375(9721):1137–1138.

Governance Challenges in Global Health
Julio Frenk
and Suerie Moon

Global health is at the threshold of a new era. Few times in history has the world faced challenges as complex as those now posed by a trio of threats: first, the unfinished agenda of infections, undernutrition, and reproductive health problems; second, the rising global burden of noncommunicable diseases and their associated risk factors, such as smoking and obesity; and third, the challenges arising from globalization itself, such as the health effects of climate change and trade policies, which demand engagement outside the traditional health sector.[1] These threats are evolving within a multifaceted and dynamic global context characterized by great diversity among societies in norms, values, and interests, as well as by large inequalities in the distribution of health risks and the resources to address them.

A robust response to this complex picture requires improved governance of health systems—certainly at the national level but also at a worldwide level in what could be thought of as the "global health system." However, the concept of governance is still poorly understood despite its growing visibility in current debates about global health. In this article, we define and discuss the importance of good global governance for health, outline major challenges to such governance, and describe the necessary functions of a global health system.

Understanding Global Health and Governance

There are many working definitions of global health. Some emphasize certain types of health problems (e.g., communicable diseases), whereas others emphasize certain populations of interest (e.g., the poor), focus on a geographic area (e.g., the Global South), or have a specific mission (e.g., equity). Global health encompasses all these dimensions, but each of them in isolation offers only a partial perspective. In our view, global health should be defined by two key elements: its level of analysis, which involves the entire population of the world, and

the relationships of interdependence that bind together the units of social organization that make up the global population (e.g., nation states, private organizations, ethnic groups, and civil society movements).

When thinking about health in populations, we must analyze two essential dimensions: health conditions (e.g., diseases and risk factors) and the way in which a society responds to those conditions. This framework can be applied at both the national level and the global level. Faced with a set of health conditions, a country articulates a response through its national health system. At the global level, the key concept in understanding the pattern of health conditions is the international transfer of health risks—that is, the way in which the movement of people, products, resources, and lifestyles across borders can contribute to the spread of disease.[2] Globalization has intensified cross-border health threats,[3] leading to a situation of health interdependence—the notion that no nation or organization is able to address single-handedly the health threats it faces but instead must rely to some degree on others to mount an effective response.[4] The organized social response to health conditions at the global level is what we call the global health system, and the way in which the system is managed is what we refer to as governance.

The notion of governance goes beyond the formal mechanisms of government and refers to the totality of ways in which a society organizes and collectively manages its affairs.[5] Global governance is the extension of this notion to the world as a whole.[6-8] It can refer to the formal decision-making processes of the United Nations Security Council, for example, or to less formal ways of influencing behavior, such as voluntary codes of conduct for multinational corporations. It includes the myriad processes that shape the way we collectively address issues of global significance, such as financial stability, environmental sustainability, peace and security, human rights, and public health.[8]

Global governance is distinct from national governance in one critical respect: there is no government at the global level. Populations are organized into sovereign nation states, but there is no hierarchical political authority, or world government, that has jurisdiction over these nation states. Traditional instruments for mobilizing collective action at the national level—such as taxation, routine law enforcement, and democratic decision-making procedures—are mostly absent at the global level. As a result, societies face enduring challenges to agree on and enforce rules, coordinate action, achieve policy coherence, and ensure accountability. In the aftermath of World War II, governments created multilateral institutions, such as the United Nations system, to help coordinate actions for shared social objectives, including public health. Thus was born, in 1948, the World Health Organization (WHO), the public health authority within the United Nations. The WHO is now governed by 194 member states and is charged with organizing international responses to shared health challenges. However, there is widespread consensus that the current institutional architecture, now more than 60 years old, is unable to respond effectively to contemporary global health threats. Today, the WHO stands on a crowded stage; though once seen as the sole authority on global health, the WHO is now surrounded by many diverse actors.

The Global Health System: The New Reality of Pluralism

The global health system is the group of actors whose primary intent is to improve health, along with the rules and norms governing their interactions.[9] At the core of the system are national governments, with their specialized health ministries, departments, or agencies, and, in the case of donor nations, the health programs of their respective bilateral development cooperation agencies (Table 18.1). National governments coordinate their responses to common health challenges through a variety of mechanisms. The WHO is the only actor in the global health system that is built on the universal membership of all recognized sovereign nation states (though it is often identified only with its secretariat), and it therefore is central to the system. Also important to the system are other United Nations and multilateral agencies that have health components (e.g., the United Nations Children's Fund [UNICEF], the World Bank, and the regional development banks), along with a diverse set of civil society organizations, multinational corporations, foundations, and academic institutions. This pluralistic landscape has been enriched by a set of innovative and influential hybrid organizations, such as the GAVI Alliance (formerly the Global Alliance for Vaccines and Immunization), UNITAID (which works to improve the functioning of global markets for commodities for the acquired immunodeficiency syndrome [AIDS], tuberculosis, and malaria), and the Global Fund to Fight AIDS, Tuberculosis, and Malaria, which are governed by representatives both from within and from outside national governments. During the past decade, there has been a population explosion in the system, and there are now more than 175 initiatives, funds, agencies, and donors.[30]

To make matters even more complex, health is increasingly influenced by decisions that are made in other global policymaking arenas, such as those governing international trade, migration, and the environment (see interactive graphic available at NEJM.org).[31-33] Actors in these arenas influence health, even though that is not their primary intent. A major example of such an institution is the World Trade Organization, which has profoundly shaped domestic and global intellectual property rules relating to pharmaceuticals, among other health-related trade issues. These policymaking institutions are not part of the global health system; instead, they represent critical policy arenas in which global health actors must learn to exert influence. The importance of these arenas is the reason why we prefer the term "global governance for health," rather than the more restrictive notion of "global health governance," which tends to focus only on entities specializing in health matters.

The challenge of achieving good governance among the diverse group of actors (Table 18.1) has drawn increased political attention.[34-38] Thus far, however, too little attention has been given to the problem of protecting and promoting health in governance processes outside the global health system.[39] "Good" global governance for health should exhibit at least the following key traits: effectiveness, equity, and efficiency in achieving outcomes, as well as credibility and legitimacy in decision-making processes. However, the achievement of these goals is hampered by three persistent governance challenges that are embedded in the

TABLE 18.1 Primary Types of Actors in the Global Health System, with Examples

Type of Actor and Examples	Annual Expenditures* millions of U.S. dollars (year)
National governments	
Ministries of health[†]	ND
Ministries of foreign affairs[†]	ND
Public research funders	
U.S. National Institutes of Health	30,860 (2010)[10]
Bilateral development cooperation agencies	
U.S. Agency for International Development and U.S. Department of State (global health and child survival)	7,779 (2010)[11]
U.K. Department for International Development (global health)	585 (2011)[12]
Norwegian Agency for Development Cooperation (health and social services)	329 (2010)[13]
United Nations system	
World Health Organization	2,000 (2010)[14]
United Nations Children's Fund	3,653 (2010)[15]
United Nations Population Fund	801 (2010)[16]
Joint United Nations Program on HIV/AIDS	242 (2009)[17]
Multilateral development banks	
World Bank (health and other social services lending)	6,707 (2011)[18]
Regional development banks	NA
Global health initiatives (hybrids)	
Global Fund to Fight AIDS, Tuberculosis, and Malaria	3,475 (2010)[19]
GAVI Alliance	934 (2010)[20]
UNITAID	269 (2010)[21]
Philanthropic organizations	
Bill and Melinda Gates Foundation (global health)	1,485 (2010)[22]
Rockefeller Foundation (all sectors)	173 (2009)[23]
Wellcome Trust	1,114 (2010)[24]
Global civil society organizations and nongovernmental organizations	
Doctors without Borders (Médecins sans Frontières)	1,080 (2010)[25]
Oxfam International	1,210 (2010)[26]
CARE International	805 (2010)[27]
Private industry	
Pharmaceutical companies (global market)	856,000 (2010)[28]
Professional associations	
World Medical Association	NA
Academic institutions	
Postsecondary educational institutions for health professionals	100,000[29‡]

* All conversions of currency to U.S. dollars were based on average exchange rates for the year cited. NA denotes not available, and ND no data.

[†]Ministries of health and ministries of foreign affairs are the parts of national governments that are likely to be particularly relevant for the global health system. Expenditures are not included, since the relevant data are generally not disaggregated or reported in this way.

[‡]This value represents a worldwide estimate.

structure of the global system: the sovereignty challenge, the sectoral challenge, and the accountability challenge.

Major Governance Challenges for Global Health

THE SOVEREIGNTY CHALLENGE

In a world of sovereign nation states, health continues to be primarily a national responsibility; however, the intensified transfer of health risks across borders means that the determinants of health and the means to fulfill that responsibility lie increasingly beyond the control of any one nation state.[40] In the absence of a world government, there is an inherent tension between the reality of national sovereignty and the imperative of international collective action to properly manage interdependence. Sovereignty can confound attempts at transnational coordination, rulemaking, and adjudication. These tasks become even more difficult given the highly unequal distribution of health risks and resources, the opposing interests of various actors, the diversity of cultures and histories, and the rapidly changing distribution of power among countries in the global system. In a context of deepening health interdependence, it becomes more urgent and yet more difficult for countries to agree on their respective responsibilities, obligations, rights, and duties, hampering effective responses to common health threats.

THE SECTORAL CHALLENGE

Global health is increasingly the product of cross-sector interdependence—that is, the outcome of policymaking processes across multiple sectors.[41,42] However, global health actors today are largely unequipped to ensure that health concerns are adequately taken into account in crucial policymaking arenas such as trade, investment, security, the environment, migration, and education.

THE ACCOUNTABILITY CHALLENGE

The formal institutions of global governance, such as the United Nations system, are built on the principle that governments of nation states are the primary decision makers and representatives of their population's interests at the international level. However, new forms of social organization are challenging the primacy of the nation state in the global arena through what David Fidler calls the "unstructured plurality" of nonstate actors.[36] For example, civil society networks, experts, foundations, multinational corporations, and journalists all wield power in processes of global governance independently of their home-country governments. Two types of accountability problems arise in the current context. The first relates to the legitimacy of intergovernmental organizations, which are formally accountable to the governments of member states rather than directly to the people whose universal rights they are supposed to uphold. This situation too

often leads to a "democratic deficit" in the way the organizations operate. This is particularly problematic when people consider their own national governance processes to be illegitimate, such as when governments restrict democratic participation, fail to represent marginalized groups, or otherwise violate the human rights of their own populations.

The second type of problem is the lack of clear mechanisms for the accountability of nonstate actors. Although the lines of accountability that stretch from intergovernmental organizations to member states to populations are clear, albeit problematic, the mechanisms for demanding that nonstate actors operating in the global arena—corporations, civil society organizations, foundations, experts, and journalists—be accountable for the global effects of their actions are relatively vague, at best. We lack effective institutions to govern the many powerful nonstate actors that influence global health today.

Four Functions of the Global Health System

These three governance challenges impede the performance of the global health system, which must carry out a number of functions to achieve common goals. Here we describe four key functions of the global health system and briefly illustrate the ways in which governance challenges can hinder attempts to carry them out (Table 18.2).

The first function is the production of global public goods, especially knowledge-related goods.[43] Examples include tools for international standardization (e.g., the International Classification of Diseases), guidelines regarding best practice (e.g., the WHO Model List of Essential Medicines), research and development of new technologies,[44] and comparative analyses and evaluation of policies and programs with respect to design and implementation. The production of global public goods requires sufficient and sustainable resources, which can be difficult to generate when sovereign states can benefit from investments made by others without contributing themselves (a situation known as free-riding).[45] Effective governance arrangements among sovereign states, such

TABLE 18.2 Four Essential Functions of the Global Health System

Function	Subfunctions
Production of global public goods	Research and development, standards and guidelines, and comparative evidence and analyses
Management of externalities across countries	Surveillance and information sharing and coordination for preparedness and response
Mobilization of global solidarity	Development financing, technical cooperation, humanitarian assistance, and agency for the dispossessed
Stewardship	Convening for negotiation and consensus building, priority setting, rule setting, evaluation for mutual accountability, and cross-sector health advocacy

as core funding for the WHO or binding legal instruments, may be needed to overcome the free-rider problem and ensure sufficient production of global public goods.[46]

The second function is the management of externalities to prevent or mitigate the negative health effects that situations or decisions originating in one country might have on others. It involves the deployment of instruments (e.g., surveillance systems, coordination mechanisms, and information-sharing channels) that are essential for controlling the international transfer of risks and ensuring a timely response to threats that spread across borders (e.g., drug resistance, pandemics, environmental pollutants, and marketing of unhealthful products such as tobacco). However, sovereignty and weak accountability mechanisms make managing externalities difficult. For example, a government may delay the disclosure of a disease outbreak for fear of economic repercussions or it could refuse to tighten regulations on an industry that pollutes the air or water flowing into a neighboring country. In both cases, there is no supranational body with authority to stop such a government from generating negative externalities.

The third function is the mobilization of global solidarity, which has been the predominant focus of traditional approaches to global health, mostly through the provision of aid. (We use the term "solidarity" in the context of classical sociological theory, rather than of any particular political ideology.[47]) The need for this function arises from the unequal distribution of both health problems and the resources to address them. The broad concept of solidarity encompasses four major subfunctions: development financing; technical cooperation, including capacity strengthening; humanitarian assistance to provide relief during natural or man-made disasters; and agency for the dispossessed,[40] in which the global community takes responsibility for protecting the rights of specific groups (e.g., displaced populations or minorities) when their own governments are not willing or able to do so. There is a clear case for global solidarity when the health system of a country is chronically incapable of addressing the needs of its population or when it is acutely overwhelmed by a crisis. However, carrying out this function can be difficult in a system of sovereign states with few accountability mechanisms. For example, if a state objects when the global community takes an interest in its marginalized groups or if it chooses not to contribute to international humanitarian relief efforts, there are few options to make that state do otherwise. Even if a state commits to providing development assistance, there are few mechanisms for accountability if it reneges.

The fourth function is stewardship, which provides overall strategic direction to the global health system so that all other functions can be performed adequately.[48] Stewardship includes the following subfunctions: convening for negotiation and consensus building (e.g., regarding policy frameworks such as Health for All through primary health care), setting priorities (e.g., among disease categories or intervention strategies), setting rules to manage the many dimensions of health interdependence (e.g., through the Framework Convention on Tobacco Control), evaluating actors and actions to ensure mutual accountability, and advocating for health across sectors. This last subfunction requires

health actors to manage the sectoral challenge by learning to advocate effectively
for health considerations in the other policy arenas that influence global health.
Stewardship requires trusted leadership, credible and legitimate processes, and
sufficient political space to protect public health in the face of powerful competing
interests. Yet all these factors can be undermined when mechanisms for accountability are weak or when sovereign states put narrowly conceived self-interests
before global health.

Implications for Policy

Strengthening the global health system will require managing persistent governance challenges to ensure that key functions are performed. It will also require
increased clarity regarding which actors should carry out which functions to
avoid a situation in which there is inefficient overlap on some functions while others are overlooked. Consensus regarding the core functions of each major actor
should determine institutional arrangements: form should follow function. This
endeavor has become even more urgent given the slowdown in funding for global
health.[49]

In current debates about WHO reform, attention should be paid to the functions this institution performs within the larger global health system and the governance challenges that must be addressed for it to perform them successfully.
For example, the WHO plays a unique and irreplaceable role in providing certain
global public goods and in fulfilling most elements of the stewardship function.
This core work must be protected and strengthened in any reform of the institution. Focusing on strong stewardship would also help to address the sectoral
challenge, especially by developing stronger competencies in the WHO and other
agencies for cross-sectoral health advocacy.

These governance challenges are not new. The past decade has shown that
the health arena can be fertile ground for institutional innovation. For example,
there have been attempts to strengthen accountability and legitimacy by according formal decision-making roles to a broader range of actors; the governing
boards of the GAVI Alliance, UNITAID, and the Global Fund to Fight AIDS,
Tuberculosis, and Malaria include nonstate representatives, such as civil society
organizations, communities of people affected by target diseases, and foundations, reflecting an attempt at more inclusive governance. Furthermore, global
norms on intellectual property have evolved to become more sensitive to concerns about access to medicines as health advocates have gained some influence
in trade policymaking.[50]

However, these encouraging innovations remain limited to a handful of institutions and are largely in their infancy. The global health system is still ham-
strung by the structural governance challenges presented here. Innovative global
governance arrangements should continue to be tested, evaluated, improved,
and—where successful—replicated. Rigorous research and analysis of the
achievements and shortfalls of past experiments in governance arrangements are

needed and merit greater attention from the academic community. Leaders of governments, multilateral institutions, civil society organizations, firms, foundations, and other influential actors should identify new governance arrangements that are more effective, equitable, and accountable.

Governance challenges will continue to complicate our best efforts to respond to urgent, complex, and serious global health problems. Any effort to strengthen the global health system will require recognition and management of these tensions so that the system can better face the realities of interdependence in the 21st century.

References

1. Frenk J, Gómez-Dantés O, Chacón F. Global health in transition. In: Parker RG, Sommer M, eds. Routledge handbook of global public health. New York: Routledge, 2011:11–17.

2. Frenk J, Sepúlveda J, Gómez-Dantés O, McGuiness MJ, Knaul F. The New World order and international health. BMJ 1997;314:1404–407.

3. Keohane RO, Nye JS. Interdependence in world politics. In: Crane GT, Amawi A, eds. The theoretical evolution of international political economy: a reader. New York: Oxford University Press, 1997:122–32.

4. Chen L, Bell D, Bates L. World health and institutional change. In: Pocantico Retreat—enhancing the performance of international health institutions. Cambridge, MA: The Rockefeller Foundation, Social Science Research Council, Harvard School of Public Health, 1996:9–21.

5. United Nations Development Programme (UNDP). Governance for sustainable human development. New York: UNDP, 1997.

6. Weiss TG. Governance, good governance and global governance: conceptual and actual challenges. Third World Q 2000;21:795–814.

7. Finkelstein LS. What is global governance? Global Governance 1995;1:367–72.

8. Commission on Global Governance. Our global neighbourhood. Oxford, United Kingdom: Oxford University Press, 1995.

9. Szlezák NA, Bloom BR, Jamison DT, et al. The global health system: actors, norms, and expectations in transition. PLoS Med 2010;7(1):e1000183.

10. The NIH almanac: appropriations 2011. Rockville, MD: National Institutes of Health (http://www.nih.gov/about/almanac/appropriations/part2.htm).

11. Congressional Budget Office. Congressional budget justification volume 2: foreign operations fiscal year 2011. Washington, DC: Department of State, 2011.

12. Provost C. The future of UK aid 2010–2015—get the data. The Guardian. October 5, 2011 (http://www.guardian.co.uk/global-development/datablog/2011/oct/05/datablog-future-plans-uk-aid).

13. Norwegian aid statistics. Oslo: Norwegian Agency for Development Cooperation (Norad), 2011 (http://www.norad.no/en/tools-and-publications/norwegian-aid-statistics).

14. World Health Organization. Unaudited interim financial report for the year 2010: financial period 2010–2011 (report A64/29). Geneva: World Health Organization, 2011.

15. United Nations Children's Fund (UNICEF). Annual report 2010. New York: UNICEF, 2011 (http://www.unicef.org/publications/index_58840.html).

16. United Nations Population Fund (UNFPA). Annual report 2010. New York: UNFPA, 2011 (http://unfpa.org/public/home/publications/pid/7797).

17. Joint United Nations Programme on HIV/AIDS (UNAIDS). Annual report 2009. Geneva: UNAIDS, 2010 (http://data.unaids.org/pub/Report/2010/2009_annual_report_en.pdf).

18. The World Bank. The World Bank annual report 2011. Washington, DC: World Bank, 2011.

19. Bernescut B, Grubb I, Jurgens R, Hacopian P. The Global Fund annual report 2010. Geneva: The Global Fund to Fight AIDS, Tuberculosis and Malaria, 2011 (http://www.theglobalfund.org/en/library/publications/annualreports).

20. Global Alliance for Vaccines and Immunization (GAVI). GAVI Alliance annual financial report 2010. Geneva: The GAVI Alliance, 2011.

21. UNITAID. UNITAID annual report 2010. Geneva: World Health Organization, Secretariat of UNITAID, 2011 (http://www.unitaid.eu/images/NewWeb/documents/AR10/unitaid_ar2010_web.pdf).

22. Bill and Melinda Gates Foundation. Bill & Melinda Gates Foundation 2010 annual report. Seattle: Bill & Melinda Gates Foundation, 2011 (http://www.gatesfoundation.org/annualreport/2010/Pages/overview.aspx).

23. The Rockefeller Foundation. The Rockefeller Foundation 2009 annual report. New York: The Rockefeller Foundation, 2010 (http://2009annualreport.rockefellerfoundation.org).

24. The Wellcome Trust. Wellcome Trust annual report and financial statements 2010. London: Wellcome Trust, 2011 (http://www.wellcome.ac.uk/stellent/groups/corporatesite/@msh_publishing_group/documents/web_document/wtx063982.pdf).

25. Medecins Sans Frontieres. Médecins Sans Frontières (MSF) activity report 2010. Geneva: Médecins Sans Frontières (MSF), 2011 (http://www.doctorswithoutborders.org/publications/ar/report.cfm?id=5457&cat=activity-report).

26. Oxfam International. Oxfam International annual report 2010–2011. Oxford, United Kingdom: Oxfam, 2011 (http://www.oxfam.org/sites/www.oxfam.org/files/oxfam-annual-report-2010-11.pdf).

27. CARE International. CARE International annual report 2010. Geneva: CARE International, 2011 (http://www.care-international.org/Media-Releases/care-launches-2010-annual-report.html).

28. IMS Institute for Healthcare Informatics. Global use of medicines: outlook through 2015. IMS Health, 2011 (http://www.imshealth.com/deployedfiles/ims/Global/Content/Insights/IMS%20Institute%20for%20Healthcare%20Informatics/Global_Use_of_Medicines_Report.pdf).

29. Frenk J, Chen L, Bhutta ZA, et al. Health professionals for a new century: transforming education to strengthen health systems in an interdependent world. Lancet 2010;376:1923–58.

30. McColl K. Europe told to deliver more aid for health. Lancet 2008;371:2072–73.

31. Costello A, Abbas M, Allen A, et al. Managing the health effects of climate change: Lancet and University College London Institute for Global Health Commission. Lancet 2009;373:1693–733. [Erratum, Lancet 2009;373:2200.]

32. Lee K, Sridhar D, Patel M. Bridging the divide: global governance of trade and health. Lancet 2009;373:416–22.

33. Smith RD, Correa C, Oh C. Trade, TRIPS, and pharmaceuticals. Lancet 2009;373:684–91.
34. Moon S, Szlezák NA, Michaud C, et al. The global health system: lessons for a stronger institutional framework. PLoS Med 2010;7(1):e1000193.
35. Lee K, Fidler D. Avian and pandemic influenza: progress and problems with global health governance. Glob Public Health 2007;2:215–34.
36. Fidler D. Architecture amidst anarchy: global health's quest for governance. Global Health Governance 2007;1:1–17.
37. Fidler D. The challenges of global health governance. New York: Council on Foreign Relations, 2010.
38. Bloom BR. WHO needs change. Nature 2011;473:143–45.
39. Ottersen OP, Frenk J, Horton R. The Lancet–University of Oslo Commission on Global Governance for Health, in collaboration with the Harvard Global Health Institute. Lancet 2011;378:1612–13.
40. Jamison DT, Frenk J, Knaul F. International collective action in health: objectives, functions and rationale. Lancet 1998;351:514–17.
41. Kickbusch I, Gleicher D. Governance for health in the 21st century: a study conducted for the WHO Regional Office for Europe. Copenhagen: World Health Organization Regional Office for Europe, 2011.
42. Commission on Social Determinants of Health. Closing the gap in a generation: health equity through action on the social determinants of health: final report of the Commission on Social Determinants of Health. Geneva: World Health Organization, 2008.
43. WHO Consultative Expert Working Group on Research and Development (CEWG). Research and development to meet health needs in developing countries: strengthening global financing and coordination. Geneva: World Health Organization, 2012.
44. Stiglitz J. Knowledge as a global public good. In: Kaul I, Grunberg I, Stern MA, eds. Global public goods: international cooperation in the 21st century. Oxford, United Kingdom: Oxford University Press, 1999:308–25.
45. Barrett S. Why cooperate? The incentive to supply global public goods. Oxford, United Kingdom: Oxford University Press, 2007.
46. Moon S, Bermudez J, 't Hoen E. Innovation and access to medicines for neglected populations: could a treaty address a broken pharmaceutical R&D system? PLoS Med 2012;9(5):e1001218.
47. Durkheim E. The division of labor in society. Glencoe, IL: Free Press, 1964.
48. Murray CJ, Frenk J. A framework for assessing the performance of health systems. Bull World Health Organ 2000;78:717–31.
49. Leach-Kemon K, Chou DP, Schneider MP, et al. The global financial crisis has led to a slowdown in growth of funding to improve health in many developing countries. Health Aff (Millwood) 2012;31:228–35.
50. Moon S. Embedding neoliberalism: global health and the evolution of the global intellectual property regime (1994–2009). (Ph.D. dissertation. Cambridge, MA: Harvard University, 2010.)

Global Health and the Law

Lawrence O. Gostin and Devi Sridhar

The past two decades have brought revolutionary changes in global health, driven by popular concern over the acquired immunodeficiency syndrome (AIDS), new strains of influenza, and maternal mortality.[1] International development assistance for health—a crucial aspect of health cooperation—increased by a factor of five, from $5.6 billion in 1990 to $28.1 billion in 2012, with the private and voluntary sectors taking on an ever-increasing share of the total.[2] Given the rapid globalization that is a defining feature of today's world, the need for a robust system of global health law has never been greater.

Global health law is not an organized legal system, with a unified treaty-monitoring body, such as the World Trade Organization. However, there is a network of treaties and so-called "soft" law instruments that powerfully affect global health, many of which have arisen under the auspices of the World Health Organization (WHO). Global health law has been defined as the legal norms, processes, and institutions that are designed primarily to attain the highest possible standard of physical and mental health for the world's population.[3]

Global health law can affect multiple spheres, ranging from national security, economic prosperity, and sustainable development to human rights and social justice. Each global health problem is shaped by the language of rights, duties, and rules for engagement used in the law (see Box 19.1).

Understanding the Law and Global Health

Safeguarding the population's health traditionally occurs at the national level, with a web of laws and regulations governing health services, injury and disease prevention, and health promotion.[4] However, in a globalized world in which pathogens and lifestyle risks span borders, the need for collective action has intensified interest in international legal solutions.[5]

The law relating to global health rests primarily within the domain of public international law, which can be broadly characterized as the rules that govern

BOX 19.1 **Glossary: Terminology in Global Health Law**

International Law

Treaty: A binding agreement between countries that is intended to create legal rights and duties. Treaties can often have substantial effects on private parties, such as corporations (e.g., trade law) and individuals (e.g., human rights).

Customary international law: Legal norms established by consistent practice among countries.

WHO Treaty-Making Powers

Convention: An international agreement under Article 19 of the WHO Constitution, which empowers the World Health Assembly to "adopt conventions or agreements" by a two-thirds vote on "any matter within the competence of the Organization." The Framework Convention on Tobacco Control (adopted in 2003) is the Assembly's only convention.

Regulation: An international rule under Article 21, which empowers the World Health Assembly to adopt regulations on a range of health topics. The two Assembly regulations are the Nomenclature with Respect to Diseases and Causes of Death (adopted in 1948) and the International Health Regulations (revised in 2005).

WHO "Soft" Law

"Soft" law: An instrument that creates health norms without the binding nature of international law. Article 23 empowers the WHO to issue formal recommendations, but the organization has developed norms through a range of soft instruments, such as global strategies, action plans, and guidelines.

Recommendations: Norms under Article 23, which empowers the World Health Assembly "to make recommendations to members." Two Assembly recommendations are the International Code of Marketing of Breast-Milk Substitutes (adopted in 1981) and the Global Code of Practice on the International Recruitment of Health Personnel (adopted in 2010).

Global strategies: Proposals that offer a strategic vision of how to tackle health challenges, listing specific objectives and guidance to stakeholders—for example, the WHO Global Health Sector Strategy for HIV/AIDS, 2011–2015. Global strategies often stress the comparative advantages of the WHO, such as its ability to leverage its strengths through partnerships and coordination.

Global action plans: Proposals that outline specific steps or activities for a strategy to succeed—for example, the Global Action Plan for the Prevention and Control of Noncommunicable Diseases, 2013–2020. Global plans often specify detailed tasks, time horizons, and resources.

Guidelines: Policies or methods of professional practice that are approved by the Guidelines Review Committee and designed to promote evidence-based health policies or clinical interventions—for example, guidelines on patient safety.

International Human Rights Law

International Covenant on Civil and Political Rights: An agreement that requires governments to safeguard civil and political rights, including the freedom of expression and religion, freedom from slavery and torture, and rights to privacy.

International Covenant on Economic, Social, and Cultural Rights: An agreement that guarantees "the right of everyone to the enjoyment of the highest attainable standard of physical and mental health," as well as capturing social determinants: "an adequate standard of living...including adequate food, clothing and housing, and to the continuous improvement of living conditions."

General Comment 14: The interpretation of the Committee on Economic, Social, and Cultural Rights of the right to health, including health goods, services, and facilities that should be available, accessible, acceptable, and of good quality.

the conduct and relations of countries, including their rights and obligations. Countries remain the major subjects of international law, but international organizations and (through human rights law) individuals are also considered to be subjects of international law.

There is a complex array of international norms, including those that are binding, or "hard" (e.g., treaties), and those that are nonbinding, or "soft" (e.g., codes of practice). Hard and soft legal instruments have many similarities and often take similar forms, since both forms of instruments are negotiated and adopted by countries, are administered by international organizations, and have similar compliance mechanisms, such as setting targets, monitoring progress, and reporting to governmental agencies. Soft instruments can influence domestic law and policy and are often viewed as part of the corpus of international law (Fig. 19.1; and the interactive timeline, available at NEJM.org).[6]

In recent years, the international community has moved toward a new language of global governance.[7] Neither global health law nor governance is well defined, but the central feature of global health law is the negotiation, adoption, and monitoring of normative rules among countries. Both law and broader governance require institutions to do much of the work, including creating norms, mobilizing resources, guiding multiple stakeholders to work collaboratively, and ensuring accountability for results. The WHO is the most important institution for negotiating international health agreements.[8]

WHO as a Normative Agency

The WHO has constitutional authority to negotiate and monitor normative instruments—both treaties and soft instruments, such as recommendations. The constitution of the WHO enunciates the universal value of the right to health—a widely adopted international legal entitlement.[9,10]

The WHO uses a variety of policy tools to set soft norms, with varying levels of institutional support. A World Health Assembly resolution expresses the will of 194 member countries. The agency has constitutional authority to adopt formal recommendations; the two most prominent are the International Code of Marketing of Breast-Milk Substitutes (adopted in 1981)[11] and the Global Code of Practice on the International Recruitment of Health Personnel (adopted in 2010).[12] The Assembly has also adopted influential global strategies and action plans.

The treaty-making powers of the WHO are extraordinary, with separate processes for negotiating agreements, or conventions, and regulations. Member countries must accept or reject a convention within 18 months after its adoption by the Assembly.[10] This is a powerful mechanism requiring countries to consider the treaty in accordance with national constitutional processes. The WHO, however, lacks the authority to enforce compliance and thus relies on governmental implementation through domestic law and policy.

The WHO can negotiate regulations on a range of health topics, including sanitation and quarantine, nomenclatures of diseases, and standards for the

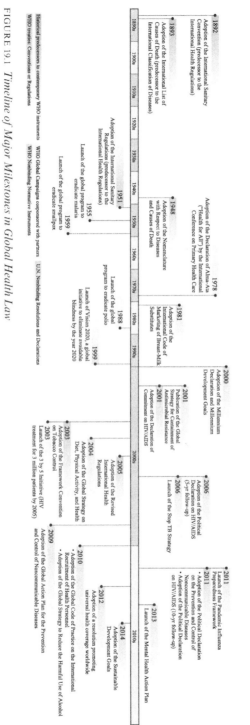

FIGURE 19.1 *Timeline of Major Milestones in Global Health Law*

safety, purity, and potency of pharmaceuticals. Regulations enter into force after adoption by the Assembly, except for members that notify the director-general within a specified time.[10] Consequently, countries must proactively opt out or they are automatically bound. The first WHO regulations—on nomenclature for diseases—date back to the late 19th century as the International List of Causes of Death; these regulations are now implemented through the International Classification of Diseases.[13] The second WHO regulations date back to 1892, when European countries adopted the International Sanitary Convention, a predecessor to the International Sanitary Regulations (now called the International Health Regulations).[3]

The constitution of the WHO creates ongoing governmental obligations to report annually on actions taken on recommendations, conventions, and regulations.[10] Despite the normative powers of the WHO, modern international health law is remarkably thin, with only two major treaties adopted since the creation of the agency.

FRAMEWORK CONVENTION ON TOBACCO CONTROL

The WHO did not negotiate a convention until the Framework Convention on Tobacco Control (FCTC), which was adopted in 2003.[14] The FCTC, which remains the only convention adopted by the World Health Assembly, was ratified by 177 countries that are home to 88% of the world's population, although the convention was not ratified by 2 countries, the United States and Indonesia, which have the third and fourth largest populations, respectively, worldwide.[15] In 2012, the Secretariat of the FCTC estimated that nearly 80% of the 159 countries that submitted reports had strengthened national tobacco-control laws after ratification.[16] However, overall progress masks unequal performance—for example, China showed "an alarming lack of progress," whereas India's implementation was "slow."[16]

The FCTC created binding norms to reduce the demand for, and supply of, tobacco products and to share information and resources. Efforts to reduce demand include taxing and pricing guided by health objectives, the provision of 100% smoke-free environments, disclosures of contents and emissions of tobacco products, large warning labels on packaging of tobacco products, comprehensive marketing bans, and tobacco cessation and treatment programs. Reducing the supply of tobacco focuses on illicit trade (e.g., smuggling and counterfeiting), which was estimated to account for 11.6% of global cigarette consumption in 2009, resulting in lost tax revenues of $30 to $50 billion per year.[17]

Despite the success of the FCTC in mobilizing governmental action and civil-society engagement, the treaty has major weaknesses. First, it contains ambiguous language, affording countries broad discretion in implementation. Second, it does not provide resources to give low- and middle-income countries sufficient capacity to implement and enforce policies outlined in the convention. In addition, the tobacco industry has fought back against the FCTC, bringing cases under the World Trade Organization and investment treaties against

Australia and Uruguay for their use of plain packaging of tobacco products and adoption of tobacco-control legislation—a classic conflict between health and commerce regimes.[18,19]

INTERNATIONAL HEALTH REGULATIONS

The World Health Assembly adopted a substantially revised version of the International Health Regulations in 2005 in the aftermath of the severe acute respiratory syndrome (SARS) outbreak, establishing a framework for global health security.[20] The aim of the regulations is to enhance the monitoring and reporting of international health threats and to improve the coordination of the response while avoiding unnecessary interference with traffic and trade.[21] The regulations govern surveillance and containment of disease within countries, at borders, and in international travel.[22]

The regulations encompass a broad spectrum of health hazards of international concern, regardless of their origin or source—biologic, chemical, or radionuclear. Using a decision instrument as a guide, governments must monitor health hazards and notify the WHO within 24 hours after events that may constitute a public health emergency of international concern. The director-general has the exclusive power to declare an emergency and has done so only once—during the 2009 influenza A (H1N1) pandemic. The regulations permit the WHO to take into account unofficial sources, such as nongovernmental organizations, scientists, and social networks in print and electronic media. Countries also agreed to develop core capacities—including legislation, national focal points, and pandemic planning—to implement the regulations.

PANDEMIC INFLUENZA PREPAREDNESS (PIP) FRAMEWORK

Although not a treaty, the WHO PIP Framework is an innovative hybrid—a soft law instrument that nonetheless can create binding obligations. Adopted in May 2011, the PIP Framework resolved the nearly 5-year controversy that erupted when Indonesia refused to share samples of influenza A (H5N1) virus with WHO collaborating centers. Claiming sovereignty over a virus that was identified in their territory, Indonesian officials expressed concern that their country would not receive a fair share of the benefits of scientific discoveries.[23,24]

The PIP Framework facilitates sharing of influenza viruses that have human pandemic potential and increases access to vaccines and antiviral medications in developing countries. The agreement incorporates "standard material transfer agreements" between the WHO and biotechnology companies or universities. When such agreements are signed, they create contractual duties to provide certain benefits in exchange for access to biologic materials. Recipients of such materials make monetary and in-kind commitments, including commitments to donate vaccines to WHO stockpiles, offer products at affordable prices, and make intellectual-property rights available. Sharing the benefits of scientific progress

is a vital aspect of global security and justice. However, the intellectual-property controversy associated with the novel corona-virus that causes the Middle East respiratory syndrome (MERS) reminds the international community that the PIP Framework applies only to pandemic influenza, with no WHO-negotiated agreement covering other emerging diseases.[25]

International Human Rights Law

The constitution of the WHO proclaims, "The enjoyment of the highest attainable standard of health is one of the fundamental rights of every human being."[10] Reflecting the same sentiment, the International Covenant on Economic, Social, and Cultural Rights, which complements the International Covenant on Civil and Political Rights and which 161 countries have accepted as binding international law, guarantees "the right of everyone to the enjoyment of the highest attainable standard of physical and mental health." It also spells out governmental obligations to reduce infant mortality, promote the development of healthy children, improve environmental and industrial hygiene, prevent and treat diseases, and ensure the provision of medical services.[26] In a demonstration of the universal value of such provisions, all countries except South Sudan have joined at least one treaty recognizing the right to health.[27]

The right to health requires that governments meet "minimum core obligations," including the provision of health facilities, goods, and services, without discrimination and distributed equitably; nutritious and safe food; shelter, housing, sanitation, and safe and potable water; and essential medicines. Health goods, services, and facilities must be available in sufficient quantity, with public accessibility, ethnic and cultural acceptability, and good quality, as outlined in General Comment 14 of the U.N. Committee on Economic, Social, and Cultural Rights.[28]

Whether human rights law influences governmental practices is disputed.[29] However, health rights are incorporated into statutes and constitutions in many countries and have formed the basis for landmark judicial rulings.[3] The real-world effect of human rights law depends on an active civil society, which can highlight governmental violations, lobby parliaments, and litigate health rights.[30] The most successful national litigation has involved access to essential medicines. For example, in 2002, the Constitutional Court in South Africa struck down government limits on access to nevirapine for pregnant women with human immunodeficiency virus (HIV) infection. As a result of this ruling, the government had to begin to realize the rights of mothers and infants to HIV prevention.[31]

Judicial decisions are increasing access to underlying determinants of health, such as food, water, and housing. In 2001, the Indian Supreme Court held that nutrition programs were legal entitlements and required that cooked meals be provided for primary school children. In later orders, the court set timetables for action on subsidized grain, maternal and child health, and food for the homeless and rural poor.[3] Table 19.1 shows country-level court cases that illustrate the effect of human rights law on health policy.

TABLE 19.1 Human Rights Court Cases Showing the Influence of International Law on Domestic Health Policy

Case	Year	Country	Basis for Decision	Court Decision
Cruz del Valle Bermúdez v. Ministerio de Sanidad y Asistencia Social	1999	Venezuela	Freedom from discrimination; rights to health, security, life, and the benefits of scientific progress	Requires government to cover treatment expenses for persons living with HIV and to develop information campaigns
People's Union for Civil Liberties v. Union of India	2001	India	Rights to health, food, and life	Requires free and universal nutrition programs (midday meal), setting standards and timetables for action
Minister of Health v. Treatment Action Campaign	2002	South Africa	Right to health	Strikes down government limits on access to nevirapine for pregnant women
A.V. et al. v. Estado Nacional	2004	Argentina	Rights to bodily integrity, health, and life	Mandates universal, free treatment for persons living with HIV
Roa Lopez v. Colombia	2006	Colombia	Rights to life and health	Finds unconstitutional a prohibition on abortions to protect the life or health of the mother or in cases of rape, even when the fetus is not viable
Judgment T-760/08	2008	Colombia	Right to health	Requires the government to unify two insurance plans with fewer benefits for indigent persons into a single plan with equal benefits for all
Lindiwe Mazibuko v. City of Johannesburg	2009	South Africa	Rights to water and sanitation	Finds no immediate duty to provide a specific amount of water but only reasonable measures within the country's resources
Caceres Corrales v. Colombia	2010	Colombia	Rights to life and heath	Upholds a complete ban on tobacco advertising and sponsorship
Canada (Attorney General) v. PHS Community Services Society	2011	Canada	Right to liberty and security of person, right to life	Finds unconstitutional the failure to exempt drug users and staff at a supervised safe-injection site from bans on possession of and trafficking in illicit drugs
Matsipane Mosetlhanyane et al. v. The Attorney General	2011	Botswana	Freedom from torture and cruel, inhuman, or degrading treatment; right to water and sanitation	Protects water rights of an indigenous community living in the Kalahari desert

TABLE 19.1 Human

Case	Year	Country	Basis for Decision	Court Decision
5000 Citizens v. Article 3 of Law No. 28705	2011	Peru	Right to health	Upholds a ban on smoking in all public places
British American Tobacco South Africa v. Minister of Health	2012	South Africa	Freedom of expression; rights to information, a clean environment, and health	Upholds the constitutionality of restrictions on tobacco advertising and marketing
Novartis AG v. Union of India	2013	India	Rights to health and life	Invalidates the patent for Gleevec because it was not materially better than the existing drug

Challenges in Global Health Law

Despite the potential of soft and hard instruments to set norms and mobilize multiple actors, global health laws have major limitations (Table 19.2). First, governments are loath to constrain themselves and, therefore, often reject international law or agree only to weak norms. Second, high-income countries are reluctant to finance capacity building in lower-income countries or to provide funding to the WHO without specific earmarks. And third, compliance mechanisms for such laws are often weak or nonexistent.

Because international law primarily addresses the rights and duties of countries, it cannot easily govern nonstate actors, which range from individuals and civil-society groups to foundations and private enterprises. Although newer global health institutions (e.g., UNAIDS, Global Fund, and GAVI Alliance) include civil-society representatives on their governing boards, the WHO has resisted nonstate participation in its governing structures.[32]

The harmonization of governmental interests, moreover, can be difficult because of the disparate perspectives.[33] Although high-income countries often favor trade liberalization, low- and middle-income countries seek greater access to drugs and the fruits of technological progress. In 2001, World Trade Organization members adopted the Doha Declaration on TRIPS (the Agreement on Trade-Related Aspects of Intellectual Property Rights) and Public Health, which allowed countries to issue a compulsory license during a public health emergency, granting to itself or a third party the right to produce or import a patented drug without authorization from the patent holder.[34] So-called "TRIPS flexibilities" were designed to ensure that intellectual property should not prevent countries from providing affordable access to essential medications in a public health emergency.

Increasingly, the reconciliation of these interests occurs at the national level. For example, in 2013, the Supreme Court of India held that Novartis did not have a valid patent in India on the lucrative cancer drug Gleevec.[35] The court ruled that Indian law grants patents only to new compounds and that modified drugs

TABLE 19.2 Limitations of Global Health Law.

Challenge	Description	Example
National sovereignty	Countries are reluctant to forgo self-governance or cede authority to international actors.	The Global Code of Practice on the International Recruitment of Health Personnel is voluntary, despite active recruitment from high-income countries.
Rise of nongovernmental actors	Businesses, foundations, and civil-society groups have major effects on health but are hard to govern at the international level.	The Global Strategy on Diet, Physical Activity, and Health does not govern marketing of food.
Divergent interests of emerging economies and high-income countries	High-income countries defend trade liberalization (e.g., intellectual property), whereas low- and middle-income countries focus on health justice (e.g., access to medicines and fair allocation of scientific benefits).	The Pandemic Influenza Preparedness Framework struggled to reconcile Indonesia's claim for fair sharing of benefits with the desire of high-income countries to receive viral samples.
Funding earmarked by private donors for specific sectors, diseases, or regions through multilateral agencies ("multi-bi" financing)	Countries route assistance through the WHO and other multilateral agencies but hold tight control over its use, limiting WHO control of its resources and ability to set priorities and diminishing the perceived independence of the WHO.	Approximately 80% of the WHO's funding is voluntary, with targets that are incongruent with the priorities of the World Health Assembly and the major causes of disability and death.
Funding for capacity building	Global health law rarely requires high-income countries to build capacities in lower-income countries to fulfill international obligations.	A committee on functioning of the International Health Regulations (2011) found that many countries lacked capacity and could not fulfill their obligations.
Compliance and incentives	WHO norms (whether soft or hard) rarely contain effective methods for holding countries and stakeholders accountable.	The Global Strategy to Reduce Harmful Use of Alcohol does not require governmental action or prevent industry from lobbying against alcohol control.
Adjudication and enforcement of norms	The WHO lacks power to adjudicate most disputes and enforce norms.	The tobacco industry uses the World Trade Organi-zation and investment treaties to challenge plain packaging of tobacco products and the initiation of tobacco-control campaigns.

must improve treatment for patients. The decision could embolden other emerging economies to reject similar intellectual-property claims. At the same time, developed countries are seeking stricter intellectual-property protection in trade agreements, such as the Trans-Pacific Partnership, which seeks to promote trade and investment among the partner countries.[36]

Trust in international organizations to act impartially and demonstrate leadership is crucial to the future of global health law. As new health security challenges arise, the integrity and efficient functioning of the WHO becomes ever more important. The WHO, however, is struggling with a small group of donors that contribute approximately 80% of its total budget.[37] The term for this type of financing is "multi-bi" aid—donors' earmarking of noncore funding for specific sectors, diseases, or regions through multilateral agencies.[38] Since the leadership of the WHO is unable to control most of its budget, these aid arrangements endanger the perceived independence and normative influence of the WHO.

Financing is intricately related to the challenge of building capacity to fulfill duties created by global health law. The 2011 review committee on the functioning of the International Health Regulations stressed that many countries lacked capacity and were not on a path to fulfill their obligations.[39] The same failure to mobilize resources has plagued WHO normative development in such areas as achieving ambitious goals set forth in action plans on noncommunicable diseases and mental health.[40–42]

Strategy for Global Health Laws

Given the undoubted need for global cooperation, international norms are accepted as important global health tools. The more difficult question is whether to pursue hard or soft routes to address health challenges. This debate plays out in international forums ranging from alcohol control and biomedical research to broader reforms such as the Framework Convention on Global Health.[30,43–45] However, there are strengths and weaknesses to both approaches.

Soft agreements are easier to negotiate, with countries more likely to accede to far-reaching norms if there is no formal obligation to comply. Countries can assent to a soft norm without the national constitutional processes entailed in ratifying a treaty. In addition, soft norms can be negotiated more quickly with the use of fewer resources. Resolutions of the WHO Health Assembly represent a major expression of political will and can lead to progressive deepening of norms—enacted into domestic law, referenced by treaty bodies, or incorporated into international law. The WHO, moreover, is building accountability mechanisms into soft agreements, with targets, monitoring, and timelines for compliance.

However, national governments can largely ignore soft instruments, and as a result, civil society often urges treaty development.[30] No hard norms have been enacted, for example, relating to food, alcohol, physical activity, injuries, pain medication, or mental health. If the WHO acts principally through voluntary agreements, while other sectors develop hard law, this weakens and sidelines the agency. Civil society often points to the obligatory nature of international trade law and its binding dispute-settlement mechanism, which often trumps WHO norms.[46]

Even with all the funding and celebrity power that has entered the global health space, key health indicators lag, whereas the health gap between rich and poor has barely abated.[47,48] A renewed attention to lawmaking efforts by the WHO and

the human right to health are crucial elements of progress. It is only through law that individuals and populations can claim entitlements to health services and that corresponding governmental obligations can be established and enforced. It is through law that norms can be set, fragmented activities coordinated, and good governance ensured, including stewardship, transparency, participation, and accountability. Global health law, despite its limitations, remains vital to achieving global health with justice.

References

1. Brandt AM. How AIDS invented global health. N Engl J Med 2013;368:2149–52.
2. Institute for Health Metrics and Evaluation. Financing global health: the end of the golden age. Seattle: Institute for Health Metrics and Evaluation, 2012.
3. Gostin LO. Global health law. Cambridge: Harvard University Press, 2014.
4. *Idem*. Public health law: power, duty, restraint. 2nd ed. Berkeley: University of California Press, 2008.
5. Cohen IG. The globalization of health care: legal and ethical issues. New York: Oxford University Press, 2013.
6. Abbot K, Snidal D. Hard and soft law in international governance. Int Organ 2000;54:421–56.
7. Frenk J, Moon S. Governance challenges in global health. N Engl J Med 2013;368:936–42.
8. Burci GL, Vignes C-H. World Health Organization. The Hague, the Netherlands: Kluwer Law International, 2004.
9. Friedman EA, Gostin LO. Pillars for progress on the right to health: harnessing the potential of human rights through a Framework Convention on Global Health. Health Hum Rights 2012;14(1):E4–19.
10. World Health Organization. WHO Constitution. Geneva: World Health Organization (http://www.who.int/governance/eb/constitution/en).
11. World Health Organization. International code of marketing of breast-milk substitutes. Geneva: World Health Organization, 1981 (http://www.who.int/nutrition/publications/infantfeeding/9241541601/en).
12. World Health Organization. WHO global code of practice on the international recruitment of health personnel. Geneva: World Health Organization, 2010 (http://www.who.int/hrh/migration/code/full_text/en).
13. World Health Organization. International statistical classification of diseases. Vol. 2. 10th rev. Geneva: World Health Organization, 2010 (http://www.who.int/classifications/icd/ICD10Volume2_en_2010.pdf).
14. Roemer R, Taylor A, Lariviere J. Origins of the WHO framework convention on tobacco control. Am J Public Health 2005;95:936–38.
15. World Health Organization. Parties to the WHO Framework Convention on Tobacco Control. Geneva: World Health Organization (http://www.who.int/fctc/signatories_parties/en).

16. World Health Organization. Global progress report on implementation of the WHO Framework Convention on Tobacco Control. Geneva: World Health Organization, 2012 (http://www.who.int/fctc/reporting/2012_global_progress_report_en.pdf).

17. Joossens L, Merriman D, Ross H, Raw M. The impact of eliminating the global illicit cigarette trade on health and revenue. Addiction 2010;105:1640–49.

18. McGrady B. Implications of ongoing trade and investment disputes concerning tobacco: Philip Morris v. Uruguay 2012. In: Voon T, Mitchell A, Liberman J, Ayres G, eds. Public health and plain packaging of cigarettes: legal issues. Northampton, MA: Edward Elgar, 2012 (http://papers.ssrn.com/sol3/papers.cfm?abstract_id=2046261).

19. Voon T, Mitchell A. Time to quit? Assessing international investment claims against plain tobacco packaging in Australia. J Int Econ Law 2012;14:515–52.

20. Fidler DP. SARS, governance and the globalization of disease. Houndmills, United Kingdom: Palgrave Macmillan, 2004.

21. World Health Organization. International Health Regulations: Article 2. Geneva: World Health Organization (http://www.who.int/ihr/publications/9789241596664/en/index.html).

22. Fidler DP. From international sanitary conventions to global health security: the new international health regulations. Chin J Int Law 2005;4:325–92.

23. Fidler DP, Gostin LO. The WHO pandemic influenza preparedness framework: a milestone in global governance for health. JAMA 2011;306:200–201.

24. Kamradt-Scott A, Lee K. The 2011 pandemic influenza preparedness framework: global health secured or a missed opportunity? Polit Stud 2011;59:831–47.

25. Fidler DP. Who owns MERS? The intellectual property controversy surrounding the latest pandemic. Foreign Affairs. June 7, 2013 (http://www.foreignaffairs.com/articles/139443/david-p-fidler/who-owns-mers).

26. World Health Organization. International covenant on economic, social and cultural rights. Geneva: World Health Organization (http://www.who.int/hhr/Economic_social_cultural.pdf).

27. Zuniga J, Marks SP, Gostin LO. Advancing the human right to health. Oxford, United Kingdom: Oxford University Press, 2013.

28. United Nations, Office of the High Commissioner for Human Rights. General comment 14L: the right to the highest attainable standard of health. Adopted at the 22nd Session of the Committee on Economic, Social, and Cultural Rights, Geneva, August 11, 2000.

29. Singh JA, Govender M, Mills EJ. Do human rights matter to health? Lancet 2007;370:521–27. [Erratum, Lancet 2007;370:1686.]

30. Gostin LO, Friedman EA, Buse K, et al. Towards a framework convention on global health. Bull World Health Organ 2013;91:790–93.

31. Minister of Health v. Treatment Action Campaign, 2002 (5) SA 721 (CC) (S. Afr.).

32. Silberschmidt G, Matheson D, Kickbusch I. Creating a committee C of the World Health Assembly. Lancet 2008;371:1483–86.

33. Feldbaum H, Michaud J. Health diplomacy and the enduring relevance of foreign policy interests. PLoS Med 2010;7(4):e1000226.

34. World Trade Organization. Doha WTO Ministerial 2001: TRIPS, WT/MIN(01)/ DEC/2, 20 November 2001: Declaration on the TRIPS agreement and public health, adopted 14 November 2001 (http://www.wto.org/english/thewto_e/minist_e/ min01_e/mindecl_trips_e.htm).

35. Kapczynski A. Engineered in India—patent law 2.0. N Engl J Med 2013;369:497–99.

36. Bollyky T. Regulatory coherence in the TPP talks. In: Lim CL, Elms D, Low P, eds. Trans-Pacific Partnership: a quest for a twenty-first century agreement. New York: Cambridge University Press, 2012.

37. Sridhar D, Gostin LO. Reforming the World Health Organization. JAMA 2011;305:1585–86.

38. Sridhar D. Who sets the global health research agenda? The challenge of multi-bi financing. PLoS Med 2012;9(9):e1001312.

39. World Health Organization. Implementation of the International Health Regulations (2005): report of the Review Committee on the Functioning of the International Health Regulations (2005) in relation to pandemic (H1N1) 2009. Geneva: World Health Organization, 2011 (http://apps.who.int/gb/ebwha/pdf_files/ WHA64/A64_10-en.pdf).

40. Magnusson RS. Non-communicable diseases and global health governance: enhancing global processes to improve health development. Global Health 2007;3:2.

41. Morain S, Mello MM. Survey finds public support for legal interventions directed at health behavior to fight noncommunicable disease. Health Aff (Millwood) 2013;32:486–96.

42. Becker AE, Kleinman A. Mental health and the global agenda. N Engl J Med 2013;369:66–73.

43. Taylor AL, Dhillon IS. An international legal strategy for alcohol control: not a framework convention—at least not yet. Addiction 2013;108:450–55.

44. Sridhar D. Health policy: regulate alcohol for global health. Nature 2012;482:302.

45. Røttingen JA, Chamas C. A new deal for global health R&D? The recommendations of the Consultative Expert Working Group on Research and Development (CEWG). PLoS Med 2012;9(5):e1001219.

46. Friedman EF, Gostin LO, Buse K. Advancing the right to health through global organizations: the potential role of a Framework Convention on Global Health. Health Hum Rights 2013;15:71–86.

47. Garay J. Global health (GH)=GH equity=GH justice=global social justice: the opportunities of joining EU and US forces together. Berkeley: University of California, European Union of Excellence, 2012 (http://eucenter.berkeley.edu).

48. Garrett L. Money or die: a watershed moment for global public health. Foreign Affairs. March 6, 2012 (http://www.foreignaffairs.com/articles/137312/laurie-garrett/ money-or-die).

Global Supply of Health Professionals
Nigel Crisp and Lincoln Chen

There is a global crisis of severe shortages and marked maldistribution of health professionals that is exacerbated by three great global transitions—demographic changes, epidemiologic shifts, and redistribution of the disability burden. Each of these transitions exerts a powerful force for change in health care systems, the roles of health professionals, and the design of health professional education.[1-5] Every country will have to respond to these global pressures for change.

There are many other reasons that it is important to think globally about the education and role of health professionals.[6] The knowledge base of the profession is global in scope, and there is increasing cross-national transfer of technology, expertise, and services. Health professionals are migrating in what is now effectively a global market for their talent, while patients are also traveling for treatment. One quarter of the doctors in the United States come from abroad, and the "medical tourism" market for travel to such countries as Thailand and Singapore is growing at a rate of 20% annually.[7,8] All people worldwide are threatened by risks such as global infectious epidemics and climate change. Health professionals globally are interlinked and interdependent, facing shared challenges.

Global diversity characterizes the way health professionals are defined, educated, and deployed.[5] The U.S. pattern of 4 years of college followed by 4 years of medical school is unusual. The United Kingdom requires 5 or 6 years of post–high-school education, and China is moving to consolidate its education of doctors to two levels of 5 or 8 years after high school. Nursing education is more varied, ranging from vocational high-school training to doctoral programs.

There are also large differences among countries and regions in numbers of health workers and their skill mix. Table 20.1 shows that there are 9.2 million doctors and 18.1 million nurses worldwide.[9] The United States, with 4% of the world's population, has 8% of the doctors and 17% of the nurses. Among world regions, the density of health workers can vary by a factor of 10, and there is great variability in the skill mix. The United States has a nurse-to-doctor ratio of 4, whereas the ratios in China and India are close to 1.

TABLE 20.1 Workforce of Doctors and Nurses According to Country or Region in 2010*

Country or Region	Population	Doctors	Nurses	Doctors and Nurses/1000 Population	Nurse-to-Doctor Ratio
	in millions	in thousands			
Country					
China	1338	1915	1,864	2.8	0.97
India	1225	768	1,179	1.6	1.54
United States	309	756	3,064	12.3	4.05
Brazil	195	338	1,278	8.3	3.78
United Kingdom	62	166	626	12.7	3.77
South Africa	50	37	198	4.7	5.30
Region					
Americas	937	1974	4,947	7.4	2.5
Europe	899	2744	5,870	9.6	2.1
Middle East and North Africa	590	654	894	2.6	1.4
Southeast Asia	1795	997	1,810	1.6	1.8
Sub-Saharan Africa	847	150	778	1.1	5.2
Western Pacific	1821	2696	3,814	3.6	1.4
World	6888	9216	18,114	4.0	2.0

*A doctor or nurse is defined as a person with the appropriate qualifications recognized in his or her own country. In this table, the nurse workforce includes nurses and midwives. Data are from the World Health Organization.[9]

The World Health Organization has underscored the alarming global shortage of approximately 4.3 million doctors and nurses, which constitutes a shortfall of 15% of the total number of doctors and nurses worldwide. It is estimated that 57 poor countries are facing a severe crisis in that they have insufficient human resources to meet minimum needs.[3] The shortage is worsened by a global imbalance between the availability of health workers and the burden of disease. Figure 20.1 shows countries according to the density of doctors, nurses, and midwives. Figure 20.2 shows that sub-Saharan Africa, with the lowest density of doctors and nurses, has the highest disease burden.

These problems are made worse by migration. The 2010 WHO Global Code of Practice on the International Recruitment of Health Personnel highlighted these issues, aiming to bring awareness to richer countries of the importance of reducing recruitment from poorer nations that have health worker shortages.[11] However, wider measures, including increased investment, improved training, and better human-resources management, are needed to address the shortfalls in both rich and poor countries.[12]

International imbalances are mirrored by inequitable distribution within nearly all countries. Remote rural and poor populations are often not able to attract or retain health professionals. There is evidence that an increased number of professionals can be retained in rural areas through improved policies in

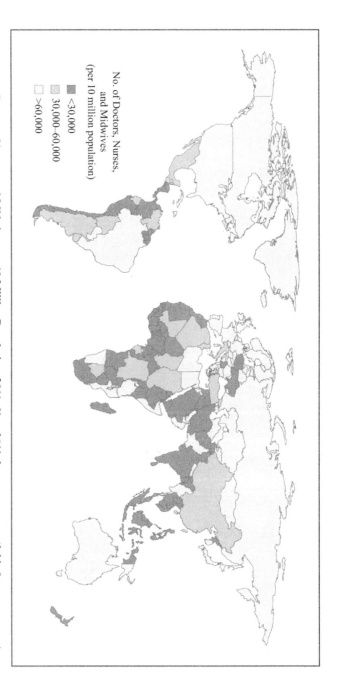

No. of Doctors, Nurses,
and Midwives
(per 10 million population)

▨ <30,000
▨ 30,000–60,000
☐ >60,000

FIGURE 20.1 **Doctors, Nurses, and Midwives per 10 Million Population, 2011** *Year 2011 data were not available for some countries; in those cases, the most recent available data are shown. Data are from the World Health Organization (WHO) Global Health Workforce Statistics.*[9]

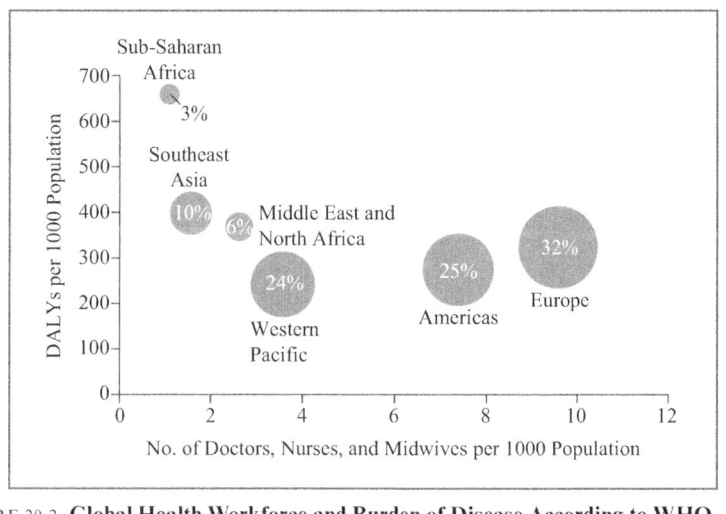

FIGURE 20.2 **Global Health Workforce and Burden of Disease According to WHO
Region** *The sizes of circles reflect the percentage share of the total global health workforce
of doctors and nurses. Health workforce data are from WHO Global Health Workforce
Statistics,[9] and data on the burden of disease, expressed as disability-adjusted life-years
(DALYs) for all causes and both sexes, are from the Institute for Health Metrics and
Evaluation.[10]*

the education sector (medical and nursing school locations, admissions policies,
scholarships, and "bonding" [requiring a period of service in a rural area after
training is complete]) and health sector (hardship pay, schooling for children,
and professional career development).[13] Many countries either do not recognize
the need for these policies or are unable to implement them. Consequently, a
practical option in disadvantaged areas is to train community health workers,
nurse practitioners, or other health professionals without medical degrees who
perform many tasks typically performed by physicians in the United States. The
obverse of this rural neglect is excessive urban concentrations of health professionals, which can generate other problems, such as unnecessary, wasteful, and
costly medical procedures.[14]

Despite widespread assertions of the right to health, it is estimated that at
least 1 billion people do not have access to a trained health worker. Millions
of people operate as unpaid caretakers—mostly women whose contribution and
human rights are often ignored.

Forces Driving Global Change

There is growing demand and competition for health workers globally. The say-
ing, "no health without a workforce"[15] is increasingly recognized as a universal
truth. Although there is no consensus on the subject, some researchers in the

United States are projecting shortages of 85,000 doctors by 2020 and 260,000 nurses by 2025.[16,17] Countries with fast-growing economies, such as India, China, Brazil, and South Africa, want more trained health workers, and critical shortages remain in the world's poorest countries.

At least five forces are shaping global supply and demand. The first are the major transitions—demographic and epidemiologic changes and shifts in disability burden—that are sweeping across many countries. Demographically, populations are aging and becoming more urbanized and more mobile. Epidemiologically, noncommunicable diseases are displacing the earlier infectious, nutrition-related, and maternity-related causes of death.[4] The disability burden attributable to mental health disorders, musculoskeletal impairment, and chronic diseases is growing rapidly. There is an urgent need to redesign most health systems to meet these challenges.

Second, people today are better educated and more assertive and enjoy greater access to information.[18] Professionals are no longer the sole source of medical or health knowledge; consequently, their relationship with their patients is changing. The shift is toward shared medical decision making and health responsibility. Some have labeled this the "coproduction of health."[19] Evidence shows that patient engagement can lead to better use of resources and improved quality of health care.[20] Remarkable stories of patient-led care are emerging, such as the report of patients with renal disease in Jonköping, Sweden, who deliver their own dialysis treatment, coming and going from the unit as they choose, with the result that quality of care is improved and costs are reduced at the same time.[21]

Third, the revolution in biosciences and information-communications technologies will continue to generate many new diagnostics, vaccines, and drugs. Expansion of the toolkit is likely to usher in greater professional specialization. At the same time, new technologies can also open opportunities for deprofessionalization and decentralization. Many diagnostic and therapeutic regimens may not require professionals to be involved in real time, and mobile technologies could enable lay workers and even patients to function more effectively at a distance from the medical professional.

Finally, two contrasting policy forces will affect all aspects of the work of health professionals. Market forces are intrinsically part of the health care system, with health expenditures now amounting to 10.1% of the world's gross domestic product and the health care industry turning over more than $6.6 trillion annually.[9] Individuals and consumers are linked to health markets, and there is a premium on the capability and willingness of health professionals with business and management skills to work in markets, devise incentives, control processes, and deliver outcomes to consumers in managed systems.

There are also countervailing forces of social justice pushing for health equity as a basic human right. There is growing social demand for fairness in health, including universal health coverage.[22] The ethos that no one, however poor, should suffer unnecessarily from preventable pain or should die prematurely is gaining consensus worldwide. Such social forces will engage citizens

and communities to influence the wider social and environmental determinants of health.

Effect on Health Professionals

All these forces ensure that future demand for health professionals will not simply be more of the same. Each force will make demands for different types of workers with relevant competencies.

The demographic and epidemiologic transitions and the shifts in disability burden mean that health systems and health professionals will have to reach into homes and communities. Teamwork involving nonprofessionals and lay people will become even more important. Better communication with an increasingly educated and informed public will be essential, so that measures for promoting health and preventing disease can influence individual behavior and lifestyle, as well as shape macro policies such as the restriction of salt or trans-fat content in foods.

Therapeutic systems will have to manage new biotechnologies delivered in the context of changing doctor–patient relationships. Technology will enable monitoring and intervention at a distance. Although health professionals will have the enhanced support of information technology, new skills will be needed to validate, synthesize, and practically apply decisions that are derived from an overload of available information.

Finally, all professional work will be embedded in complex market and social environments, with all their ambiguities and tensions. The social justice rationale, for example, emphasizes the importance of understanding social issues, leading to new demand for public health workers who are able to manage collaboration across sectors.[23] Commercial goals, on the other hand, require business and managerial qualities and the ability and willingness to work in market-based systems.

Frontiers of Educational Reform

All these changes have come together in the ferment of new ideas and actions around the education of health workers. The Commission on the Education of Health Professionals for the 21st Century, of which both of us were members, has brought many of these ideas of shared competencies, systems thinking, and social purpose together in a framework of instructional and institutional changes.[5] The commission proposes that we move into a third generation of "system-based" education. The Flexner Report, written by Abraham Flexner in 1910, introduced a scientific basis into medical education in North America that had previously been absent and resulted in the closure of many medical schools. Building on Flexner's first generation of science-based curricular reform in universities and moving through the second generation of problem-based learning with the growth of academic centers, the commission proposes a third generation

of reforms that are competency-based in academic health systems (i.e., health systems that provide professional education in a variety of service settings). The emphasis on competencies moves beyond pedagogy to reexamining the skills required for a changing health care system. Synchronizing academic educational and health systems can improve horizontal integration of training from the undergraduate to the clinical-practical level and vertical integration from tertiary care to primary care teaching sites.

COMPETENCY-BASED SKILLS

Given all these impending changes, continuous reassessment of competencies relevant to local contexts should drive a learning process that preserves valuable old skills, discards outdated procedures, and adds new capabilities. Although there have been efforts at establishing a single universal competency, there cannot be only one standard for all health professionals in a world of 200 countries among which the burden of disease and the capacity of health systems vary enormously.[5] The average national income in the richest and the poorest countries differs by a factor of more than 300 (from $271 in Burundi to $98,081 in Norway), and expenditures in health care vary by a factor of more than 600 (from $14 in Eritrea to $8,608 in the United States).[9] Recognition of these differences does not imply that we should discard requirements for core competencies; there are those that can and should be required of health professionals, regardless of country. Although the emphasis on disease, technology, service systems, and financing will necessarily vary across countries and regions, all local competencies must draw on the common pool of global knowledge, and all professional learning must progress along the continuum from basic science education to the application of knowledge in academic health systems, which combine the educational and health systems.

CHANGING ROLES

New roles are already evolving among different cadres of health workers. The demarcation of the responsibility and authority of different professions is not fixed. New technologies and practices will enable some health workers—imaging technologists, nurse endoscopists, physician assistants, and the like—to take on work previously performed by those with higher qualifications. Much innovation in such roles is taking place in low-income and middle-income countries in which the scarcity of resources has prompted some remarkable innovations to flourish.[24] In Mozambique, *técnicos do cirurgia*—mainly nurses with extra training—perform nearly all cesarean sections, with outcomes that are as good as those observed when the procedure is performed by physicians, and at a much lower cost,[25] and Pakistan's "Lady Health Workers" have shown the ability to influence health promotion and treatment in villages.[26] Community health workers, such as those in Bangladesh, are contributing to better child survival in many countries.[27] Figure 20.3 shows the numbers of such paraprofessionals, community

health workers, and health workers trained in accordance with local standards in comparison with the numbers of doctors and nurses in various countries. In some low-income countries, the former can be more numerous than the latter. Some of the lessons about community health workers that have been learned from poorer countries are now being applied in richer countries (see, for example, the efforts to incorporate community health workers in the New York City health care system[34]).

TEAMWORK

Teamwork will be essential for the successful management of health care systems. A reasonable hypothesis is that insular training for individual professions does not sufficiently promote understanding, respect, and knowledge of allied professions in a health team. The current model of professional training—in which members of each health profession are trained in isolation from the others until

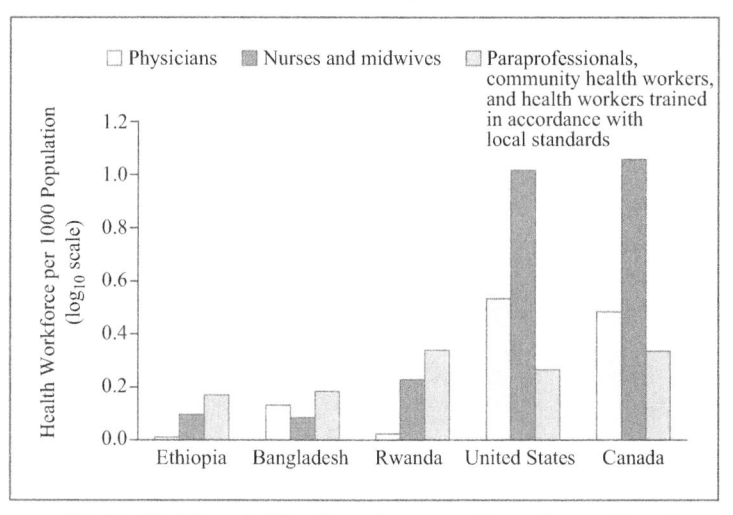

FIGURE 20.3 **Health Workforce in Five Countries, According to Type of Health Worker, 2011** *Year 2011 data were not available for some countries; in those cases, the most recent available data are shown. Data are from WHO Global Health Workforce Statistics,[9] with the following exceptions: the number of community health workers in Ethiopia, which includes numbers of Health Extension Program workers and their supervisors, is from Belatchew[28]; the number of community health workers in Bangladesh is from Standing et al.[29] and Reichenberg et al.[30]; the number of paraprofessionals in the United States, which includes nurse practitioners and physician assistants, is from the Henry J. Kaiser Family Foundation[31,32]; and the number of paraprofessionals in Canada, which includes midwives, nurse practitioners, and social workers, is from the Canadian Institute for Health Information.[33] Because the absolute number of workers per 1000 population in some cases was less than 1, which resulted in negative values when converted to a logarithmic scale, 1 was added to each value before conversion.*

they join the workplace, where they are expected to perform as teams—needs to be reexamined with the aim of inculcating cooperative and collaborative skills, through interprofessional and transprofessional education, as professionals are trained to be members of health teams.

INNOVATIONS IN LEARNING

We are at the leading edge of a wave of innovations in the education of health professionals. Recently, massive open online courses (MOOCs), provided by companies such as Coursera, MIT–Harvard edX, Udacity, and iTunes U, have captured much attention.[35] Information technology–based mass online courses can expand time for new approaches to teaching, such as the "flipped classroom," in which the sequence of lecture and homework is reversed. Online materials can be taken as homework before peer and mentored interactions, with an aim toward enhancing the learning process in classrooms. Some of the innovations are coming from outside the health field; for example, the Khan Academy, an online educational organization that began by teaching online middle-school and high-school math, has now partnered with the Stanford School of Medicine "to provide free health and medicine content to anyone, anywhere" (www.khanacademy.org/partner-content/stanford-medicine). Other innovations come from the health field, such as Peoples-uni and the Institute for Healthcare Improvement Open School, a student-led initiative that in 3 years has grown to include 628 chapters in 65 countries.[36,37] Hospital groups, such as North Shore–Long Island Jewish Health System in New York State, have set up new medical schools. A study of African medical schools has shown how much innovation is emerging.[38] The large number of new private medical schools in Brazil and India is an additional development—one that is driven by commercial purposes but that nevertheless meets the aspirations of many young people.[5]

Not all these educational reforms will proceed smoothly. There are great concerns about the quality of skills and service delivery systems around the world. These concerns are magnified by commercial incentives that prioritize profit rather than health goals. The explosive growth of private medical education (more than three quarters of new medical schools that were opened in the year 2000 were private rather than public) harkens back to the pre-Flexner era, during which many low-quality schools were eventually forced to close. Another concern is that changes in professional roles—referred to as "task shifting," "task sharing," or "skill-mix changes"—have frequently not succeeded in the past, sometimes compromising health care quality and safety. Moreover, there may be instances in which new knowledge dictates that tasks need to be shifted to specialists rather than to less-trained workers. There is, however, already evidence regarding the factors that make for success—such as whether roles are well defined and whether workers are well trained, have access to retraining, and can refer patients to more skilled colleagues.[39] Teamwork is a desirable process and outcome, but we have little evidence about the kinds of medical school curricula, role modeling, or extracurricular

activities that can nurture qualities that promote teamwork. The wave of new learning methods and new medical schools is too recent to allow us to draw conclusions about their effect.

Most important, the education of health professionals must reflect the different yet complementary roles that professionals play in the health care system. Beyond simply producing functionaries to serve a given health care system, education also produces researchers and scientists, leaders and change agents, and health policymakers and managers. That is why the commission argued for a third educational stage of "transformative learning." The first, informative stage provides information and may be expected to create an expert. The second, formative stage inculcates values and behavior for producing members of a profession. Transformative learning, the third stage, promotes the development of leaders and change agents who are able to engage in the transformation of health care systems. It may be hypothesized that the blended learning process introduced by MOOCs, involving flipped classrooms, peer interaction, individual mentoring, and interactive problem identification and problem solving, promises to help accelerate the transition of learning from informative and formative to transformative. While many professionals perform routinized work, others must also rise above functionality to serve as leaders in navigating the changes of the existing health system.

To do so, the professions will have to navigate the underlying tension between social and market forces. For example, there is a movement to instill the "social accountability" of medical education in schools. In the same vein, commercial schools must achieve acceptable levels of competency. The social mission is important to societies and governments seeking to improve the health of all people. However, health is also a financial business. The pressing health issues—access, quality, and costs—must all be tackled by health professionals with these wider perspectives in their hearts and minds.

Resistance to change may be expected. After all, millions earn their living from the status quo. That may be why policymakers in the past have found it easier to redesign services than to redesign roles. There are powerful forces demarcating responsibility, privilege, and authority.

Change, however, is already under way, and there is great energy and impetus for more. Educators of health professionals must grasp the opportunity to produce transformative leaders who have the motivation and capability to shape the future—or themselves be shaped by it.

We thank Catherine Michaud and Zhihui Li for their assistance with the research for and preparation of this article.

References

1. Joint Learning Initiative. Human resources for health: overcoming the crisis. Cambridge, MA: Harvard University Press, 2004.
2. Crisp N, Gawanas B. Scaling up, saving lives. Geneva: World Health Organization, 2008.

3. World health report 2006: working together for health. Geneva: World Health Organization, 2006.

4. Murray CJL, Vos T, Lozano R, et al. Disability-adjusted life years (DALYs) for 291 diseases and injuries in 21 regions, 1990-2010: a systematic analysis for the Global Burden of Disease Study 2010. Lancet 2012;380:2197–223.

5. Frenk J, Chen L, Bhutta ZA, et al. Health professionals for a new century: transforming education to strengthen health systems in an interdependent world. Lancet 2010;376:1923–58.

6. Crisp N. Global health capacity and workforce development: turning the world upside down. Infect Dis Clin North Am 2011;25:359–67.

7. Mullan F. The metrics of the physician brain drain. N Engl J Med 2005;353:1810–18.

8. Kanchanachitra C, Lindelow M, Johnston T, et al. Human resources for health in southeast Asia: shortages, distributional challenges, and international trade in health services. Lancet 2011;377:769–81.

9. World Health Organization. WHO global health workforce statistics (http://www.who.int/hrh/statistics/hwfstats).

10. Institute for Health Metrics and Evaluation. Search GBD data (http://www.healthmetricsandevaluation.org/search-gbd-data).

11. The WHO global code of practice on the international recruitment of health personnel (http://www.who.int/hrh/migration/code/code_en.pdf).

12. Chen LC, Boufford JI. Fatal flows—doctors on the move. N Engl J Med 2005;353:1850–52.

13. Chen LC. Striking the right balance: health workforce retention in remote and rural areas. Bull World Health Organ 2010;88:323.

14. Goodman DC, Fisher ES. Physician workforce crisis? Wrong diagnosis, wrong prescription. N Engl J Med 2008;358:1658–61.

15. World Health Organization. A universal truth: no health without a workforce: Third Global Forum on Human Resources for Health report. November 2013 (http://www.who.int/workforcealliance/knowledge/resources/hrhreport2013/en/).

16. AMA marks National Doctors' Day with an eye to the future. News release of the American Medical Association, Chicago, March 12, 2009.

17. Buerhaus PI, Auerbach DI, Staiger DO. The recent surge in nurse employment: causes and implications. Health Aff (Millwood) 2009;28:w657–68.

18. Horton R. The neglected epidemic of chronic disease. Lancet 2005;366:1514.

19. Hyde P, Davies HTO. Service design, culture and performance: collusion and co-production in health care. Hum Relat 2004;57:1407–426.

20. Bjorkman M, Svensson J. Power to the people: evidence from a randomized field experiment on community-based monitoring in Uganda. Q J Econ 2009;124:735–69.

21. Progress report 2012. Cambridge, MA: Institute for Healthcare Improvement, 2012.

22. Savedoff WD, de Ferranti D, Smith AL, Fan V. Political and economic aspects of the transition to universal health coverage. Lancet 2012;380:924–32.

23. Tulchinsky TH, McKee M. Education for a public health workforce in Europe and globally. Public Health Rev 2011;33:7–15.

24. Crisp N. Turning the world upside down: the search for global health in the 21st century. Boca Raton, FL: CRC Press, 2010:107–125.

25. Pereira C, Bugalho A, Bergström S, Vaz F, Cotiro MA. A comparative study of caesarean deliveries by assistant medical officers and obstetricians in Mozambique. Br J Obstet Gynaecol 1996;103:508–512.

26. External evaluation of the National Programme for Family Planning and Primary Health Care: quantitative survey report. Lady Health Workers Programme, Pakistan. Oxford, England: Oxford Policy Management, 2002.

27. Haines A, Sanders D, Lehmann U, et al. Achieving child survival goals: potential contribution of community health workers. Lancet 2007;369:2121–31.

28. Belatchew M. Retaining community health workers in Ethiopia. March 2011 (http://www.capacityplus.org/community-health-workers-ethiopia).

29. Standing H, Chowdhury AM. Producing effective knowledge agents in a pluralistic environment: what future for community health workers? Soc Sci Med 2008;66:2096–107.

30. Reichenbach L, Shimul SN. Sustaining health: the role of BRAC's community health volunteers in Bangladesh, Afghanistan and Uganda. Research monograph series no. 49. Dhaka, Bangladesh: BRAC Centre, September 2011.

31. Henry J. Kaiser Family Foundation. Total nurse practitioners. 2011 (http://kff.org/other/state-indicator/total-nurse-practitioners).

32. *Idem.* Physician assistants by primary state of employment. 2010 (http://kff.org/other/state-indicator/total-physician-assistants).

33. Canadian Institute for Health Information. Canada's health care providers (https://secure.cihi.ca/estore/productSeries.htm?pc=PCC56).

34. Sachs J, Singh P. We are already applying lessons from Africa in New York's Harlem (http://www.ttwud.org/commentary/we-are-already-applying-lessons-africa-new-yorks-harlem#.UoZyyxbFCDk).

35. Lewin T. Instruction for masses knocks down campus walls. New York Times. March 4, 2012 (http://www.nytimes.com/2012/03/05/education/moocs-large-courses-open-to-all-topple-campus-walls.html?_r=4&hpw&).

36. People's Open Access Education Initiative: peoples-uni (http://www.peoples-uni.org).

37. Institute for Healthcare Improvement. IHI open school (http://www.ihi.org/offerings/IHIOpenSchool/Pages/default.aspx).

38. Mullan F, Frehywot S, Omaswa F, et al. Medical schools in sub-Saharan Africa. Lancet 2011;377:1113–21. [Erratum, Lancet 2011;377:1076.]

39. Africa All-Party Parliamentary Group. How new roles and better teamwork can release potential and improve health services. London: All-Party Parliamentary Group on Global Health, July 2012.

Convergence to Common Purpose in Global Health

David J. Hunter
and Harvey V. Fineberg

Health and disease are, to a large extent, effects of local environmental conditions, and the work of health professionals is still largely performed one patient at a time, facilitated or constrained by local resources. So does it make sense to conceptualize "global health" on a worldwide basis rather than as a patchwork of national and local jurisdictions and responses? In examining the contributions to this series, we see five major forces and trends suggesting that as the 21st century progresses, a global perspective on public health will be increasingly critical.

First, the demographic transition from high birth and death rates to low birth and death rates in most countries, leading to a doubling of life expectancy in the 20th century and a quadrupling of the world population, is associated with the epidemiologic transition from infectious causes of death to noncommunicable diseases as the primary causes of death. In terms of morbidity, mental illness now accounts for a large proportion of years lived with a disability. Between 2010 and 2050, the proportion of the world's population older than 65 years of age will almost double, and the proportion older than 85 will be three and a half times as large.[1] This dramatic reshaping of the age structure of the world population predicts an equally dramatic reshaping of disease patterns, which will challenge health systems to adjust across the spectrum of preventive and therapeutic services. Although the transition will be completed in some countries, people in many low- or middle-income countries will face a "double burden" of disease—the "unfinished agenda" of persisting common infections, undernutrition, and maternal mortality, plus a growing burden of noncommunicable diseases.

The second major trend relates to the health consequences of globalization. The tripling of world merchandise exports since 1980, a result of economic liberalization and cheaper transport, has had manifold effects on health. Economic growth and countries' movement from low-income to middle-income status have

led to decreased poverty rates in countries such as China and India, along with an ability to invest more in health infrastructure and to plan for, or at least debate, approaches to implementation of universal health coverage. By 2030, India will probably have the world's largest population, and China will probably be the largest economy; decisions made in New Delhi and Beijing are arguably already more important to global health than those made in Washington, Brussels, or Geneva. Jamison et al.[2] have proposed that by 2035, a "grand convergence in health" is possible, as mortality patterns equilibrate in many countries.

Economic growth, however, has been accompanied by rapid urbanization, reduced physical activity, increased tobacco and alcohol consumption, and adverse changes in dietary patterns. Increases in the volume and speed of travel will enable pandemics to spread more rapidly—but there has been no corresponding acceleration in the development and manufacturing of drugs and vaccines. Diseases such as polio, which had been limited to a handful of countries and attended by hopes for worldwide eradication, can recrudesce when conditions favor the virus and a pool of unimmunized children is present. These changes in lifestyle and habitation and in the numbers of people traveling are predicted to increase, along with the consequences for human health. International disease-control regulations and other global governance mechanisms are rudimentary when compared with the size of the challenges.

Third, environmental threats are destabilizing long-standing agricultural and residential patterns and access to clean air and water, setting off unpredictable changes that affect all regions of the globe. The most obvious threat comes from climate change; related threats include the cross-border spread of air and water pollution and the export of toxic wastes. Global solutions to these problems will require unprecedented global solidarity and coordinated responses. The multilateral actions aimed at reducing atmospheric chlorofluorocarbons set a promising precedent, but the actions needed to reduce the effects of climate change are far more complex, and the delay between action and mitigation longer—all of which suggest that scaling up capacities for humanitarian response to address the increased incidence of weather-related disasters will be a necessary activity for several decades.

The fourth major trend is the internationalization of medical knowledge and the globalization of the health workforce. As little as 30 years ago, medical knowledge traveled slowly, if at all, in the pages of journals, sometimes in "airmail editions" printed on lightweight paper. Now, key articles appear online a month or two before publication in print and are available around the world instantaneously. But because drugs and devices are far from universally available and affordable, there are growing inequities in doctors' ability to treat their patients using the latest medical knowledge. These limitations are particularly unfortunate now that medical knowledge flows in multiple directions and innovations borne of necessity in poor countries may hold the key to reducing the cost of health care in rich countries.[3] New educational opportunities, such as massive open online courses, or MOOCs, hold the promise of training more health

workers more quickly than can possibly be done in standard brick-and-mortar classrooms.

The globalization of the health workforce has many benefits, but rich countries' importing of health professionals from poorer countries, a result of poor workforce planning, strips poorer countries of precious health professionals and reduces their populations' access to care.[4] We must not let the communications revolution, which should lead to more up-to-date and better-trained health professionals and more globally engaged and collegial interactions around the world, become a Trojan horse for accelerated medical migration from poorer countries. To the extent that such migration is fed by frustration with inadequate infrastructure for practicing medicine to the highest standards, those problems could be mitigated by relatively modest investments in improving health facilities.[2]

The final trend is the globalization of medical science. Since the report in the late 1980s of the Commission on Health Research for Development,[5] the number of countries engaged in what the commission referred to as "essential national health research" has increased substantially; China, a developing country at the time, is now second in the number of articles published annually and listed in the Science Citation Index. Countries can increasingly decide for themselves what medical science they wish to pursue, instead of relying on the interests of scientists in other countries.

How we handle these five trends will do much to determine the quality of health and health services in the world in the coming decades. The environmental community uses the concept of "local to global" to remind us that individuals and communities have a role in environmental impact worldwide. Although the individual patient encounter is a local event, and global health institutions may constitute a patchwork of entities, each patient encounter takes place in a global tapestry of influences that constitute "global public health."

References

1. World population prospects: the 2012 revision. New York: United Nations, Department of Economic and Social Affairs, 2012 (http://esa.un.org/unpd/wpp).
2. Jamison DT, Summers LH, Alleyne G, et al. Global health 2035: a world converging within a generation. Lancet 2013;382:1898–955.
3. Learning from low-end middle-income countries. In: Crisp N. Turning the world upside down: the search for global health in the 21st century. Boca Raton, FL: CRC Press, 2010:107–25.
4. A universal truth: no health without a workforce—Third Global Forum on Human Resources for Health report. Global Health Workforce Alliance and World Health Organization, 2013 (http://www.who.int/workforcealliance/knowledge/resources/hrhreport2013/en).
5. Evans JR. Essential national health research: a key to equity in development. N Engl J Med 1990;323:913–15.

{ INDEX }

Page numbers followed by *f* or *t* indicate figures or tables. Page numbers followed by *b* indicate boxes.

Printed by Amazon Italia Logistica S.r.l.
Torrazza Piemonte (TO), Italy

12568122R00190